ADVANCES IN

Pharmacology and Chemotherapy

VOLUME 8

ADVANCES IN

Pharmacology and Chemotherapy

EDITED BY

Silvio Garattini
Istituto di Ricerche Farmacologiche "Mario Negri" Milano, Italy

A. Goldin
National Cancer Institute Bethesda, Maryland

F. Hawking
National Institute for Medical Research London, England

I. J. Kopin
National Institute of Mental Health Bethesda, Maryland

VOLUME 8

ACADEMIC PRESS New York and London 1970

ACADEMIC PRESS, INC.
111 Fifth Avenue, New York, New York 10003

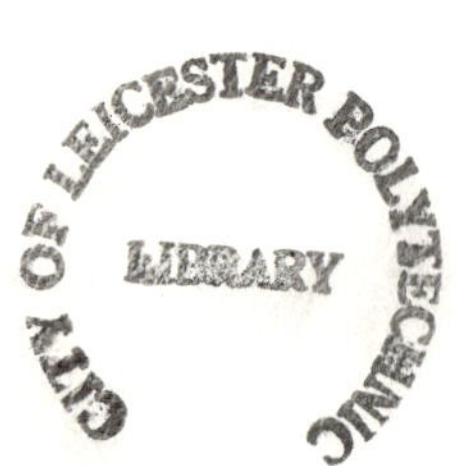

United Kingdom Edition published by
ACADEMIC PRESS, INC. (LONDON) LTD.
Berkeley Square House, London WIX 6BA

Library of Congress Catalog Card Number: 61-18298

PRINTED IN THE UNITED STATES OF AMERICA

CONTENTS

The Combined Action of Pyrimidines and Sulfonamides or Sulfones in the Chemotherapy of Malaria and Other Protozoal Infections

W. H. G. Richards

Chemotherapeutic Compounds Affecting DNA Structure and Function

B. A. Newton

Interactions of Monoamine Oxidase Inhibitors, Amines, and Foodstuffs

E. Marley and B. Blackwell

CONTRIBUTORS TO THIS VOLUME

Numbers in parentheses indicate the pages on which the authors' contributions begin.

ALAN C. AISENBERG (31), *The John Collins Warren Laboratories, Huntington Memorial Hospital of Harvard University at the Massachusetts General Hospital, Boston, Massachusetts*

B. BLACKWELL* (185), *Institute of Psychiatry, De Crespigny Park, London, England*

S. K. CARTER (57), *National Cancer Institute, Bethesda, Maryland*

THOMAS N. CHASE (1), *Laboratory of Clinical Science, National Institute of Mental Health, Bethesda, Maryland*

D. A. COONEY (57), *National Cancer Institute, Bethesda, Maryland*

RICHARD I. KATZ (1), *Laboratory of Clinical Science, National Institute of Mental Health, Bethesda, Maryland*

R. B. LIVINGSTON (57), *National Cancer Institute, Bethesda, Maryland*

E. MARLEY (185), *Institute of Psychiatry, De Crespigny Park, London, England*

B. A. NEWTON (149), *Medical Research Council Biochemical Parasitology Unit, The Molteno Institute, University of Cambridge, Cambridge, England*

W. H. G. RICHARDS (121), *Wellcome Laboratories of Tropical Medicine, Langley Court, Beckenham, Kent, England*

J. M. VENDITTI (57), *National Cancer Institute, Bethesda, Maryland*

* Present address: Department of Psychiatry and Pharmacology, University of Cincinnati, Cincinnati, Ohio.

ADVANCES IN

Pharmacology and Chemotherapy

VOLUME 8

Neurohumoral Mechanisms in the Brain Slice

RICHARD I. KATZ AND THOMAS N. CHASE

Laboratory of Clinical Science
National Institute of Mental Health
Bethesda, Maryland

I. Introduction

Our understanding of the biochemical and physiological effects of drugs within the central nervous system (CNS) has lagged behind that of drug actions in peripheral nervous structures. This situation derives as much from the prodigious heterogeneity of CNS tissues as from their physical and chemical inaccessibility. Among the approaches employed to circumvent the inherent difficulties of studying CNS function *in vivo* is the use of the brain slice. The rapidly expanding application of this preparation to investigations of drug actions on substances which may serve as mediators of central synaptic transmission is the subject of this review.

While the brain slice presents such problems as the presence of damaged cells [estimated by Hill (1932) to involve only about 0.2% of the total cell surface], lack of circulating fluid, loss of normal innervation and heterogeneity of cellular constitutents, the preparation affords a unique opportunity to study a complex tissue in isolation and in a precisely controlled environment (cf. McIlwain, 1966). When incubated in a suitable medium, brain slices retain many of the *in vivo* attributes of cerebral tissue for several hours. These include (1) respiration and glycolysis (McIlwain, 1966); (2) uptake and metabolism of a broad range of compounds; (3) recovery and maintenance of normal intra- and extracellular ionic concentration gradients (McIlwain, 1966); and (4) maintenance of resting membrane potentials which may be reversibly displaced by appropriate electrical stimulation (Hillman *et al.*, 1963; Richards and McIlwain, 1967). Studies employing brain slices have specific advantages over *in vivo* investigations of the metabolism of compounds believed to mediate central neurotransmission. Not only is the problem of penetration of these substances across the blood-brain barrier (Weil-Malherbe *et al.*, 1961; Bertler *et al.*, 1966) circumvented, but quantitative estimates of catabolite formation become feasible. Such estimates cannot be carried out *in vivo* because these compounds pass from the CNS into the general circulation at differing rates (Glowinski and Baldessarini, 1966; Werdinius, 1967).

For more than a century (cf. Bernard, 1856), it has been recognized that synaptic transmission is peculiarly sensitive to modification by drugs, possibly owing to the fact that the process is mediated by specific chemical substances. The influence of pharmacological agents on compounds presumed to play a role in central neurotransmission may be studied in brain slices at one or more of the following stages (cf. Bloom and Giarman, 1968; Glowinski and Baldessarini, 1966; Carlsson, 1965, 1966): (1) precursor uptake, (2) sequential biosynthesis of the substance, (3) storage of the active compound, (4) release of the substance upon neuronal depolarization, and (5) termination of action of the substance by reuptake into the presynaptic neuron or by enzymatic degradation. The literature pertaining to the use of brain slices for studies of putative neurotransmitters will be discussed in relation to these stages. Although a number of compounds have been implicated in the mediation of neurotransmission within the CNS, this review will be limited to a consideration of the biogenic amines (norepinephrine, dopamine, and serotonin), certain amino acids (especially γ-aminobutyric acid), and acetylcholine.

II. Uptake and Storage

The availability of radioactively labeled acetylcholine (ACh), biogenic amines, and amino acids (AA) of high specific activity has facilitated *in vitro* studies of the accumulation of these pharmacologically active substances by cerebral tissue. Although simple diffusion dominates the uptake process when the substances are added in high concentrations to the incubation medium, active mechanisms may be demonstrated when lesser concentrations are employed. Under the latter circumstances a portion of the accumulation appears to occur in nerve terminal structures normally containing the endogenous material. The use of brain slices has enabled studies of the ionic requirements for the uptake of putative neurotransmitters into CNS tissue and provided insight into drug effects on reuptake mechanisms which may play a role in terminating the postsynaptic action of neurotransmitters released into the synaptic cleft.

A. Catecholamine Uptake

The ability of mammalian cerebral slices to actively accumulate norepinephrine (NE) from a suitable incubation medium is now well established (Dengler *et al.*, 1961, 1962; Dengler, 1965; Hamberger and Masuoka, 1965; Haggendal and Hamberger, 1967; Snyder *et al.*, 1968; Ross and Renyi, 1966a; Jonason and Rutledge, 1968a). It would appear that the exogenous amine is largely taken up by noradrenergic terminals within CNS tissues. Dengler *et al.* (1962) have shown that slices of cat brain, heart, and spleen, organs which are rich in adrenergic nerve endings, attain a 4:1 tissue-to-medium ratio of NE-^{3}H, whereas slices prepared from adrenergic-poor organs such as liver, kidney, or skeletal muscle fail to achieve concentrations of labeled NE greater than those in the medium. Hamberger and Masuoka (1965) and Hamberger (1967) have applied the fluorescent histochemical technique of Falck (1962) to study the uptake of the monoamine into rat cerebral cortex slices. They observed that NE was largely confined to varicose axons, indistinguishable from those which contain endogenous NE, as well as to nonvaricose, more proximal portions of the axon. Lenn (1967) using electron microscopic radioautography to localize NE-^{3}H accumulated by brain slices, concluded that most of the tritium was taken up in relation to small unmyelinated axons (40%), nerve endings (30%), and axons (10%). The radioautographic study of Ishii and Friede (1968) performed in human cerebral autopsy specimens, which showed strong binding of NE-^{3}H to membrane sites known to contain high endogenous NE levels, further supports the contention that exogenous NE is accumulated at central adrenergic terminals. Considerably more binding of NE was found at the surface membrane of pigmented neurons in substantia nigra, nucleus coeruleus, and nucleus dorsalis vagi than at various nonpigmented nuclei. Some accumulation may, however, occur in nonadrenergic structures inasmuch as the amount of labeled NE taken into slices from various brain regions (Snyder *et al.*, 1968; Iversen and Snyder, 1968) does not correspond precisely to endogenous NE levels or to NE accumulations after intraventricular injection of the labeled amine (Glowinski and Iversen, 1966).

Although the analysis of NE uptake into brain slices is complicated by ongoing metabolism and varying rates of efflux of the accumulated catecholamine, two components may be identified: an active process which approximates Michaelis-Menten kinetics and simple diffusion (Dengler *et al.*, 1961, 1962; Titus and Dengler, 1966; Ross and Renyi, 1966b; Snyder *et al.*, 1968; Iversen and Snyder, 1968; Haggendal and Hamberger, 1967; Jonason and Rutledge, 1968a). Dengler *et al.* (1962) observed that the accumulation of NE exhibited the characteristics of active uptake at amine concentrations in the incubation medium of about 10^{-7} M, but that simple diffusion predominated at higher concentrations. The view that the accumulation of NE by brain slices occurs by an active process derives from the observations that uptake is temperature dependent, requires oxygen and glucose, is retarded by inhibitors of cell metabolism, occurs against a concentration gradient, and depends on sodium in the external medium (Dengler *et al.*, 1961, 1962; Dengler, 1965; Ross and Renyi, 1964, 1966a). Omission of calcium or magnesium ions from the incubation medium has little effect on NE uptake in brain slices (Hamberger, 1967).

Drugs which inhibit the uptake and storage of labeled NE in the brain of the living animal usually have a similar effect on the accumulation of NE by CNS tissues *in vitro* (Dengler *et al.*, 1961, 1962; Dengler, 1965; Hamberger and Masuoka, 1965; Hamberger, 1967; Ross and Renyi, 1964, 1966a). These drugs include ouabain, cocaine, phenoxybenzamine, chlorpromazine, imipramine, desmethylimipramine, reserpine, amphetamine, and related sympathomimetic amines. Most of these agents are effective at concentrations of the order of 10^{-4} M. Lysergic acid diethylamide and haloperidol are without effect at this concentration. Drugs such as cocaine, and desmethylimipramine, which are thought to impair NE uptake by inhibiting the cell membrane pump, exert a greater effect on uptake when a short incubation period is used (Ross and Renyi, 1966a). This observation suggests that uptake by the neuronal membrane is the initial dominant factor at a time when storage mechanisms play a minor role. Prolongation of incubation time leads to an increasing effect of reserpine, presumably due to a time-dependent increase in the importance of storage mechanisms. Although it cannot be excluded that binding of amines to intraneuronal storage sites may have some significance for the initial uptake of amines by brain slices, it seems probable that the results of kinetic analysis of cocaine sensitive uptake (Ross and Renyi, 1966a; Dengler *et al.*, 1962; Snyder *et al.*, 1968) reflect mainly the cell membrane pump.

The uptake of the NE precursors tyrosine, dopa, and dopamine (DA) has been described (Neame, 1961a; Guroff *et al.*, 1961; Dengler *et al*, 1962; Ross and Renyi, 1966b; Yoshida *et al.*, 1963a,b, 1965). The active accumulation of DA into brain slices resembles that of NE (Ross and Renyi, 1964, 1966a), although differences have been described regarding regional variations in uptake as well as in the catabolism of the two catecholamines (Jonason and

Rutledge, 1968a). Guroff *et al.* (1961) have shown that rat brain slices actively concentrate tyrosine from the suspending medium and can attain intracellular concentrations more than four times that of the medium. Tyramine and α-methyl-*m*-tyrosine are also concentrated, while *p*-hydroxyphenylacetic acid appears to be taken up only passively. The uptake of tyrosine is impaired by a variety of metabolic inhibitors and enhanced by glucose and other hexoses; excess calcium or magnesium increases uptake whereas potassium decreases it. Differences in the accumulation of catecholamine precursors between brain slices and cerebral tissue *in vivo* are suggested by the finding that L-tyrosine enters the brain of the living animal more rapidly than D-tyrosine, while in brain slices D- and L-tyrosine are concentrated at equal rates (Chirigos *et al.*, 1960).

The accumulation of L-dihydroxyphenylalanine (L-dopa) by brain slices by an energy-dependent process has also been reported (Yoshida *et al.*, 1963a,b). As with other active uptake systems, this uptake has been shown to be temperature dependent, to require oxygen and glucose, and to be impaired by metabolic inhibitors. Omission of sodium, potassium, or magnesium retards the accumulation of dopa by brain slices, but calcium omission enhances it. Ouabain and proveratrine (Yoshida *et al.*, 1963a,b) as well as protamine (Yoshida *et al.*, 1965) reduce dopa uptake.

B. Serotonin Uptake

Studies of the accumulation of serotonin (5-HT) by cerebral slices (Schanberg, 1963; Ross and Renyi, 1967; Blackburn *et al.*, 1967; Pletscher and Bartholini, 1967) illustrate the dependence of uptake mechanisms on the concentration of the exogenous amine. Although Schanberg (1963) and Pletscher and Bartholini (1967) were unable to demonstrate active transport of 5-HT into brain slices, the maximum amount of amine entering the tissue by a carrier mechanism at the high incubation medium concentrations used (above 10^{-7} *M*) would be small in comparison to that entering by passive diffusion. It is thus not surprising that at these concentrations, little difference between the uptake of labeled 5-HT into brain slices or slices of kidney, liver, or spleen, could be demonstrated. Blackburn *et al.* (1967), however, observed that brain slices incubated with 5-HT-^{14}C at a concentration of 2×10^{-8} *M* accumulated the labeled amine by a mechanism showing all the characteristics of active transport. The kinetic constant (K_m) estimated by Blackburn *et al.* (1967) for 5-HT uptake by rat brain slices resembles that for 5-HT uptake by platelets (Hughes and Brodie, 1959; Weissbach *et al.*, 1960) and choroid plexus (Tochino and Schanker, 1965) and for NE uptake by brain slices (Dengler *et al.*, 1962; Snyder *et al.*, 1968). Approximately 60% of the 5-HT accumulated in the experiments reported by Blackburn *et al.* (1967)

was recovered in the nerve ending (synaptosomal) fraction and 40% in the supernatant after fractionation of the tissue homogenates on a sucrose density gradient. The subcellular distribution of 5-HT-^{14}C taken up into brain slices is thus similar to that of endogenous 5-HT (Schanberg and Giarman, 1962) and NE (Potter and Axelrod, 1963).

A number of drugs have been found to alter the uptake of 5-HT into brain slices. Imipramine, desmethylimipramine, ouabain, cocaine, and chlorpromazine substantially inhibit 5-HT-^{14}C uptake at a concentration of 10^{-5} *M* (Blackburn *et al.*, 1967; Ross and Renyi, 1967). Reserpine does not appear to influence the transport of 5-HT-^{14}C into cerebral slices, but, as with other amines, it does act to reduce their capacity for binding 5-HT (Schanberg, 1963; Ross and Renyi, 1966b, 1967; Blackburn *et al.*, 1967). Iproniazid, which has no effect on 5-HT uptake, inhibits the reserpine-induced depletion of 5-HT-^{14}C from brain slices by blocking serotonin degradation (Ross and Renyi, 1967). These findings agree with previous evidence that reserpine produces a depletion of biogenic amines *in vivo* by interfering with vesicular storage rather than by inhibition at the membrane pump (Carlsson, 1965) and that reserpine pretreatment does not alter transport of 5-HT into brain *in vivo* (Palaic *et al.*, 1967).

D,L-Amphetamine, a potent inhibitor of the accumulation of NE by brain slices (Hillarp and Malmfors, 1964; Dengler *et al.*, 1961), exerts a less powerful inhibitory influence on the accumulation of 5-HT (Ross and Renyi, 1967; Schanberg, 1963). The impairment of 5-HT uptake by drugs which also inhibit the uptake of NE suggests a similarity between uptake mechanisms for the two biogenic amines. NE interferes with 5-HT uptake, but inasmuch as the concentration of NE required to produce significant inhibition is approximately 100 times greater than the K_m for NE uptake (Titus and Dengler, 1966; Dengler *et al.*, 1962), it would seem that 5-HT and NE are normally accumulated at different sites. This is in contrast to results of experiments performed with rabbit choroid plexus, where there appears to be a common mechanism for the active accumulation of relatively large amounts of NE and 5-HT (Tochino and Schanker, 1965).

The uptake of 5-HT-^{3}H into brain slices is also inhibited by several tryptamine derivatives (Ross and Renyi, 1967). One of the most potent of these compounds is bufotenine which is effective at concentrations as low as 3×10^{-6} *M*. *N,N*-Dimethyltryptamine is somewhat less active, while lysergic acid diethylamide, when given intraperitoneally one hour prior to the experiment, had a negligible effect. In the studies of Blackburn *et al.* (1967) uptake of 5-HT-^{14}C was inhibited by tryptamine (10^{-5} *M*); dopamine was a less effective inhibitor and L-NE or D,L-5-HTP (both at 10^{-4} *M*) had relatively little effect.

Facilitated transport of 5-hydroxytryptophan (5-HTP), the immediate stereospecificity (Lajtha and Toth, 1963), energy requirements (Elliott and van Gelder, 1958; Neame, 1961b; Abadom and Scholefield, 1962a; Lajtha, 1967), kinetic constants, and drug effects (Lajtha and Toth, 1965) have been examined in detail.

It is generally agreed that brain slices accumulate labeled AA from an incubation medium until a concentration gradient is established such that intracellular levels are severalfold those of the medium. Since there appears to be relatively little metabolism of AA taken up into brain slices during a 30–60-minute period of incubation (Blasberg and Lajtha, 1965; Oversen and Neal, 1968), transport rather than metabolism is probably the major determinant of this steady state. Transport constants for the influx of amino acids into brain slices must, however, be determined in short-term experiments which essentially measure the initial unidirectional flux; transport constants for influx cannot be derived from steady state experiments inasmuch as amino acid exodus from brain cells is also a mediated process and demonstrates saturation kinetics. Both the rate of AA uptake and release are concentration dependent (Levi *et al.*, 1965), influx depending on AA concentration in medium and efflux on AA concentration in the intracellular water. Net amino acid accumulation will continue until an intracellular concentration is attained at which influx and efflux are equal and a new steady state is attained.

Amino acid transport in brain slices appears to involve a number of carrier systems which may be partially characterized by the particular group of AA they predominantly mediate across the cell membrane. Comparison of representative small neutral, large neutral, large basic and acidic amino acids (α-aminoisobutyric acid, L-phenylalanine, L-arginine, and L-aspartate, respectively) indicates that at least four transport systems are involved with the passage of AA across brain cell membranes (Blasberg, 1968). These systems evidently do not possess absolute specificity because a number of AA seem to have some capacity for transport by carrier systems other than those which primarily mediate their passage into the cell.

Regional differences in the concentration of endogenous free AA have been compared with AA uptake by slices from the same brain areas (Levi and Lajtha, 1965; Kandera *et al.*, 1968). The distribution pattern of the free pool varies with the AA and with the region analyzed. Similarly the uptake of AA into slices prepared from various regions of brain vary with the AA tested. In general, steady state accumulations attained *in vitro* parallel the physiological levels found in the living animal. Amino acids occurring at high concentrations *in vivo* are usually accumulated to higher levels in brain slices (Levi *et al.*, 1967). It thus appears that transport mechanisms play a major although not exclusive role in determining the regional distribution of AA in living brain.

The site of accumulation of exogenous AA by brain slices remains uncertain. Since uptake decreases upon slice swelling, at a time when the extracellular precursor of serotonin, has been demonstrated in cerebral slices fr species (Wartburg, 1962; Schanberg, 1963; Smith, 1963). The acc of 5-HTP does not appear to be associated with the activity of 5-H boxylase, since α-methyldopa, a potent inhibitor of this enzyme fa the uptake of 5-HTP (Schanberg, 1963). That the mechanism of up slices and the decarboxylating enzyme are not linked is further by the observation of Smith (1963) that under optimal conditions brain homogenates will decarboxylate about 20 times more 5-HT decarboxylated by brain slices. Only a small portion of the 5-HT cumulated by rat brain slices is decarboxylated to the amine (Smith

The uptake of 5-HTP into slices of cerebral tissue is retarded by the n occurring neutral amino acids L-tryptophan (although not by its D- L-phenylalanine, L-tryrosine, L-dopa, L-leucine, L-isoleucine, and L when added to the incubation medium at a concentration of 2 × (Schanberg, 1963). Since in brain the transport of an AA is generally in by structurally related analogs (Neame, 1968; Blasberg, 1968), it would that 5-HTP fits the classification of a neutral amino acid. The upt 5-HTP-^{14}C into brain slices is not influenced by the presence of other bi amines such as histamine (10^{-6} *M*), NE (10^{-6} *M*), epinephrine (10^{-6} *M*), γ-aminobutyric acid (GABA) (5×10^{-2} *M*) (Schanberg, 1963). Althou already noted dopa partially blocks 5-HTP uptake, α-methyldopa, given to rats (400 mg/kg) 45 minutes prior to sacrifice and added to the me (10^{-4} *M*), fails to reduce 5-HTP-^{14}C uptake into brain slices. This lo inhibitory activity by α-methyl analogs was also observed in the trypto series (Schanberg, 1963).

Many drugs which exert profound central actions, when administere rats in concentrations sufficient to influence behavior, fail to alter 5-H uptake into brain slices subsequently prepared from these animals. Th agents include lysergic acid diethylamide, chlorpromazine, imipram iproniazid, pheniprazine, morphine, phenobarbital, and reserpine (Schanbe 1963; Wartburg, 1962), suggesting that the possible influences of these dru on serotonergic mechanisms do not derive from an effect on precursor uptal

C. Amino Acid Uptake

The extensive literature describing the movement of AA into mammalia brain slices has been the subject of several recent reviews (Lajtha, 1968; Blasberg, 1968; Neame, 1968). At low bath concentrations AA flux occurs mostly through mediated transport mechanisms rather than by simple diffusion (Chirigos *et al.*, 1960; Lajtha, 1964; Lajtha and Toth, 1961, 1963). Many properties of these transport mechanisms such as substrate specificity (Neame, 1961a; Abadom and Scholefield, 1962b; Blasberg and Lajtha, 1966), space presumably increases, it is more probably intracellular than extracellular (Lahiri and Lajtha, 1964). Furthermore, nonspecific binding does not appear to be involved since omission of sodium from the incubation medium, which abolishes concentrative uptake, is unlikely to affect all specific binding sites (Lahiri and Lajtha, 1964).

Uptake sites for GABA may be unique to central nervous tissue (cf. Curtis and Watkins, 1965), because slices of rat liver under similar conditions fail to accumulate GABA-^{3}H (Iverson and Neal, 1968; Elliott and van Gelder, 1958). Varon *et al.* (1965) have shown that a considerable portion of the labeled GABA taken up by mouse brain particulate preparations is contained in synaptosomal particles, suggesting that GABA uptake sites may be associated with nerve terminals in brain. Iversen and Snyder (1968) have recently examined different synaptosomal populations storing exogenous catecholamines and GABA in homogenates prepared from rat brain slices. Slices from hypothalamus and striatum were incubated with labeled NE, DA, or GABA, homogenized and placed on sucrose gradients. Each of these labeled substances was found in the soluble supernatant fraction and in a particulate fraction having the density characteristics of synaptosomal particles. The peak of NE-^{14}C, however, occurred at a denser level of sucrose than that of GABA-^{3}H. A similar contrast between DA-^{3}H and GABA-^{14}C was observed, while DA-^{3}H and NE-^{14}C were found in the same particulate fraction. These observations suggest the existence of different populations of brain synaptosomes subserving different putative transmitters. Overlapping populations of synaptosomes remain to be separated.

The effects of the ionic composition of the incubation medium on AA uptake have been the subject of several investigations. An absolute requirement for sodium has been demonstrated for GABA uptake into cerebral slices (Iversen and Neal, 1968; Lajtha, 1968). The absence of potassium, calcium, magnesium, or phosphate ions inhibit uptake of GABA only slightly, while excess potassium or phosphate are strongly inhibitory. In their studies of AA in mouse brain slices, Lahiri and Lajtha (1964) noted that slices swelled greatly in the absence of sodium, but not if sodium was replaced by lithium or choline. Tsukada *et al.* (1963) observed that the uptake of D- or L-glutamatic acid was accompanied by marked potassium accumulation and cell swelling. In contrast, GABA or β-alanine, neutral amino acids, were accumulated actively without changes in electrolyte distribution or concomitant swelling of cells. In these studies, omission of potassium inhibited, while omission of calcium ions tended to enhance, AA uptake. In a potassium-rich media, GABA and β-alanine uptake was slightly inhibited, while that of D- and L-glutamic acid was markedly increased.

The effects of various substrates on uptake of GABA, L-glutamic acid, L-histidine, and glycine have been compared by Barborosa *et al.* (1968).

The presence of glucose, pyruvate, lactate, and oxaloacetate favored maximal uptake of these AA into brain slices, while in the presence of succinate and fumarate, uptake was only slightly higher than in the absence of substrate. Hypoxia and metabolic inhibitors diminished uptake, confirming the dependence of uptake on oxidative metabolism.

Several drugs have been reported by Lajtha and Toth (1965) to influence the accumulation of AA by brain slices. The uptake of L-lysine or cycloleucine is markedly reduced by ouabain (10^{-5} *M*), reserpine (10^{-3} *M*), and pentobarbital (10^{-3} *M*). Chlorpromazine exerts a diphasic effect; relatively high concentrations (2×10^{-3} *M*) strongly inhibit while lower concentrations (2×10^{-5} *M*) slightly enhance uptake. Morphine (10^{-3} *M*) has only a mild inhibitory action, while pentylenetetrazole (10^{-3} *M*) and cocaine (10^{-3} *M*) have no significant influence on the accumulation of L-lysine or cycloleucine. The uptake of α-aminoisobutyric acid was also found to be reduced by ouabain (10^{-5} *M*) and chlorpromazine (2×10^{-3} *M*). Presumably these drug effects on AA transport *in vitro* are mediated by more than one mechanism.

D. Acetylcholine Uptake

Although a variety of early studies failed to demonstrate a significant accumulation of ACh by brain slices, it is now apparent that the active uptake of this substance into cerebral tissue does occur *in vitro* in the presence of a suitable cholinesterase inhibitor. In brain slices as well as in nerve ending particles, Burton (1964) and Guth (1962) found negligible uptake of ACh in the absence of anticholinesterase agents. Similarly, uptake experiments in which eserine (physostigmine) was used to inactivate cholinesterase yielded negative or nearly negative results (Mann *et al.*, 1938; Elliott and Henderson, 1951; Schuberth and Sundwall, 1967), due to the strong inhibitory action of this drug on ACh uptake mechanisms (Polak and Meeuws, 1966). In the presence of the irreversible organophosphorus inhibitors, soman (pinacolyl methylphosphonofluoridate), sarin (isopropyl methylphosphonofluoridate), or paraoxon (diethyl-4-nitrophenyl phosphate), however, a significant accumulation of ACh has been observed (Polak and Meeuws, 1966; Schuberth and Sundwall, 1967; Liang and Quastel, 1969a; Polak, 1969; Heilbronn, 1969). The major fraction of this uptake occurs against a concentration gradient, requires oxygen, and is impaired by substances interfering with energy metabolism. The role of active uptake appears to depend on the concentration of ACh in the incubation medium according to Michaelis-Menten kinetics (Schuberth and Sundwall, 1967; Polak and Meeuws, 1966; Lang and Quastel, 1969a).

Preliminary experiments reported by Schuberth and Sundwall (1967) on the subcellular distribution of ACh-^{3}H actively accumulated in brain slices suggest that 75% is located in the supernatant while 25% is in the nerve ending fraction. Thus, the main part of the structurally bound ACh-^{3}H is concentrated in the nerve ending fraction. The relatively large amount of unbound ACh-^{3}H may in part be an artifact of the separation techniques employed. On the other hand, autoradiography carried out on sections of rat cortical slices incubated with ACh-^{3}H reveal a diffuse labeling with no apparent preference for certain cell types or cell structures (Polak, 1969).

Striatal tissues, which contain high concentrations of cholinergic terminals and of choline acetyltransferase (Hebb and Whittaker, 1958), exhibit a surprising avidity for exogenous ACh (Sattin, 1966). Even in the absence of a cholinesterase inhibitor, rat striatal slices appear to accumulate six times the concentration of ACh found *in vivo*. Of this, Sattin (1966) characterized 45% as the osmotically labile and 20% the osmotically stable form of bound ACh; 35% was free ACh. Evidence was given to suggest that this distribution depends on intact cellular structure and that the labile form of ACh may be most intimately related to cholinergic transmission systems in brain. Eserine failed to preserve maximal extractable ACh in incubated slices, and it was proposed that eserine may act to release ACh from bound stores (Sattin, 1966). When compared with the findings of Whittaker *et al.* (1964) in synaptosomes, these observations support the proposal that ACh is synthesized in the cytoplasm of nerve endings and is secondarily taken up into synaptic vesicles.

The ionic requirements for ACh uptake *in vitro* have been the subject of several recent studies. Although replacement of sodium in the incubation medium by lithium failed to alter ACh uptake, replacement by rubidium or cesium exerted a marked inhibitory action (Schuberth and Sundwall, 1967). The rate of ACh accumulation declined in the absence of potassium (Liang and Quastel, 1969a) but was not affected by magnesium omission (Schuberth and Sunwall, 1967); reports of the effect of calcium ion omission on ACh uptake are in conflict (Schuberth and Sundwall, 1967; Liang and Quastel, 1969a). In the presence of relatively high concentrations of potassium, calcium, or magnesium, the accumulation of ACh is reduced (Schuberth and Sundwall, 1967; Liang and Quastel, 1969a; Polak, 1969).

Active accumulation of choline, the immediate precursor of ACh, has also been demonstrated in brain slices (Schuberth *et al.*, 1966). At low external concentrations, choline uptake occurs against a concentration gradient, requires oxygen and glucose, and is impaired by metabolic inhibitors. The maximum rate of choline transport exceeds that of ACh by more than 50%. Choline is also concentrated by active mechanisms in slices of rat kidney cortex (Sung and Johnstone, 1965). In kidney slices, however, choline is largely converted to betaine, while in brain slices nearly all of the labeled choline remains unmetabolized (Schuberth *et al.*, 1966).

The effects of drugs on the uptake of ACh into brain slices have been the subject of several recent studies. All were carried out in the presence of an organophosphorus cholinesterase inhibitor. The ability of the reversible anticholinesterase agent, eserine, to interfere with ACh uptake contrasts with the action of such irreversible, organophosphorus compounds as DFP (diisopropyl phosphofluoridate), tabun, sarin, soman, or paraoxon (Schuberth and Sundwall, 1967; Liang and Quastel, 1969b; Polak 1969). These latter agents are thought to react with an ester binding group on the enzyme, while eserine combines also with a negative group. The inhibitory effect on ACh uptake may relate to an affinity for anionic sites (Polak, 1969). Other drugs known to act on cholinergic transmission which competitively inhibit the accumulation of ACh include hemicholinium-3, atropine, *d*-tubocurarine, succinyl choline, nicotine, methacholine, tetraethylammonium chloride (TEA), hexamethonium, and strychnine (Schuberth and Sundwall, 1967; Liang and Quastel, 1969b; Polak, 1969). In addition morphine (Schuberth and Sundwall, 1967), as well as several local anesthetics including cocaine, procaine, and lidocaine (Liang and Quastel, 1969b), have been found to act competitively to inhibit ACh uptake. A comparison of the inhibitor constants of several drugs which competitively inhibit the accumulation of ACh, with the inhibitor constants toward acetylcholin esterase or certain ACh receptor sites has lead to the suggestion that the chemical structure of the transport carrier site for ACh is not identical with the anionic site of acetylcholinesterase or with the receptor sites for ACh (Liang and Quastel, 1969b).

Drugs found to interfere noncompetitively with ACh uptake include amphetamine and chlorpromazine (Liang and Quastel, 1969b). Pentobarbitone (10^{-4} *M*), tetrodotoxin (10^{-5} *M*), reserpine (10^{-5} *M*), epinephrine (10^{-4} *M*), and NE (5×10^{-5} *M*) have no effect on the accumulation of ACh (Schuberth and Sundwall, 1967; Liang and Quastel, 1969b). Although ouabain (10^{-5} *M*) inhibits ACh uptake into cortical slices incubated at physiological potassium concentrations in the presence of paraoxon (Liang and Quastel, 1969a), no such effect was observed in slices incubated with soman at relatively high potassium concentrations (Polak, 1969). Certain differences in the activity of drugs on the transport of ACh and choline into brain slices have been noted by Schuberth and Sundwall (1967). Hemicholinium-3 exerts a ten-times greater inhibitory effect against ACh than against choline uptake. In further contrast to the effects on ACh uptake, the active accumulation of choline is not materially effected by eserine, atropine, or oxotremorine, although sarin appears to enhance choline uptake slightly. The accumulation of ACh is reduced by the presence of choline in the incubation medium (Polak, 1969).

III. Metabolism

A. Catecholamine Metabolism

The ability of brain slices to convert precursor AA to catecholamines (CA) has been demonstrated in several mammalian species including man

(Masuoka *et al.*, 1961, 1963; Kindwall and Weiner, 1966). The rate of CA formation in bovine brain slices is approximately twice that of homogenates (Kindwall and Weiner, 1966). Studies with slices from various areas of brain indicate marked regional differences in the amount of DA and NE synthesized, which in general correspond to local endogenous levels. Slices of caudate and putamen exhibit the greatest synthesis of DA-^{14}C from tyrosine-^{14}C, while lower rates are found in cerebral cortex, hypothalamus, and substantia nigra (Masuoka *et al.*, 1961, 1963; Kindwall and Weiner, 1966). NE formation is most active in hypothalamic slices, while little or none is produced in slices of caudate nucleus (Kindwall and Weiner, 1966). A similar difference in the rate of DA versus NE formation in striatal slices has also been observed in studies using labeled tyrosine *in vivo* (Glowinski and Axelrod, 1966). Since substantial activity of dopamine β-oxidase, the enzyme which mediates the conversion of DA to NE, has been found in supplemented homogenates of caudate nucleus (Udenfriend and Creveling, 1959), conceivably DA and the enzyme are confined to separate compartments.

Drugs known to influence the synthesis of CA *in vivo* have also been studied in brain slices. The enzymatic conversion of tyrosine to dopa and CA by rat subcortical slices is favored by ATP and NADPH and inhibited by the addition of pyridoxal phosphate to the bathing medium (Iyer *et al.*, 1963). The formation of CA by brain slices is substantially less than that found under comparable conditions in rat adrenal medulla slices. Furthermore, in brain slices there is a relatively greater increase in dopa than in DA or NE. These results are in accord with the observation that brain normally contains a much higher ratio of dopa and DA to NE than does adrenal medulla (von Euler, 1956). Although the metabolism of endogenous CA in rat hypothalamic slices is unaffected by pretreatment with the dopa decarboxylase inhibitor decarborane, *de novo* synthesis of NE from tyrosine in slices is impaired (Merritt and Schutz, 1966). Exposure to this drug produces a slight diminution in dopa and a marked decrease in DA and NE, suggesting that decarborane acts by blocking the conversion of dopa to DA through inhibition of dopa decarboxylase. Synthesis of CA in brain slices is also inhibited by 5×10^{-4} M α-methyltyrosine methyl ester (H 44/68) (Udenfriend and Creveling, 1959).

Both oxidative deamination and *O*-methylation, the two enzymatic routes by which CA may be catabolized *in vivo*, are operative in brain slices. Rutledge and Jonason (1967) incubated rabbit cortex slices with similar concentrations of DA-^{14}C or NE-^{3}H to quantify the catabolites formed. They observed that DA was converted mainly to the two phenolic acids, 3,4-dihydroxyphenylacetic acid and homovanillic acid, whereas NE was catabolized primarily to the two phenolic glycols, 3-methoxy-4-hydroxyphenyglycol and 3,4-dihydroxyphenylglycol. Only negligible amounts of 3-methoxy-4-hydroxyphenylethanol and 3,4-dihydroxyphenylethanol were detected after incubation with DA. Although considerable quantities of normetanephrine were produced from exogenous NE, none could be detected from NE formed from exogenous DA. This observation suggested that newly formed NE may initially be catabolized by intraneuronal monoamine oxidase (MAO) and subsequently by extraneuronal catechol-*O*-methyltransferase, whereas exogenously added NE can be catabolized initially by either enzyme.

In further studies of the metabolism of CA in slices of rabbit cortex, Jonason and Rutledge (1968b) found that pretreatment of animals with the tricyclic antidepressant protryptiline reduced the catabolism of DA and NE to 58 and 33% of normal, respectively, using the same substrate concentration. Interestingly, protryptiline pretreatment inhibited retention of each amine correspondingly, whereas the MAO activity of brain cortex homogenates was unchanged. They suggested that protryptiline inhibits CA metabolism, in part at least, by interfering with amine uptake by cell membranes. When DA was used as the substrate, protryptiline caused a marked reduction of 3,4-dihydroxyphenylacetic acid, a slight reduction of homovanillic acid, and an increase in methoxytryptamine. On the other hand, a marked reduction of 3,4-dihydroxyphenylglycol and dihydroxymandelic acid, a smaller reduction of both vanillylmandelic acid and 3-methoxy-4-hydroxyphenylglycol with no effect on normetanephrine was observed when NE was used as the substrate. Pretreatment with protryptiline inhibited total synthesis of NE from DA, an effect antagonized by increasing the substrate concentration. These findings support the view that dopamine-β-hydroxylase is localized within monoaminergic neurons in cerebral cortex. Pretreatment of rabbits with the MAO inhibitor nialamide markedly reduces the formation of deaminated catabolites of both NE and DA but leads to a six-fold increase in methoxytyramine after incubation with DA or a 1.5-fold rise in normetanephrine after incubation with NE. High doses of nialamide increase the net synthesis of NE as well as its total synthesis (NE plus catabolites) (Rutledge and Jonason, 1968b).

Differences in metabolic fate of phenylethylamine compounds may relate to the presence of the β-hydroxyl group (Breese *et al.*, 1969). In rat brain slices, phenylethylamine derivatives such as DA, 3-methoxytyramine, or tyramine are converted predominantly to acidic metabolites while their β-hydroxylated analogs (NE, normetanephrine, octopamine) are catabolized primarily to neutral derivatives. In the guinea pig this difference may be specific to cerebral tissue inasmuch as brain slices convert normetanephrine mainly to 3-methoxy-4-hydroxyphenylglycol, while in liver slices normetanephrine is largely metabolized to 3-methoxy-4-hydroxymandelic acid. Results with 3-methoxy-4-hydroxyphenylglycol and 3,4-dihydroxyphenylglycol suggest that the mechanism of glycol formation involves direct reduction of intermediate aldehyde and not keto alcohol formation. Studies comparing the metabolism of intravenously and intracisternally injected normetanephrine-^{3}H indicate that reduction of the intermediate aldehyde is the predominant route of cerebral metabolism of β-hydroxylated phenylethylamines *in vivo* as well as *in vitro*. The finding of mostly glycol derivatives from β-hydroxylated amines is also in good agreement with the results of experiments in which these amines were injected intracisternally (Schanberg *et al.*, 1968). In the *in vivo* studies, however, the glycol derivatives were largely conjugated while minimal conjugation could be demonstrated in brain slices.

B. Serotonin Metabolism

The conversion of 5-HTP to 5-HT occurs in brain slices (Smith, 1963; Wartburg, 1962) although at a rate severalfold slower than that found in homogenates of cerebral tissue (Graham-Smith, 1964; Smith, 1963). 5-HTP decarboxylation in brain slices is inhibited by methyldopa, D,L-dopa, and D,L-methyl-*m*-tyrosine (Smith, 1963). The MAO inhibitor pheniprazine also suppresses the conversion of 5-HTP to 5-HT as does chlorpromazine in the presence of 5 or 105 m*M* potassium chloride (Wartburg, 1962).

The catabolism of 5-HT to 5-hydroxyindoleacetic acid (5-HIAA) or 5-5-hydroxytryptophol, probably through an intermediate aldehyde, has been demonstrated in rat and human brain homogenates (Eccleston *et al.*, 1966) well as in rat brain slices (Eccleston *et al.*, 1969). Under the usual incubation conditions a relatively greater amount of 5-hydroxytryptophol is found in brain slices after incubation with 5-HT than may be identified in the brain of the living animal. The formation of 5-hydroxytryptophol, which does not appear to be conjugated by brain slices (Eccleston *et al.*, 1966), evidently requires reduced NADP in contrast to liver where reduced NAD is required (Eccleston *et al.*, 1966; Feldstein and Wong, 1965). Whether oxidation of 5-hydroxyindolealdehyde depends primarily on NADP (Eccleston *et al.*, 1966) or NAD (Deitrich, 1966; Feldstein and Williamson, 1968) has not yet been resolved.

Reserpine acts to expose 5-HT to rapid degradation both *in vitro* and *in vivo*. In brain slices, the drug reduces the total accumulation of 5-HT-^{14}C from the incubation medium but does not affect 5-HIAA-^{14}C levels (Pletscher and Bartholini, 1967). Monoamine oxidase inhibition by iproniazid reverses this effect on 5-HT-^{14}C in slices from reserpinized brains. These findings are compatible with the generally accepted view that reserpine reduces the binding of 5-HT and other amines to intraneuronal storage granules, thus accelerating the metabolism of amines accumulated in reserpinized tissue. In slices incubated with 5-HT-^{14}C, amphetamines markedly diminish the formation of 5-HIAA-^{14}C while slightly increasing the accumulation of 5-HT-^{14}C. The addition of tyramine to the incubation medium leads to a decrease of 5-HT-^{14}C in slices and of 5-HIAA-^{14}C in the incubation medium (Pletscher and Bartholini, 1967). These observations suggest that monoamine-depleting drugs may affect 5-HT metabolism in brain slices by different mechanisms: (1) impairment of intracellular storage; (2) competitive inhibition of MAO; or (3) inhibition of amine uptake.

Studies of the effects of ethanol on 5-HT metabolism in brain are of interest in view of the marked changes in the urinary excretion of 5-HIAA and 5-hydroxytryptophol produced by ethanol administration to human subjects (Davis *et al.*, 1967). Preliminary *in vitro* data reported by Eccleston *et al.* (1969) suggest that 5-HT utilization is slightly reduced by high ethanol concentrations in brain but not in liver. The rate of 5-HIAA or 5-hydroxytryptophol formation in brain slices was not significantly influenced by ethanol. In liver slices, however, ethanol (10^{-1} *M*) increased 5-hydroxytryptophol fifteen times while 5-HIAA formation decreased to about one-third the normal rate. Differences in the effect of ethanol on 5-HT utilization in these tissues may relate to diverse coenzyme requirements or substrate affinities of the alcohol dehydrogenases responsible for the oxidation of ethanol and the formation of 5-hydroxytryptophol (Koen and Shaw, 1966; Eccleston *et al.*, 1966). The findings of Eccleston *et al.* (1969) suggest that the changes in urinary excretion of 5-hydroxyindoles following ethanol ingestion in man may largely if not exclusively reflect metabolic events occurring in peripheral rather than central structures.

C. Amino Acid Metabolism

In general, there appears to be relatively little retention of the metabolic products of AA taken up by mammalian brain tissue *in vitro*. Scheparty (1963) found that less than 0.1% of ^{14}C-labeled AA incubated with mouse brain homogenates were incorporated into protein. Most of the radioactivity recovered from extracts of mouse brain slices incubated for 70 minutes at 37°C in a physiological medium containing representative acidic, neutral, or basic AA (2×10^{-3} *M*) was in the form of the unchanged AA (Blasberg and Lajtha, 1965). In this latter study, L-glutamine appeared to be metabolized to a greater extent than any of the other AA tested; about 25% of the radioactivity recovered from slices incubated with this AA was in the form of metabolic products, principally glutamic acid. The decarboxylation of glutamate to form GABA has been demonstrated in brain tissue preparations (Awapara *et al.*, 1950; Roberts and Frankel, 1950). Cerebral cortex slices incubated with glutamate may increase their GABA content to three times endogenous levels (Elliott and van Gelder, 1958). As *in vivo*, this reaction is dependent on the presence of pyridoxal phosphate as coenzyme (Roberts and Frankel, 1950, 1951). By means of isotope tracer techniques, the ability of rat cerebral cortex slices to convert glucose-^{14}C into labeled glutamate and aspartate as well as into GABA has been demonstrated (Beloff-Chain *et al.*, 1955; Kini and Quastel, 1959). In the presence of glucose, increased concentrations of potassium enhance the formation of GABA and glutamate, probably by accelerating the conversion of pyruvate to acetyl coenzyme A (Kini and Quastel, 1959; Machiyama *et al.*, 1967).

Evidence of the catabolism of exogenous GABA by brain tissue *in vitro* has been reported. Following incubation of rat cortical slices with GABA-^{3}H for 10 minutes in a relatively small volume of medium, labeled metabolites accounted for over half the radioactivity in the medium (Iversen and Neal, 1968). Despite the accumulation of metabolites in the incubation medium, only unchanged GABA-^{3}H was detectable in the tissues. GABA degradation by means of the reversible transamination reaction between GABA and α-ketoglutarate to yield succinic semialdehyde and glutamate has been observed in whole brain homogenates (Bessman *et al.*, 1953; Roberts and Bregoff, 1953). The ability of guinea pig brain slices to evolve $^{14}CO_2$ from GABA labeled in the carboxyl group as well as to transaminate exogenous GABA has also been demonstrated (Tsukada *et al.*, 1957).

D. Acetylcholine Metabolism

In 1936, Quastel *et al.* reported that brain cortex slices allowed to respire in a medium containing eserine formed a substance which produced a powerful contraction of an eserinized leech muscle preparation. The substance, considered to be a choline ester, was in all probability ACh formed as a result of metabolic processes in the tissue slice. Its rate of synthesis was accelerated by glucose in a phosphate or bicarbonate medium when potassium or calcium ions were absent. Addition of these cations decreased synthesis of the substance in a bicarbonate medium but enhanced it in a phosphate-glucose medium. L-Lactate, pyruvate, or glutamate substituted poorly for glucose, and the addition of choline did not measurably increase synthesis. Kidney, spleen, liver, or testis had no measurable activity in forming the choline ester under conditions most favorable for its production in brain. There was no correlation between the cholinesterase activity of these organs and their ability to produce the choline ester *in vitro*.

Observations on the requirements for *in vitro* synthesis of ACh by brain were extended by Mann *et al.* (1938) who defined a "combined" inactive form and a "free," pharmacologically active, form. They demonstrated that the presence of choline enhances ester formation under optimal conditions and advanced a reasonably accurate scheme of ACh synthesis from its choline precursor. The formation of "free" ACh was found to be enhanced by the addition of 27 m*M* potassium to the incubation medium. The accelerating effect of potassium could be neutralized by calcium or magnesium ions and failed to occur in substrate-free media. Although Mann *et al.* (1938) considered these effects of potassium to be due primarily to changes in cell permeability, other workers (Welsh and Hyde, 1944) have suggested that potassium may play a role in carbohydrate metabolism and that high potassium levels may favor formation of the energy-rich phosphate compounds shown by Nachmansohn (1962) to supply energy for ACh synthesis. Thus more than one action of potassium may be responsible for its effects on ACh formation and release.

Although Quastel *et al.* (1936) demonstrated the formation of ACh by cortical slices respiring in an eserine-glucose medium, it was not established whether glucose donated carbon atoms or indirectly stimulated ACh synthesis from other sources. Using ^{14}C-labeled precursors Browning and Schulman (1968) observed that glucose-U-^{14}C and pyruvate-2-^{14}C formed similar amounts of labeled ACh in brain slices. Hydrolysis of ACh with chromatography of the resultant acetic acid showed that all the label was located in the acetyl moiety. Acetate-^{14}C did not serve as a precursor of the acetyl group of ACh. Equivalent incorporation of carbons 1 and 6 of glucose indicated that glucose metabolism occurred via the Enden-Meyerhoff pathway. Choline-^{14}C, either methyl or chain labeled, formed ACh-^{14}C while ethanolamine, serine, and methionine did not. Synthesis from radioactive choline was glucose dependent. The addition of 10^{-4} *M* hemicholinium-3 inhibited ACh formation by 90% from both glucose-U-^{14}C and choline-ME-^{14}C. Confirmation of these findings in brain slices have been provided by Chakrin and Shideman (1968) and Chakrin *et al.* (1968) who demonstrated *in vivo* synthesis of ACh from labeled choline previously injected into the cortex of the intact cat brain.

The synthesis of free ACh by brain slices under optimal conditions has been reported to be accelerated by very low concentrations and inhibited by higher concentrations of a variety of convulsant (picrotoxin, pentylenetetrazol, camphor), narcotic, or anticonvulsant (pentobarbital, amytal, phenobarbital, tribromethanol) drugs (McLennan and Elliott, 1951), More recently Polak (1967) reported that antimuscarinic drugs such as atropine, hyoscine, and especially the hallucinogenic antimuscarinic 3-quinuclidol enhance ACh synthesis in rat brain slices. It was suggested that these agents might increase synthesis by blocking a negative feedback mechanism linking synthesis with ACh levels as postulated by Mann *et al.* (1939).

IV. Release

Studies employing electrically stimulated brain slices previously incubated with labeled amines provide an alternative approach to the investigation of stimulation-induced release of central neurotransmitters. McIlwain and co-workers have been the principal contributors to our understanding of the neurophysiological properties of separated cerebral tissues. Using micro-electrodes they have found that mammalian cortical slices maintain membrane potentials of up to 60 mV (Li and McIlwain, 1957) which are sensitive to oxygen and glucose deprivation as well as to changes in the ionic composition of the incubation medium (Hillman and McIlwain, 1961; Hillman *et al.*, 1963; Gibson and McIlwain, 1965). These membrane potentials may be reversibly diminished by raising the potassium concentration of the incubation medium or by applying small quantities of potassium-rich solutions to the tissue surface (Hillman and McIlwain, 1961). Application of 0.5 to 2.0 *M* KCl in this fashion evokes a prompt change in the membrane potential which can reach complete depolarization in 5 to 10 milliseconds (Gibson and McIlwain, 1965). Spontaneous discharges, which more closely resemble neuronal spikes than the potentials associated with glial or vascular cells (Hillman *et al.*, 1963), as well as evoked electrical activity in the form of trains of spike discharges have also been demonstrated in brain slices (Richards and McIlwain, 1967).

The resting membrane potentials which are measurable in slices of cerebral tissue may also be reversibly displaced by appropriate electrical stimulation (Hillman *et al.*, 1963). Measurement of the time course of recovery of membrane potential after 10 minutes of stimulation indicates that potentials reach nearly zero and recover at the rate of about 12.5 mV per minute. A variety of metabolic responses attend such stimulation (McIlwain, 1966). These appear to be unique to slices of cerebral tissue; neither evoked electrical activity nor stimulation-induced metabolic alterations have been demonstrated in slices of liver or kidney (McIlwain, 1966). Furthermore, tissue subjected to mechanical damage fails to evidence resting or evoked membrane potentials and no response to pulse stimulation has been established in ground or homogenized tissue or in subcellular particles (Narayanaswami and McIlwain, 1954). Resting membrane potentials as well as the metabolic sequelae of electrical stimulation may be substantially modified by a variety of pharmacological agents when added to the incubation medium (Hillman *et al.*, 1963).

Electrical stimulation of mammalian brain slices previously incubated with a labeled amine or amino acid has been used to study the stimulus-induced release of several putative cerebral neurotransmitters (Baldessarini and Kopin, 1966, 1967; Chase *et al.*, 1967; Katz *et al.*, 1968, 1969; Chase *et al.*, 1969; Iversen and Neal, 1968; Mitchell *et al.*, 1968). Following incubation, the slices are transferred to individual chambers through which fresh medium is rapidly circulated. When the spontaneous efflux of radioactivity diminishes and becomes nearly steady, electrical field stimuli of low intensity and short duration is applied and the effluent superfusate collected for assay of radioactive constituents. Stimulation of brain slices, previously incubated with labeled monoamines produces a rapid rise in the efflux of radioactivity which consists mainly of the unmetabolized amine.

The specificity of release of exogenous amines by electrical field stimulation of superfused brain slices is suggested by the following observations: (1) electrical stimulation predominantly effects the efflux of the unchanged amine rather than its principal metabolites (Baldessarini and Kopin, 1967; Chase *et al.*, 1967); (2) release appears to depend on the viability and structural integrity of the brain slices (Chase *et al.*, 1969); (3) labeled substances such as urea, inulin, and 5-HIAA which are not concentrated in nerve terminals do not appear to be liberated by electrical stimulation (Baldessarini and Kopin, 1967; Chase *et al.*, 1969); (4) the amount of stimulus-evoked release of putative neurotransmitters appears to parallel the local concentration of these substances *in vivo* (Katz *et al.*, 1969; Chase *et al.*, 1969); noncerebral tissue such as liver, duodenum, or denervated salivary gland which have few, if any, monoaminergic terminals, evidence relatively small amounts of release during electrical stimulation (Baldessarini and Kopin, 1967). Presumably nonspecific uptake (Hamberger, 1967; Lenn, 1967) and release may account for much of the stimulus-evoked liberation of radioactivity from such extracerebral tissues.

A. Catecholamine Release

Spontaneous or stimulus-evoked release of exogenous amines can be influenced by altering the ionic content or by adding drugs to the superfusing medium. The demonstration that elevated external potassium concentration (25 m*M* or above) substantially enhances the rate of efflux of labeled NE (Baldessarini and Kopin, 1967) may relate to the ability of increased potassium levels to induce nerve membrane depolarization in brain slices (Hillman and McIlwain, 1961). Spontaneous efflux of exogenous NE does not appear to be affected by omission of sodium or calcium ions or by enhanced (7 m*M*) calcium levels (Katz and Kopin, 1969a).

Lithium salts appear to be effective in the treatment of mania and hypomania (Baastrup and Schou, 1967; Gershon and Yuwiler, 1960) and to influence the metabolism of NE *in vivo* (Schildkraut *et al.*, 1966). Lithium at a concentration of 2.4 meq/liter, comparable to that found in brain 8 hours after a parenteral injection of 7.5 meq/kg (Corrodi *et al.*, 1967), partially inhibits the electrically induced release of NE-^{3}H from brain slices (Katz *et al.*, 1968). When other monovalent cations (cesium, rubidium, choline, or tetramethylammonium, all 2.4 meq/liter) are substituted for lithium in the superfusate, no difference in either spontaneous or evoked release can be demonstrated. Stimulation-induced amine release from brain slices prepared from rats treated with lithium *in vivo* for 3 days (2.5 meq/kg) is also significantly diminished. The mechanism of release of NE from adrenal medulla (Douglas, 1966), peripheral sympathetic nerve (Burn and Gibbons, 1964), atria (Katz and Kopin, 1969a), and brain slice (Baldessarini and Kopin, 1967; Katz and Kopin, 1969a) is calcium dependent. Because the lithium-induced blockade of NE-^{3}H release is reversed by augmented levels of calcium in the superfusate (Katz and Kopin, 1969a), it appears that lithium may act directly or indirectly to interfere with calcium participation in stimulus-release coupling.

At concentrations which have been shown to block the uptake of monoamines into brain slices (Dengler *et al.*, 1962), ouabain significantly diminishes the evoked release of NE-^{3}H (Katz and Kopin, 1969a). This effect of ouabain, which is not reversed by augmented calcium levels, may relate to the drug's ability to interfere with sodium-dependent axonal conduction of the nerve action potential. Inhibition by tetrodotoxin of low amperage (10 mamp) induced release may also reflect an interference with impulse conduction to the nerve terminal. This view is supported by the finding that the inhibition of low amperage release produced by lithium, ouabain, tetrodotoxin, or calcium omission may be reversed through the use of higher current strengths, which may act directly to depolarize nerve terminals. Inhibition of stimulus-evoked release of NE-^{3}H from brain slices has also been demonstrated with a variety of psychoactive compounds including phenobarbital, chlorpromazine, and desipramine (Baldessarini and Kopin, 1967), bromide ions (Goodwin *et al.*, 1969), and *d*-lysergic acid diethylamide (Katz and Kopin, 1969b).

Preliminary experiments suggest that labeled DA (Baldessarini and Kopin, 1966) as well as metaraminol (Kopin, personal communication) can be released from brain slices, but studies of ionic requirements or drug effects remain to be performed.

B. Serotonin Release

Numerous studies have demonstrated that radioactively labeled 5-HT taken up by mammalian brain slices can be released during procedures which induce neuronal depolarization (Chase *et al.*, 1967, 1969; Katz *et al.*, 1968; Katz and Kopin, 1969b). Passage of a small electric current through the slice or elevating the external potassium concentration are similarly effective. Whether 5-HT-^{3}H is introduced into the brain of the living animal or incubated with cerebral tissue *in vitro* appears to make little difference in the amount of tritiated amine liberated.

In view of the regional differences in the density of 5-HT-containing nerve terminals in rat brain (Fuxe, 1965), corresponding variations in the accumulation and stimulus-evoked release of 5-HT-^{3}H might be anticipated. Chase *et al.* (1969) have shown that while there is an appreciable uptake of tritiated 5-HT into slices of frontal cortex, corpus striatum, and hypothalamus, only sparse uptake can be demonstrated in cerebellar folia. Marked regional differences in release of 5-HT-^{3}H were also found. Striatal and hypothalamic slices exhibited the largest evoked efflux of any of the regions tested. Significantly less release was obtained from frontal cortex and thalamus while release from cerebellum was negligible.

Lithium chloride (2.4 meq/liter) markedly inhibits evoked release of 5-HT-^{3}H and this diminution was unaffected by enhanced (11 m*M*) calcium levels in the superfusate (Chase *et al.*, 1969). In contrast to the inhibitory effect of low calcium on the release of NE-^{3}H from brain slices, the absence of calcium in the superfusate dose not appear to interfere with the release of 5-HT-^{3}H (Chase *et al.*, 1969; Katz and Kopin, 1969a). Thus it appears that the mechanism of release of 5-HT may differ from that of NE. The observation that the lithium-induced inhibition of the evoked release of 5-HT-^{3}H is not reversed by increased calcium levels is consistent with the view that 5-HT release is not calcium dependent. The inhibition of the noncalcium-dependent release of 5-HT suggests that lithium may not diminish NE release by a direct effect on calcium.

The disposition of 5-HT in brain slices can be altered by a variety of drugs. Bowers *et al.* (1965) have reported that the initial spontaneous release of endogenous 5-HT from whole brain slices was enhanced by addition of reserpine (2×10^{-5} *M*) to the incubation medium although it was uncertain whether the 5-HT release originated from bound stores or from synthesis as well. The former possibility would appear more likely, however, in view of the well documented influence of reserpine and related compounds to alter the binding of serotonin to particulate nerve ending fractions (Marchbanks, 1966). The addition of ouabain (10^{-4} *M*), chlorpromazine (10^{-4} *M*), tetrodotoxin (10^{-6} g/ml), *d*-LSD (10^{-6} *M*), or bromide ions (20 meq/liter) to the superfusing medium substantially inhibits the stimulus-induced release of 5-HT-^{3}H from striatal slices (Chase *et al.*, 1969; Katz and Kopin, 1969a, b).

d-LSD and related hallucinogens appear to exert a relatively selective inhibitory effect on the stimulus-induced release of 5-HT from brain slices (Chase *et al.*, 1969; Katz and Kopin, 1969b). The lowest incubation medium concentration of *d*-LSD producing significant inhibition is 10^{-6} *M*. This is considerably greater than the level of *d*-LSD which inhibits firing of serotonergic neurons (Aghajanian *et al.*, 1968), but less than that used to demonstrate changes in serotonin metabolism in brain (Rosencrans *et al.*, 1967). At this dose level, evoked release of NE is unaffected. The L-isomer of LSD as well as BOL, which are relatively impotent hallucinogens, fail to inhibit evoked release of 5-HT, while other hallucinogenic compounds, mescaline and *N*,*N*-dimethyltryptamine, inhibit release of 5-HT without influencing

NE release (Katz and Kopin, 1969b). Other psychoactive drugs such as chlorpromazine, which inhibit release of 5-HT, also inhibit release of NE to about the same extent at comparable dose levels.

The foregoing observations are of interest in view of collateral evidence suggesting an effect of hallucinogenic agents on central serotonergic mechanisms (cf. Giarman and Freedman, 1965; Appel and Freedman, 1964; Kawai and Yamamoto, 1968). Although there is considerable evidence to indicate that LSD may act directly on serotonergic receptors in brain (Aghajanian *et al.*, 1968), Rosencrans *et al.* (1967) have observed that LSD produces a small but significant elevation in brain 5-HT concentrations, while reducing levels of 5-HIAA, the principal metabolite of 5-HT. This effect could reflect a decrease in 5-HT turnover consequent to an inhibition of release (Diaz *et al.*, 1968). The observation that LSD increases the specific activity of 5-HT in brain 60 minutes after injection of 5-HTP-^{14}C (Siva Sankar *et al.*, 1962) is compatible with this view.

C. Amino Acid Release

The stimulus evoked release of exogenous GABA from brain slices has been reported (Katz *et al.*, 1969; Mitchell *et al.*, 1968). Unmetabolized GABA-^{3}H in the effluent superfusate from both stimulated or non-electrically stimulated slices accounts for about three-quarters of the total radioactivity (Katz *et al.*, 1969). The amount of spontaneous release from frontal cortex, striatum, diencephalon, and cerebellum is not significantly different. On the other hand, there are regional variations in the evoked release of GABA which to some extent parallel the local endogenous concentrations of this substance in mammalian brain (Fahn and Coté, 1968). These findings suggest that uptake into specific neurons may be essential for high level release by electrical stimulation. In addition to the results with GABA, the electrically evoked release of representative basic (L-lysine-^{14}C), neutral (L-leucine-^{14}C), and acidic (glutamic acid-^{14}C) amino acids as well as the amino acid decarboxylation product taurine-^{14}C and the synthetic amino acid analog L-amino cyclopentane-1-carboxylic acid-^{14}C have also been observed in slices of rat striatum (Katz *et al.*, 1969).

In general, the depolarization-induced release of amino acids from brain slices is similar to that occurring with exogenous NE or 5-HT. Elevating the potassium concentration of the superfusing medium produces a rapid increase in the efflux of radioactivity (Katz *et al.*, 1969; Mitchell, 1968). In contrast to NE but similar to 5-HT, the mechanism of GABA and other AA release from cerebral tissues does not appear to require ionic calcium (Katz *et al.*, 1969; Mitchell *et al.*, 1968). Furthermore, although AA are actively taken up into a variety of tissues *in vitro* (Christensen, 1962), no significant electrically induced release of GABA-^{3}H or L-glutamic acid-^{14}C could be demonstrated from slices of liver or kidney. The presence of lithium chloride (2.4 meq/liter) in the superfusate produces a significant reduction in the stimulation-induced release of labeled AA. Increasing the calcium concentration of the superfusing medium to 11 m*M* fails to reverse the lithium-induced inhibition of radioactive amino acid release. In this instance, as in the case of calcium dependence, the release of amino acids from brain slices resembles that of 5-HT more than that of NE.

The mechanism by which electrical stimulation liberates substances from brain slices remains unknown. Although there is some evidence that endogenous GABA may be stored in nerve terminal particles (Salganicoff and DeRobertis, 1965; Iversen and Snyder, 1968), the subcellular distribution of all other endogenous free amino acids appears to be mainly, if not exclusively, in the cytoplasm (Whittaker, 1965; Ryall, 1964). It would thus appear that localization to neuronal vesicles may not be necessary for depolarization-induced release under the conditions used in these experiments. Electrically induced release may merely reflect the increased permeability of cell membranes which presumably attends electrical stimulation. Unlike the uptake of AA, however, which occurs to a significant degree in nonneural tissues such as liver and kidney (Christensen, 1962), the electrically induced release of AA may be a unique property of neural tissue.

D. Acetylcholine Release

Much of the early information on release of ACh from nervous tissue derives from studies of ACh synthesis and the influence of ions or drugs on the partition of ACh between tissue and medium (Mann *et al.*, 1938, 1939; Welsh and Hyde, 1944; McLennan and Elliott, 1950; Elliott *et al.*, 1950). The bioassay techniques used in these studies have recently been questioned (Hosein *et al.*, 1965; Hosein and Orzeck, 1966) although defended by others (Strovinoha and Ryan, 1965; Crossland and Redfern, 1963; McLennan *et al.*, 1963; Pepeu *et al.*, 1963).

Recent studies of the spontaneous liberation of endogenous ACh have been reported by Bowers (1967). Incubation of rat cerebral cortex preparations for 30 minutes to 1 hour in a modified Tyrode's solution containing eserine failed to alter significantly the slice content of ACh and only small amounts of ACh were found in the bathing medium. If the potassium concentration of the incubation medium was raised tenfold in the presence of eserine, approximately half of the tissue-bound ACh was liberated into the medium during the 1-hour incubation period. Because a low rather than a high potassium concentration in the incubation medium favors the accumulation of ACh into brain slices in the presence as compared to the absence of eserine (Bowers, 1967; Elliott and Henderson, 1951), it would appear that increased levels of potassium tend to release ACh and prevent the binding of newly synthesized ACh. While ACh reuptake may occur in an eserinized, low potassium solution, this phenomenon has not been observed and the reutilization of ACh released from nerve endings remains to be demonstrated. It seems reasonable, therefore to attribute the effects of high potassium to a modification of ACh release from its bound form with only secondary effects on synthesis.

Kalant and Grose (1967) have examined the influence of ethanol and pentobarbital on the spontaneous release of ACh from guinea pig cerebral cortex *in vitro*. Ethanol (10^{-1} M) reversibly diminished ACh release from brain slices incubated in a medium containing 5 mM potassium. In the presence of 15 or 27 mM potassium, ACh release was greater but ethanol had no effect. Pentobarbital exerted a biphasic action: low concentrations stimulating and high concentrations inhibiting ACh release. Interestingly, brain slices from animals made tolerant to ethanol by daily administration of intoxicating doses were refractory to the *in vitro* effects of ethanol on ACh release.

The evoked release of ACh from brain slices from several species has been studied by Rowsell (1954). With electrical stimulation, enhanced efflux of free ACh into the incubation medium and reduced ACh content of the tissue slice was observed. Prior to stimulation, the ACh content of the brain slices was allowed to increase to levels severalfold greater than those found *in vivo*. The possibility that the stimulation itself enhanced synthesis could not be ruled out. Bowers (1967) also observed that the application of electrical stimulation to brain slices resulted in a significantly increased content of ACh in the incubation medium compared to unstimulated controls. The mean slice concentration of ACh, however, did not differ in the two groups after the stimulation period. Although there was a slight increase in total (slice plus incubate) ACh under the stimulus conditions, the change was not statistically significant.

The influence of belladonna alkaloids on the dynamics of ACh in the CNS *in vivo* and *in vitro* has been studied by several investigators. The experiments of Bowers (1967) suggest that, *in vitro*, either scopolamine or electrical stimulation increase the efflux of ACh from brain slices. These results are in general agreement with earlier findings that the output of ACh from exposed cerebral cortex is increased following the administration of atropine, scopolamine, or other anticholinergics (Mitchell, 1963; Collier and Mitchell, 1966) and that these compounds tend to reduce cerebral ACh levels (Giarman and Pepeu, 1965). The mechanism by which anticholinergics stimulate ACh release and deplete levels of this substance in CNS tissues remains uncertain. Conceivably, a blockade of postsynaptic receptors with a secondary activation of feedback mechanisms which accelerate neuronal firing (MacIntosh, 1963) or an interference with possible reuptake and reutilization of released ACh or its precursors by central neurons (Giarman and Pepeu, 1964; Szerb, 1964; Celesia and Jasper, 1966) may be responsible.

V. Conclusions

Attempts to explain the mode of action of drugs in the central nervous system in terms of their effects on neurohumoral mechanisms depends upon an array of detailed observations under controlled conditions. Despite its obvious limitations, the brain slice facilitates such observations and has already contributed to our understanding of physiological and biochemical processes in cerebral tissues. Available results, however, indicate some disparities between the uptake metabolism and release of putative general neurotransmitters *in vitro* and *in vivo*. The continued usefulness of this preparation requires a more precise delineation of the relationship between events observed in isolated cerebral tissues and those occurring in living brain.

References

Abadom, P. N., and Scholefield, P. G. (1962a). *Can. J. Biochem. Physiol.* **40**, 1575.
Abadom, P. N., and Scholefield, P. G. (1962b). *Can. J. Biochem. Physiol.* **40**, 1591.
Aghajanian, G. K., Foote, W. E., and Sheard, M. H. (1968). *Science* **161**, 706.
Appel, J. B., and Freedman, D. X. (1964). *Biochem. Pharmacol.* **13**, 861.
Awapara, J., Landau, A. J., Fuerst, R., and Seale, B. (1950). *J. Biol. Chem.* **187**, 35.
Baastrup, P., and Schou, M. (1967). *Arch. Gen. Psychiat.* **16**, 162.
Baldessarini, R. J., and Kopin, I. J. (1966). *Science* **152**, 1630.
Baldessarini, R. J., and Kopin, I. J. (1967). *J. Pharmacol. Exp. Ther.* **156**, 31.
Barborosa, E., Joanny, P., and Corriol, J. (1968). *Experientia* **24**, 1196.
Beloff-Chain, A., Cantazaro, R., Chain, E. B., Masi, I., and Pocchiari, F. (1955). *Proc. Roy Soc., Ser. B* **144**, 22.
Bernard, C. (1856). *C. R. Acad. Sci.* **43**, 825.
Bertler, A., Falck, B., Owman, C., and Rosengren, E. (1966). *Pharmacol. Rev.* **18**, 369.
Bessman, S. R., Rossen, J., and Layne, E. C. (1953). *J. Biol. Chem.* **201**, 385.
Blackburn, K. J., French, P. C., and Merrills, R. J. (1967). *Life Sci.* **6**, 1653.
Blasberg, R. (1968). *Progr. Brain Res.* **29**, 245.
Blasberg, R., and Lajtha, A. (1965). *Arch. Biochem. Biophys.* **112**, 361.
Blasberg, R., and Lajtha, A. (1966). *Brain Res.* **1**, 86.
Bloom, F. E., and Giarman, N. J. (1968). *Annu. Rev. Pharmacol.* **8**, 229.
Bowers, M. B. (1967). *Int. J. Neuropharmacol.* **6**, 399.
Bowers, M. B., Roodman, S. T., and Filbert, M. G. (1965). *Biochem. Pharmacol.* **14**, 374.
Breese, G. R., Chase, T. N., and Kopin, I. J. (1969). *J. Pharmacol. Exp. Ther.* **165**, 9.
Browning, E. T., and Schulman, M. P. (1968). *J. Neurochem.* **15**, 1391.
Burn, J. H., and Gibbons, W. R. (1964). *Brit. J. Pharmacol. Chemother.* **22**, 540.
Burton, R. M. (1964). *Int. J. Neuropharmacol.* **3**, 13.
Carlsson, A. (1965). *Handbuch. Exp. Pharmakol.* **19**, 529.

Carlsson, A. (1966). *In* "Mechanisms of Release of Biogenic Amines," Proc. Int. Wenner-Gren Symp. (U. S. von Euler, ed.), p. 331. Macmillan (Pergamon), New York.
Celesia, G. G., and Jasper, H. H. (1966). *Neurology* **16**, 1053.
Chakrin, L. W., and Shideman, F. E. (1968). *Int. J. Neuropharmacol.* **7**, 337.
Chakrin, L. W., Shideman, F. E., and Marazzi, A. S. (1968). *Int. J. Neuropharmacol.* **7**, 351.
Chase, T. N., Breese, G. R., and Kopin, I. J. (1967). *Science* **157**, 1461.
Chase, T. N., Katz, R. I., and Kopin, I. J. (1969). *J. Neurochem.* **16**, 607.
Chirigos, M. A., Greengard, P., and Udenfriend, S. (1960). *J. Biol. Chem.* **235**, 2075.
Christensen, H. N. (1962). "Biological Transport," p. 133. Benjamin, New York.
Collier, B., and Mitchell, J. F. (1966). *J. Physiol.* (*London*) **184**, 239.
Corrodi, H., Fuxe, K., Hokefelt, T., and Schou, M. (1967). *Psychopharmacologia* **11**, 345.
Crossland, J., and Redfern, P. H. (1963). *Life Sci.* **10**, 711.
Curtis, D. R., and Watkins, J. C. (1965). *Pharmacol. Rev.* **17**, 347.
Davis, J. E., Brown, H., Huff, J. A., and Cashaw, J. L. (1967). *J. Lab. Clin. Med.* **69**, 132.
Deitrich, R. A. (1966). *Biochem. Pharmacol.* **15**, 1911.
Dengler, H. J. (1965). *Proc. 2nd Int. Pharmacol. Meeting, Prague, 1963* **3**, 261.
Dengler, H. J., Spiegler, H. E., and Titus, E. (1961). *Nature* (*London*) **191**, 816.
Dengler, H. J., Michaelson, I. A., Spiegel, H. E., and Titus, E. (1962). *Int. J. Neuropharmacol.* **1**, 23.
Diaz, P. M., Ngai, S. H., and Costa, E. (1968). *Advan. Pharmacol.* **6B**, 75.
Douglas, W. W. (1966). *Pharmacol. Rev.* **18**, 471.
Eccleston, D., Moir, A. T. B., Reading, H. W., and Ritchie, I. M. (1966). *Brit. J. Pharmacol. Chemother.* **28**, 367.
Eccleston, D., Reading, H. W., and Ritchie, I. M. (1969). *J. Neurochem.* **16**, 274.
Elliott, K. A. C., and Henderson, N. (1951). *Amer. J. Physiol.* **165**, 365.
Elliott, K. A. C. and van Gelder, R. (1958). *J. Neurochem.* **3**, 28.
Elliott, K. A. C., Swank, R. L., and Henderson, N. (1950). *Amer. J. Physiol.* **162**, 469.
Fahn, S., and Coté, L. J. (1968). *J. Neurochem.* **15**, 209.
Falck, B. (1962). *Acta Physiol. Scand. Suppl.* **197**, 56.
Feldstein, A., and Williamson, O. (1968). *Brit. J. Pharmacol.* **34**, 38.
Feldstein, A., and Wong, K. (1965). *Life Sci.* **4**, 183.
Fuxe, K. (1965). *Acta Physiol. Scand. Suppl.* **247**, 39.
Gershon, S., and Yuwiler, A. (1960). *J. Neuropsychiat.* **1**, 229.
Giarman, N. J., and Freedman, D. X. (1965). *Pharmacol. Rev.* **17**, 1.
Giarman, N. J., and Pepeu, G. (1964). *Brit. J. Pharmacol. Chemother.* **23**, 123.
Gibson, I. M., and McIlwain, H. (1965). *J. Physiol.* (*London*) **176**, 261.
Glowinski, J., and Axelrod, J. (1966). *Pharmacol. Rev.* **18**, 775.
Glowinski, J., and Baldessarini, R. J. (1966). *Pharmacol. Rev.* **18**, 1201.
Glowinski, J., and Iversen, L. L. (1966). *J. Neurochem.* **13**, 655.
Goodwin, J. S., Katz, R. I., and Kopin, I. J. (1969). *Nature* (*London*) **221**, 556.
Graham-Smith, D. G. (1964). *Biochem. Biophys. Res. Commun.* **16**, 586.
Guroff, G., King, W., and Udenfriend, S. (1961). *J. Biol. Chem.* **236**, 1773.
Guth, P. S. (1962). *Fed. Proc. Fed. Amer. Soc. Exp. Biol.* **21**, 1100.
Haggendal, J., and Hamberger, B. (1967). *Acta Physiol. Scand.* **70**, 277.
Hamberger, B. (1967). *Acta Physiol. Scand. Suppl.* **295**, 1.
Hamberger, B., and Masuoka, D. (1965). *Acta Pharmacol. Toxicol.* **22**, 363.
Hebb, C., and Whittaker, V. P. (1958). *J. Physiol.* (*London*) **142**, 187.

Heilbronn, E. (1969). *J. Neurochem.* **16**, 627.

Hill, A. V. (1932). "Chemical Wave Transmission in Nerve," p. 34. Cambridge Univ. Press, London and New York.

Hillarp, N.-A., and Malmfors, T. (1964). *Life Sci.* **3**, 703.

Hillman, H. H., and McIlwain, H. (1961). *J. Physiol. (London)* **157**, 263.

Hillman, H. H., Campbell, W. J., and McIlwain, H. (1963). *J. Neurochem.* **10**, 325.

Hosein, E. A., and Orzeck, A. (1966). *Can. J. Physiol. Pharmacol.* **44**, 510.

Hosein, E. A., Rambaut, P., Chabrol, J. G., and Orzeck, A. (1965). *Arch. Biochem. Biophys.* **111**, 540.

Hughes, F. B., and Brodie, B. B. (1959). *J. Pharmacol. Exp. Ther.* **127**, 96.

Ishii, T., and Friede, R. L. (1968). *Amer. J. Anat.* **122**, 139.

Iversen, L. L., and Neal, M. J. (1968). *J. Neurochem.* **15**, 1141.

Iversen, L. L., and Snyder, S. H. (1968). *Nature (London)* **220**, 796.

Iyer, N. T., McGeer, P. L., and McGeer, E. G. (1963). *Can. J. Biochem. Physiol.* **41**, 1565.

Jonason, J., and Rutledge, C. O. (1968a). *Acta Physiol. Scand.* **73**, 411.

Jonason, J., and Rutledge, C. O. (1968b). *Acta Physiol. Scand.* **73**, 161.

Kalant, H., and Grose, W. (1967). *J. Pharmacol. Exp. Ther.* **158**, 386.

Kandera, J., Levi, G., and Lajtha, A. (1968). *Arch. Biochem. Biophys.* **126**, 249.

Katz, R. I., and Kopin, I. J. (1969a). *Biochem. Pharmacol.* **18**, 1935.

Katz, R. I., and Kopin, I. J. (1969b). *Pharmacol. Res. Commun.* **1**, 54.

Katz, R. I., Chase, T. N., and Kopin, I. J. (1968). *Science* **162**, 466.

Katz, R. I., Chase, T. N., and Kopin, I. J. (1969). *J. Neurochem.* **16**, 961.

Kawai, N., and Yamamoto, C. (1968). *Brain Res.* **7**, 325.

Kindwall, E. P., and Weiner, N. (1966). *J. Neurochem.* **13**, 1523

Kini, M. M., and Quastel, J. H. (1959). *Nature (London)* **184**, 252.

Koen, A. L., and Shaw, C. R. (1966). *Biochim. Biophys. Acta* **128**, 48.

Lahiri, S., and Lajtha, A. (1964). *J. Neurochem.* **11**, 77.

Lajtha, A. (1964). *In* "Comparative Neurochemistry" (D. Richter, ed.), p. 491. Macmillan (Pergamon) New York.

Lajtha, A. (1967). *Vopr. Biokhim. Mozga* **3**, 31.

Lajtha, A. (1968). *Progr. Brain Res.* **29**, 201.

Lajtha, A., and Toth, J. (1961). *J. Neurochem.* **9**, 199.

Lajtha, A., and Toth, J. (1963). *J. Neurochem.* **10**, 909.

Lajtha, A., and Toth, J. (1965). *Biochem. Pharmacol.* **14**, 729.

Lenn, N. J. (1967), *Amer. J. Anat.* **120**, 377.

Levi, G., and Lajtha, A. (1965). *J. Neurochem.* **12**, 639.

Levi, G., Cherayil, A., and Lajtha, A. (1965). *J. Neurochem.* **12**, 757.

Levi, G., Kandera, J., and Lajtha, A. (1967). *Arch. Biochem. Biophys.* **119**, 303.

Li, C.-H., and McIlwain, H. (1957). *J. Physiol. (London)* **139**, 178.

Liang, C. C., and Quastel, J. H. (1969a). *Biochem. Pharmacol.* **18**, 1169.

Liang, C. C., and Quastel, J. H. (1969b). *Biochem. Pharmacol.* **18**, 1187.

Machiyama, Y., Balasz, R., and Richter, D. (1967). *J. Neurochem.* **14**, 591.

McIlwain, H. (1966). *In* "Biochemistry and the Central Nervous System" (H. McIlwain, ed.), p. 49. Little, Brown, Boston, Massachusetts.

MacIntosh, F. C. (1963). *Can. J. Biochem. Physiol.* **41**, 2555.

McLennan, H., and Elliott, K. A. C. (1950). *Amer. J. Physiol.* **163**, 605.

McLennan, H., and Elliott, K. A. C. (1951). *Amer. J. Physiol.* **164**, 35.

McLennan, H., Curry, L., and Walker, R. (1963). *Biochem. J.* **89**, 163.

Mann, P. G. H., Tennenbaum, M., and Quastel, J. H. (1938). *Biochem. J.* **32**, 243.

Mann, P. G. H., Tennenbaum, M., and Quastel, J. H. (1939). *Biochem. J.* **33**, 822.
Marchbanks, R. M. (1966). *J. Neurochem.* **13**, 1481.
Masuoka, D. T., Clark, W. G., and Schott, H. F. (1961). *Rev. Can. Biol.* **20**, 1.
Masuoka, D. T., Schott, H. F., and Petriello, L. (1963). *J. Pharmacol. Exp. Ther.* **139**, 73
Merritt, J. H., and Schutz, E. J. (1966). *Life Sci.* **5**, 27.
Mitchell, J. F. (1968). *J. Physiol. (London)* **165**, 98.
Mitchell, J. F., Neal, M. J., and Srinivasan, V. (1968). *Brit. J. Pharmacol.* **34**, 661P.
Nachmansohn, D. (1962). *In* "Neurochemistry" (K. A. C. Elliott, I. H. Page, and J. H. Quastel, eds.), p. 522. Thomas, Springfield, Illinois.
Narayanaswami, A., and McIlwain, H. (1954). *Biochem. J.* **57**, 412.
Neame, K. D. (1961a). *Nature (London)* **192**, 173.
Neame, K. D. (1961b). *J. Neurochem.* **6**, 358.
Neame, K. D. (1968). *Progr. Brain Res.* **29**, 185.
Palaic, D., Page, I. H., and Khairallah, A. (1967). *J. Neurochem.* **14**, 63.
Pepeu, G., Schmidt, K. F., and Giarman, N. J. (1963). *Biochem. Pharmacol.* **12**, 385.
Pletscher, A., and Bartholini, G. (1967). *Med. Pharmacol. Exp.* **16**, 432.
Polak, R. L. (1967). *Acta Physiol. Pharmacol.* **14**, 505.
Polak, R. L. (1969). *Brit. J. Pharmacol.* **36**, 144.
Polak, R. L., and Meeuws, M. M. (1966). *Biochem. Pharmacol.* **15**, 989.
Potter, L. T., and Axelrod, J. (1963). *J. Pharmacol. Exp. Ther.* **142**, 291.
Quastel, J. H., Tennenbaum, M., and Wheatley, A. H. (1936). *Biochem. J.* **30**, 1668.
Richards, C. D., and McIlwain, H. (1967). *Nature (London)* **215**, 704.
Roberts, E., and Bregoff, H. M. (1953). *J. Biol. Chem.* **201**, 393.
Roberts, E., and Frankel, S. (1950). *J. Biol. Chem.* **187**, 55.
Roberts, E., and Frankel, S. (1951). *J. Biol. Chem.* **190**, 505.
Rosencrans, J. A., Lovell, R. A., and Freedman, D. X. (1967). *Biochem. Pharmacol.* **16**, 2011.
Ross, S. B., and Renyi, A. L. (1964). *Acta Pharmacol. Toxicol.* **21**, 226.
Ross, S. B., and Renyi, A. L. (1966a). *J. Pharm. Pharmacol.* **18**, 322.
Ross, S. B., and Renyi, A. L. (1966b). *Acta Pharmacol. Toxicol* **24**, 297.
Ross, S. B., and Renyi, A. L. (1967). *Life Sci.* **6**, 1407.
Rowsell, E. V. (1954). *Biochem. J.* **57**, 666.
Rutledge, C. O., and Jonason, J. (1967). *J. Pharmacol. Exp. Ther.* **157**, 493.
Ryall, R. W. (1964). *J. Neurochem.* **11**, 131.
Salganicoff, L., and DeRobertis, E. (1965). *J. Neurochem.* **12**, 287.
Sattin, A. (1966). *J. Neurochem.* **13**, 515.
Schanberg, S. M. (1963). *J. Pharmacol. Exp. Ther.* **139**, 191.
Schanberg, S. M., and Giarman, N. J. (1962). *Biochem. Pharmacol.* **2**, 187.
Schanberg, S. M., Schildkraut, J. J., Breese, G. R., and Kopin, I. J. (1968). *Biochem. Pharmacol.* **17**, 247.
Scheparty, B. (1963). *J. Neurochem.* **10**, 825.
Schildkraut, J. J., Schanberg, S. M., and Kopin, I. J. (1966). *Life Sci.* **5**, 1479.
Schuberth, J., and Sundwall, A. (1967). *J. Neurochem.* **14**, 807.
Schuberth, J., Sundwall, A., Sorbo, B., B., and Lindell, J.-O. (1966). *J. Neurochem.* **13**, 347.
Siva Sankar, D. V., Phipps, E., Gold, E., and Sankar, B. D. (1962). *Ann. N.Y. Acad. Sci.* **96**, 93.
Smith, S. E. (1963). *Brit. J. Pharmacol.* **20**, 178.
Snyder, S. H., Green, A. I., and Hendley, E. D. (1968). *J. Pharmacol. Exp. Ther.* **164**, 90.
Strovinoha, W. B., and Ryan, L. C. (1965). *J. Pharmacol. Exp. Ther.* **150**, 231.

Sung, C. P., and Johnstone, R. M. (1965). *Can. J. Biochem.* **43**, 1111.

Szerb, J. C. (1964). *Can. J. Physiol. Pharmacol.* **42**, 303.

Titus, E., and Dengler, H. J. (1966). *Pharmacol. Rev.* **18**, 525.

Tochino, Y., and Schanker, L. S. (1965). *Biochem. Pharmacol.* **14**, 1557.

Tsukada, Y., Nagata, Y., and Tagaki, N. (1957). *Proc. Jap. Acad.* **33**, 510.

Tsukada, Y., Nagata, Y., Hirano, S., and Matsutani, T. (1963). *J. Neurochem.* **10**, 241.

Udenfriend, S., and Creveling, C. R. (1959). *J. Neurochem.* **4**, 350.

Varon, S., Weinstein, H., Kakefude, T., and Roberts, E. (1965). *Biochem. Pharmacol.* **14**, 1213.

von Euler, U. S. (1956). "Noradrenaline: Chemistry, Physiology, Pharmacology and Clinical Aspects," p. 382. Thomas, Springfield, Illinois.

Wartburg, J. P. (1962). *Can. J. Biochem. Physiol.* **40**, 1439.

Weil-Malherbe, H., Whitby, L. G., and Axelrod, J. (1961). *J. Neurochem.* **8**, 55.

Weissbach, H., Redfield, B. G., and Titus, E. (1960). *Nature* (*London*) **185**, 99.

Welsh, J. H., and Hyde, J. E. (1944). *Amer. J. Physiol.* **142**, 512.

Werdinius, B. (1967). *Acta Pharmacol. Toxicol.* **25**, 18.

Whittaker, V. P. (1965). *Progr. Brain Res.* **8**, 90.

Whittaker, V. P., Michaelson, I. A., and Kirkland, R. J. A. (1964). *Biochem. J.* **90**, 293.

Yoshida, H., Namba, J., Kaniike, K., and Imaizumi, R. (1963a). *Jap. J. Pharmacol.* **13**, 1.

Yoshida, H., Kaniike, K., and Namba, J. (1963b). *Jap. J. Pharmacol.* **13**, 10.

Yoshida, H., Fujisawa, H., and Ohi, Y. (1965). *Can. J. Biochem.* **43**, 841.

An Introduction to Immunosuppressants

ALAN C. AISENBERG*

The John Collins Warren Laboratories
Huntington Memorial Hospital of Harvard University
at the Massachusetts General Hospital
Boston, Massachusetts

I. Introduction

While the major practical direction of classic immunology was toward enhancement of immunological responsiveness to increase resistance in infectious disease, immunology of the past decade has been principally concerned with attentuation of this responsiveness. Attenuation of immune reactions is directed toward two ends, the facilitation of organ transplantation and the control of autoimmune disease. Because these ends are of considerable clinical importance, and because immunosuppressants are the most effective

* The author's research is supported by Research Grant CA-07179 of the National Cancer Institute, United States Public Health Service, and Grant T-438 of the American Cancer Society. This is publication No. 1359 of the Cancer Commission of Harvard University.

means of diminishing immune responsiveness, a vast number of publications about these agents have appeared in the past 10 years. [One recent review includes over 900 references (Gabrielsen and Good, 1967).] The plethora of primary source material stems from the variation in immune responsiveness of different species and to different antigenic stimuli, here compounded by the variety of immunosuppressants available. The intention of this brief review is to establish underlying principles of immunosuppressive therapy rather than to catalog encyclopedic detail; other excellent and more extensive recent reviews are available (Schwartz, 1965, 1967, 1968; Berenbaum, 1965; Gabrielsen and Good, 1967; Hersh and Freireich, 1968; Parker and Vavra, 1969).

Although the interest of the nonimmunologist in immunosuppressants centers on man, unfortunately there are almost no experimental data on the action of these compounds on the immune response of normal individuals. The sparse available human data deal with diseased individuals (Levin *et al.*, 1964; Hersh *et al.*, 1965; Parker and Vavra, 1969), while the great preponderance of information comes from experimental animals. Clearly, the data from lower animals must be applied to man with considerable caution.

A few preliminary points should be made at the outset. This review is restricted to extrinsic agents which inhibit the immune response; inhibition by manipulations of antigen *alone* (specific immunological unresponsiveness or tolerance) are excluded from consideration. It should be stressed, however, that effective immunosuppression requires that, in some measure, there be specificity toward the antigen, organ, or tissue to which reactivity is to be suppressed, i.e. drug-induced immunological tolerance. Without this specificity, insufficient residual immunological reactivity would remain to cope with the variety of infectious organisms organisms to which every species is susceptible.

Successful immunosuppression also requires that the agent should not irreversibly damage any other body function. Inasmuch as the immunosuppressants are, for the most part, cytotoxic compounds which attack all rapidly dividing cells, the principal life-threatening toxicity usually involves depression of bone marrow production of the formed blood elements (polymorphonuclear leukocytes and blood platelets).

II. Immunosuppressants

Tables I and II contain, respectively, a listing of the principal immunosuppressive agents and their structual formulas. Table I is not meant to be exhaustive; it contains only those compounds with major immunosuppressive activity or those of historical or theoretical interest. Agents with a minor

TABLE I

THE PRINCIPAL IMMUNOSUPPRESSIVE AGENTS

1. Alkylating agents
   a. Nitrogen mustard
   b. Cyclophosphamide (Cytoxan)
   c. Chlorambucil (Leukeran)

2. Antimetabolites
   a. Antipurines: 6-mercaptopurine, azathioprine (Imuran), 6-thioguanine
   b. Folic acid antagonists: methotrexate
   c. Antipyrimidines: 5-fluorouracil,[a] 5-bromodeoxyuridine[a]

3. Antibiotics
   a. The actinomycins (C and D)
   b. Chloramphenicol
   c. Azaserine
   d. Mitomycin C[a]
   e. Puromysin[a]

4. Adrenal corticoids: predisone, etc.

5. Miscellaneous compounds
   a. Periwinkle alkaloids: vincristine and vinblastine
   b. Methyl hydrazine derivative: procarbazine

6. Antilymphocyte serum

7. Thoracic duct drainage

8. X-irradiation

[a] Predominant action *in vitro*.

effect in a single immunological system have been omitted. It is immediately apparent that Table I could serve equally well as a classification for cancer chemotherapeutic compounds. The reason for this will be clarified in a later section, but for the present it is obvious that a detailed consideration of the pharmacological or biochemical properties of this diverse group of complex compounds is beyond the scope of this review. Further, little would be gained by such a consideration since a number of excellent monographs in the field of cancer chemotherapy are available (Karnovsky and Clarkson, 1963; Burchenal, 1963; Calabresi and Welch, 1965; Brodsky and Kahn, 1967; Stock, 1966; Ochoa and Hirschberg, 1967).

Of the alkylating agents listed in Table I, nitrogen mustard is included largely for historical purposes. The progenitor of nitrogen mustard, sulfur mustard, was among the first materials to demonstrate significant immuno-

TABLE II

STRUCTURAL FORMULAS OF THE PRINCIPAL IMMUNOSUPPRESSIVE DRUGS

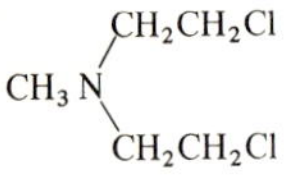
CH_2CH_2Cl
CH_3N
CH_2CH_2Cl

Methyl-bis (β-chloroethyl) amine

Nitrogen mustard

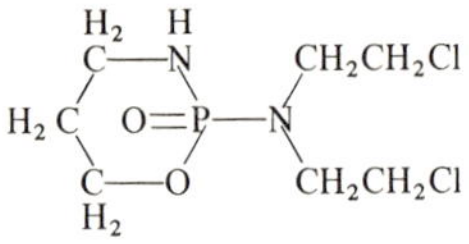
H_2 H
C—N
CH_2CH_2Cl
H_2C O=P—N
C—O
CH_2CH_2Cl
H_2

N,N-bis(β-Chloroethyl)-*N,O*-propylene phosphoric acid

Cyclophosphamide (Cytoxan)

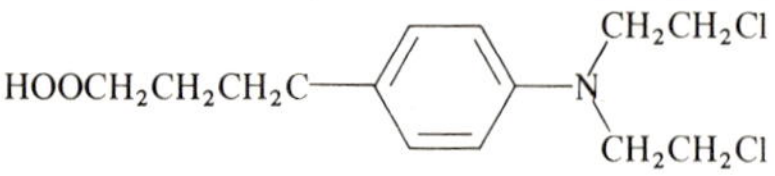
$HOOCH_2CH_2CH_2C$
N
CH_2CH_2Cl
CH_2CH_2Cl

p-di (β-Chloroethyl) aminophenylbutyric acid

Chlorambucil (Leukeran)

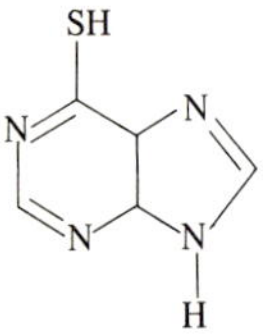
SH
N
N
N
N
H

6-Mercaptopurine

6-MP

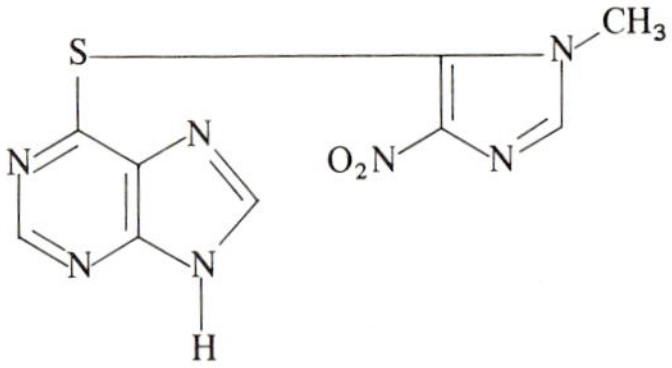
S
N
CH_3
N
N
O_2N
N
N
N
H

6-(1-Methyl-4-nitro-5-imidazoyl) thiopurine

Azathioprine (Imuran)

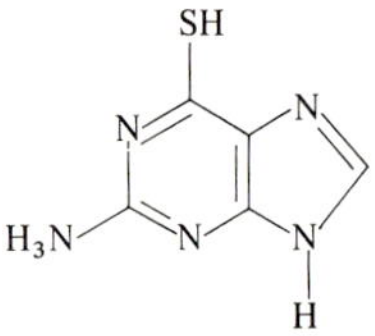
SH
N
N
H_3N
N
N
H

6-Thioquanine

6-TG

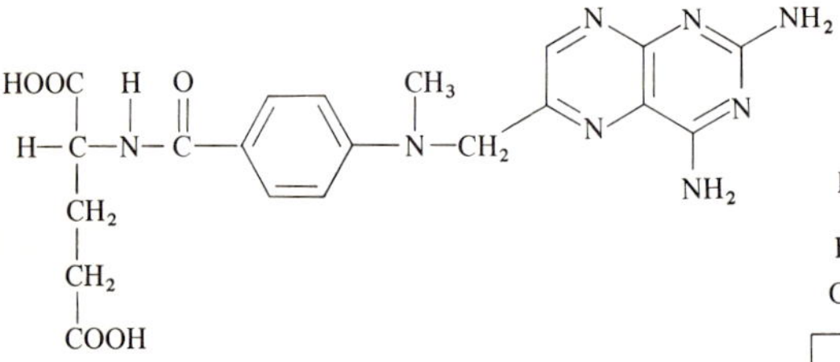
HOOC H O
H—C—N—C
CH_3
N—CH_2
N
N
NH_2
N
N
NH_2
CH_2
CH_2
COOH

4-Amino-N^{10}-methylpteroylglutamic acid

Methotrexate (Amethopterin)

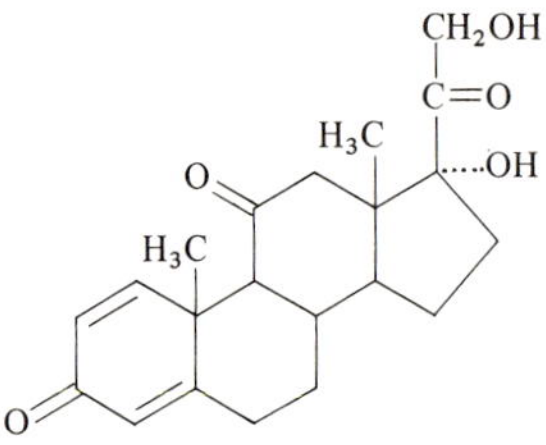
CH_2OH
C=O
H_3C
....OH
O
H_3C
O

17, 21-Dihydroxypregna-1,4-diene-3,11,20-trione

Prednisone

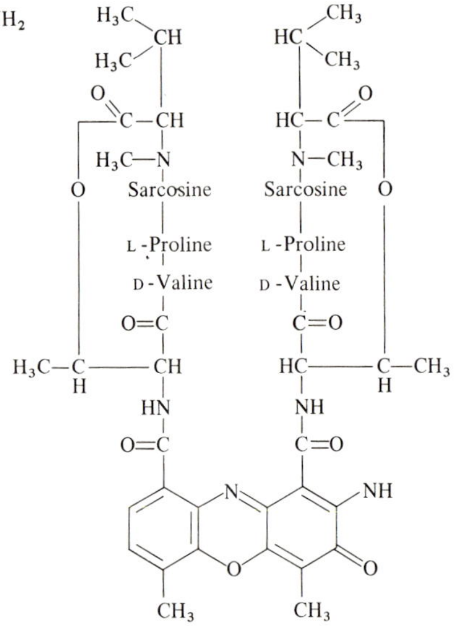
H_3C
CH
H_3C
CH_3
HC
CH_3
O
C—CH
O
HC—C
H_3C—N
N—CH_3
O
Sarcosine
Sarcosine
O
L-Proline
L-Proline
D-Valine
D-Valine
O=C
C=O
H_3C—C
H
CH
HC
C—CH_3
H
HN
NH
O=C
C=O
N
NH
O
O
CH_3
CH_3

Actinomycin D

suppression (Hektoen and Corper, 1921), and nitrogen mustard itself was the first immunosuppressive alkylating agent with controlled toxicity to receive careful investigation in experimental animals (Bukantz *et al.*, 1949; Philips *et al.*, 1956) and in man (Dubois, 1954). Cyclophosphamide is a recently developed alkylating compound which is a remarkably effective immunosuppressant in guinea pigs (Maguire and Maibach, 1961), mice (Berenbaum and Brown, 1964), and other rodents. Because of their safety and ease of administration, cyclophosphamide and chlorambucil are logical choices among the alkylating agents for trial in man.

Modern immunosuppression began slightly over a decade ago with the successful inhibition of immune responsiveness by the antimetabolite 6-mercaptopurine. Schwartz *et al.* (1958) suppressed the antibody response of rabbits to bovine serum albumin, after earlier workers (Sterzl and Holub, 1957) had suggested the use of the compound but had been unfortunate in their choice of an immune test system. Figure 1, reproduced from the original paper of Schwartz *et al.* (1958), illustrates complete inhibition of antibody formation by nontoxic levels of 6-mercaptopurine. While 6-mercaptopurine is an effective immunosuppressant in the rabbit, a derivative, azathioprine (Elion *et al.*, 1961), enjoys a somewhat more favorable ratio of therapeutic to toxic effect in man, and it has become the standard human immunosuppressant. Thioguanine, like the two preceding compounds, appears to be an effective antipurine immune inhibitor and has been employed in several human diseases (Schwartz and Dameshek, 1962; Goodman *et al.*, 1963).

The folic acid antagonist methotrexate was introduced as an immunosuppressant before the thiopurines (Haas and Stewart, 1956; Uphoff, 1958; Friedman *et al.*, 1961; Friedman and Buckler, 1963; Friedman, 1964; Turk, 1964), and this compound has proven to be a potent inhibitor of immune responses in the guinea pig. Unfortunately, because of delayed toxicity and renal excretion, methotrexate has proven to be a difficult compound to use in man, particularly for treatment of renal homograft rejection. The antipyrimidines (5-fluorouracil and 5-bromodeoxyuridine), in contrast to the antipurines and folic acid antagonists, are quite *ineffective in vivo* (Gabrielsen and Good, 1967); they are included because of their *in vitro* inhibition of immune responses (Dutton and Pearce, 1962). It is of interest that the antipyrimidines, which in cancer chemotherapy act against neoplasms of glandular epithelium, are ineffective immunosuppressants, whereas the folic acid antagonists and antipurines, which act against leukemias and squamous cell neoplasms, are among the most effective.

Of the remaining compounds in Table I, the actinomycins and the adrenal corticoid prednisone (Mannick and Egdahl, 1968) have been employed extensively in human immunosuppressive regimens, while azaserine has minor activity when used in combination with other agents (Murray *et al.*,

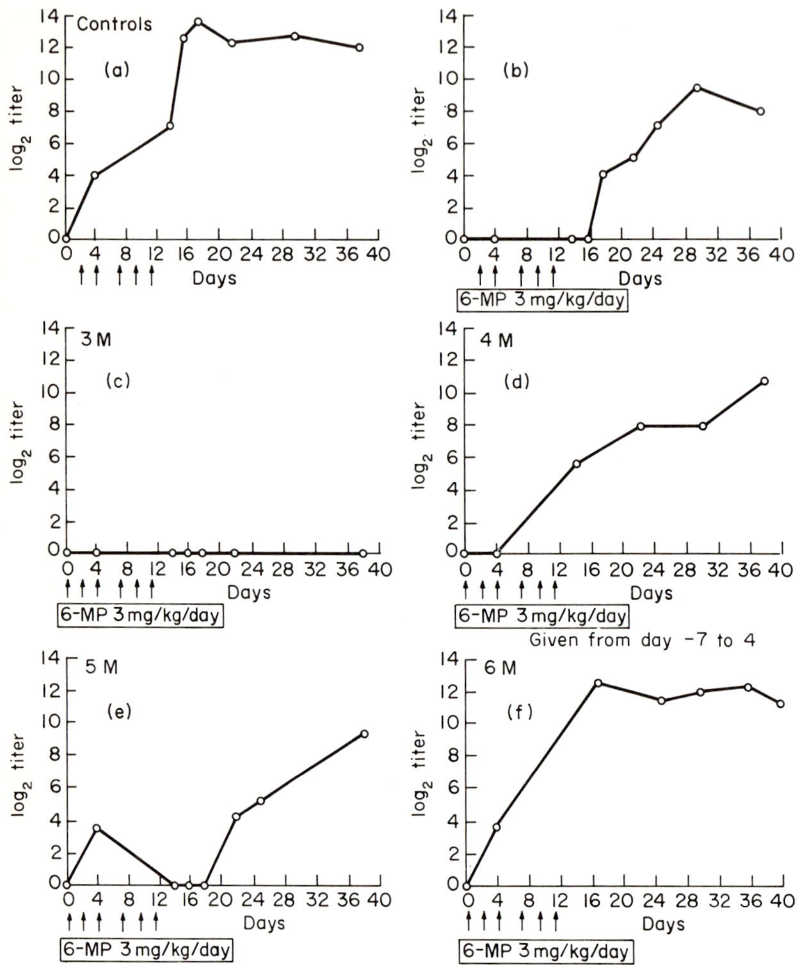

FIG. 1. Course of the immune response in control and 6-mercaptopurine (6-MP) treated rabbits. Each vertical arrow represents an injection of antigen (bovine serum albumin). The time of administration of 6-MP is represented by the clear block and each value depicted in the graph represents the average titer of five animals. (From Schwartz *et al.*, 1958.)

1963). All the antibiotics listed in Table I have displayed their most prominent inhibition on *in vitro* systems, and some like puromycin (Smiley *et al.*, 1964) and mitomycin (Bloom *et al.*, 1964) are active only *in vitro*. The periwinkle alkaloids (Aisenberg and Wilkes, 1964) and the methylhydrazine derivative procarbazine (Amiel *et al.*, 1964) are compounds which combine demonstrated immunosuppressive activity in animal systems with modest and acceptable toxicity in man, and they deserve further human trial.

Antilymphocyte serum (ALS), a recent development in the field of immunosuppressants, has proven effective both in experimental animals and man. ALS has an extensive literature of its own (Wolstenholme and O'Connor, 1967; Medawar, 1968) and will not be considered in detail in this review. Thoracic duct drainage is a new modality which is receiving initial evaluation in man (Dumont, 1968). X-irradiation is included in the table because of the many parallels between this form of ionizing irradiation and immunosuppressive drugs (Taliaferro *et al.*, 1964; Dukor and Dietrich, 1968).

III. Variables Which Determine the Success of an Immunosuppressive Regimen

The following paragraphs consider a number of factors which in large measure determine the effectiveness of an immunosuppressive program. In essence, these variables establish the relative strengths of the antigenic stimulus and the immunosuppressive counterforce. In an age when scientific terms proliferate, frequently without adequate reason, the term "immunopharmacology" may some day be coined to describe this field.

A. Drug and Dosage

The choice of drug, route of administration, and dosage is of the same obvious importance in immunosuppression as in any other branch of pharmacology. It should be stressed that in comparing results in man and experimental animals, it is important to contrast the lower human drug dosage with the near lethal levels employed in most animal systems.

B. Amount, Form, and Route of Antigen Administration

In all immunosuppressive regimens antigen must be administered in addition to immunosuppressant. The antigenic requirements are the same as those for the induction of specific immunological tolerance (Dresser and Mitchison, 1968; Leskowitz, 1967); namely, it is preferable that antigen be present in large amounts, be in soluble form, and be administered via the intravenous route.

C. Timing of Drug and Antigen

The success or failure of an immunosuppressive program rests in considerable measure on the appropriate timing of drug and antigen, the critical point being that maximum immunosuppression and maximum antigen-stimulated lymphoid proliferation must coincide closely in time. This is illustrated in Fig. 2, which depicts the suppression in mice of the response to a

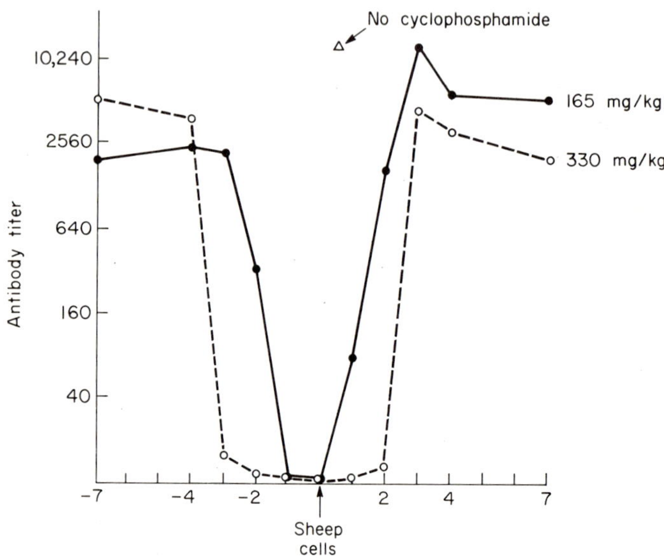

FIG. 2. Relationship of the times of antigen (sheep cells) and cyclophosphamide injection. The points represent average hemagglutination titers in mice 5 weeks after sheep cell injection. (From Aisenberg, 1967.)

nonreplicating antigen (sheep erythrocytes) with the alkylating agent cyclophosphamide. Cyclophosphamide must be given simultaneously with antigen or within the preceding 24 hours to achieve complete suppression at low drug dosage (165 mg/kg), while at higher drug levels (330 mg/kg) the agent may be given up to 48 hours before or after antigen. With a replicating antigen, the immunosuppressant must be delayed to allow the antigen to build up to the necessary level. Thus with lymphocytic choriomeningitis virus (Hotchin, 1962), it was found that maximum immunosuppression was achieved when methotrexate was delayed until 4 days after virus inoculation, the time of peak virus titer. An elegant example of meticulous timing of immunosuppressant treatment is illustrated in the work of Berenbaum and Brown (1965). These workers demonstrated that appropriately timed folic acid would "rescue" guinea pigs from the toxicity of methotrexate with marked improvement in drug mortality and skin graft survival.

Immunological Stimulus

te the strength of immunological stimuli, of achieving immunosuppression is closely ntigen. Thus, the response to weak soluble albumin or γ-globulin is much more easily strong particulate antigens (phage, viruses, Similarly, in the field of tissue transplantation, nor histoincompatibilities than major ones. The histocompatibility site (Snell and Stimpfling, ssion of skin homografts which bridge this major h difficulty, whereas homograft reactions which loci can be controlled with relative ease. In man occupies the same dominant position that the H-2 mouse (Dausset and Rapaport, 1968). It now appears uppressive regimens are adequate in man for kidney hed at the Hu-1 locus, but that the long term survival tched at this locus is less satisfactory (Patel *et al.*, 1968). sier to suppress the primary response (initial exposure to econdary (second antigen exposure in the primed animal). kers found it impossible to inhibit the secondary response purine (Schwartz *et al.*, 1959), but Fig. 3 indicates that the even the tertiary, response to a weak antigen (bovine serum e suppressed in the rabbit with very high doses of this excellent essant.

E. Nature of the Immune Response

ctrum of immunological responses is best divided into those mediated ody and those mediated by cells. Antibody is synthesized in plasma certain larger lymphocytes and subserves a variety of *classic* immune es (precipitin reaction, agglutination, opsinization, immune lysis, ement fixation, and anaphylaxis). In response to many antigens, the ody sequence is an initial formation of a macroglobulin in the 19 S range, ned IgM, followed by the protracted formation of a smaller 7 S antibody ned IgG (Uhr and Finkelstein, 1967).

Modern immunology has been particularly concerned with the cellular mmune reactions mediated by small lymphocytes (Gowans and McGregor, 1965). Responses mediated by small lymphocytes include the familiar forms of delayed hypersensitivity (bacterial and contact sensitivity), graft-versus-host reactions, and, with some reservations, the homograft reaction (Wilson and Billingham, 1967).

There appears to be a difference in the susceptibility of the of immune response to immunosuppressants. For example, wit purine, delayed hypersensitivity (cellular immunity) is more eas than the IgG antibody response, which in turn is more easily suppr

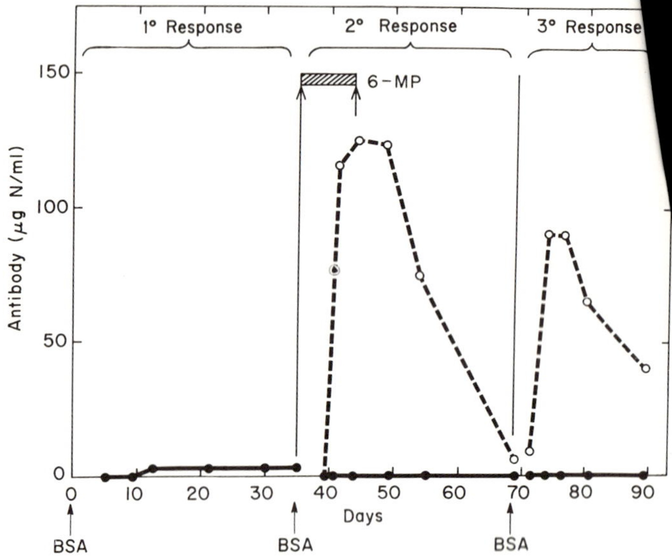

FIG. 3. Depression of primary, secondary, and tertiary response to bovine se albumin (BSA) with 6-mercaptopurine (6-MP). The solid lines are drug-treated anim and the broken lines represent controls. BSA injections are indicated by arrows and period of 6-MP injection by the cross-hatched block. Results are expressed in antib binding capacity (micrograms of nitrogen per milliliter). (Modified from Gabrielsen a Good, 1967.)

IgM response (Sahier and Schwartz, 1964; Borel *et al.*, 1965). Susceptibility t immunosuppression appears to parallel the thymus dependence of immune reactions: cellular immunity is most thymus dependent, IgG antibody formation intermediate, and IgM formation least (Taylor, 1969).

F. SPECIES

There is considerable species variability in the effectiveness of individual immunosuppressants. Examples of successful combinations are cyclophosphamide in the mouse, methotrexate in the guinea pig, 6-mercaptopurine in the rabbit, and azathioprine in the dog and man. This differential effectiveness probably reflects only minor differences in drug uptake, transport, and detoxification rather than any fundamental difference in the mode of action or the immunological mechanisms in the various species. Nonetheless, the practical importance of properly mating the drug and species should not be underestimated.

G. Innate Immunological Reactivity

Immunological responsiveness is modified by a variety of genetic and environmental factors. Among mouse strains, the C57BL animal is particularly reactive to a variety of antigenic stimuli, and it is quite difficult to suppress the immune responses of this strain. Again, the guinea pig displays particular development of delayed hypersensitivity. Furthermore, in mice (McDevitt and Sela, 1965) and in guinea pigs (Levine and Benacerraf, 1965), it has been clearly shown that reactivity to certain antigens in genetically determined. (The inherited trait may determine antigen processing.) Man, like the guinea pig, is noteworthy for extreme development of delayed hypersensitivity (Kligman and Epstein, 1959) and exhibits wide variation of responsiveness from individual to individual and a decline of reactivity with age and chronic illness.

H. Resistance to Immunological Injury

There is a wide variation among grafts of different organs and tissues in regard to the extent of immunological insult they can sustain without irreversible damage and functional failure. Thus the kidney is remarkable in its resistance to immunological injury (Murray *et al.*, 1964; Dammin, 1968), the skin quite susceptible (Medawar, 1958; Rapaport and Converse, 1968), and the heart in between (Spencer *et al.*, 1969).

I. Immunological Nature of the Phenomenon to be Suppressed

In assessing the potential benefit of an immunosuppressive program, some attention must be paid to whether or not the phenomenon to be suppressed is immunological. This applies particularly to autoimmune diseases where there is often considerable doubt about the immunological nature of the process and of the detailed mechanism involved. The matter is further complicated because immunosuppressants are agents toxic to a variety of cells, and the ability to ameliorate a process is no assurance that the process was of immune genesis.

IV. Immunosuppressive Mechanisms

A. Biochemical

Almost certainly immunosuppressive drugs act by killing lymphoid cells or preventing their proliferation through interference with the replication of deoxyribonucleic acid (DNA). The evidence for this conclusion, which is in large measure circumstantial, will be presented. First, it seems unlikely that the list of immunosuppressants would include essentially all the cytotoxic agents employed to treat human lymphoid neoplasms (acute and chronic lymphocytic leukemia and the malignant lymphomas) were this not the case. Second, a recent study has shown a close parallel between cyclophosphamide-inhibited spleen DNA synthesis and suppression of the antibody response of mice to heterologous erythrocytes (Aisenberg, 1967). Finally, the next paragraph will list the site of action of the more important immunosuppressants; in almost every instance this site involves DNA synthesis. For further details, the reader is referred to the specific references below and the reviews of cancer chemotherapy listed in Section II.

The alkylating agents react with a variety of biologically important macromolecules but the evidence is good that their primary action is to cross-link adjacent DNA chains via binding at the guanine residues (Wheeler, 1967). The mode of action of 6-mercaptopurine is quite complex and remains unsettled. This compound inhibits at least a half dozen steps in purine and pyrimidine biosynthesis, but it appears most reasonable that its principal action also is to inhibit DNA synthesis (Hitchings and Elion, 1967). Methotrexate poisons the enzyme dihydrofolate reductase, an enzyme which supplies one-carbon fragments for a number of synthetic functions including several essential steps in the synthesis of DNA (Bertino and Johns, 1967). Actinomycin D is an inhibitor of considerable biochemical interest. This antibiotic binds to DNA, and in so doing inhibits DNA-dependent RNA synthesis (Goldberg and Rabinowitz, 1962).

With two exceptions, it seems unlikely that the agents listed in Tables I and II have an important primary effect on either protein or RNA synthesis. The exceptions are chloramphenicol (Gale, 1963) and puromycin (Nathans and Lipmann, 1961), both of which are inhibitors of protein synthetic pathways.

B. Immunological Parameters

1. *Nonspecific Suppression*

Immunosuppressants frequently inhibit immune responsiveness, in part, through nonspecific damage to the lymphoid system. Such suppression is undesirable since it is unrelated to antigen and produces a parallel increase in susceptibility to infectious agents. Figure 4 illustrates this occurrence in

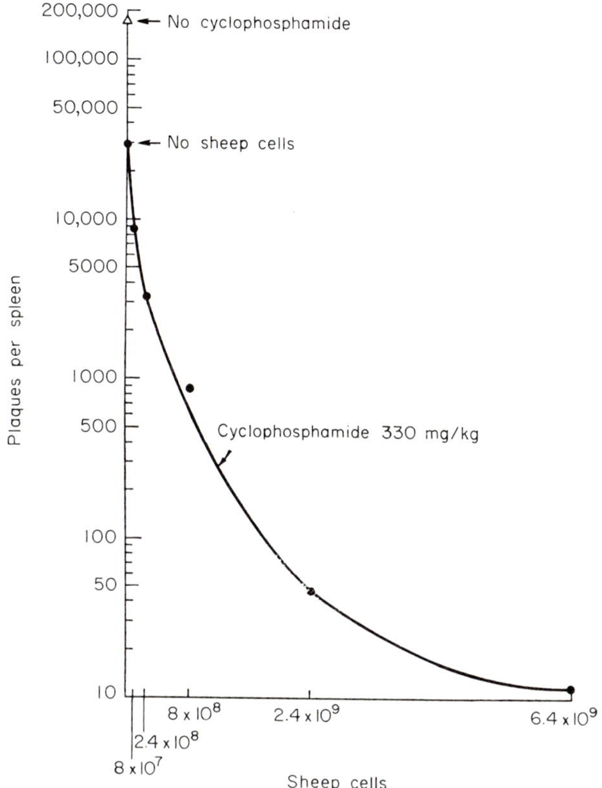

FIG. 4. Nonspecific lymphoid injury and specific immunological tolerance in cyclophosphamide-treated mice. Seventeen days before, animals had received either no cyclophosphamide and no sheep cells, or cyclophosphamide and no sheep cells, or cyclophosphamide with varying amounts of sheep cells. The results are expressed as the average number of antibody-forming cells (hemolytic plaque-forming cells) in the spleen of mice that had, in each case, received antigenic challenge with sheep cells 4 days before plaquing. (From Aisenberg, 1967.)

mice that have been treated with cyclophosphamide to inhibit their response to sheep erythrocytes. The chart indicates the number of antibody-forming cells (plaque cells) in the spleen of animals 17 days after receiving the immunosuppressant. Note that the animals that had received cyclophosphamide without sheep erythrocytes had but one sixth the number of antibody-forming cells of those that received no drug, a measure of nonspecific unresponsiveness at this time.

2. *Specific Immunological Tolerance*

The classic experiments of Billingham, Brent, and Medawar (1956), in which specific immunological unreactivity was produced by the neonatal injection of antigen, suggested that immaturity of the lymphoid system was essential for the production of tolerance. However, over the past decade an abundance of experimental data (Dresser and Mitchison, 1968) has indicated that immunological paralysis can be produced in the adult when persistent antigen levels can be achieved without provoking an antibody response. The early work of Schwartz and Dameshek (1959) established that 6-mercaptopurine was able to induce such specific unreactivity in the adult animal, an observation which has been confirmed with other immunosuppressants (Schwartz, 1965). The induction of tolerance to sheep erythrocytes (a strong antigen) is illustrated in Fig. 4, where it will be noted that very large amounts of antigen must be administered together with cyclophosphamide to produce a state of complete unreactivity (Dietrich and Dukor, 1967; Aisenberg, 1967; Aisenberg and Davis, 1968).

3. *Inhibition of Established Immunity*

Potent immunosuppressants are able to inhibit delayed hypersensitivity even when begun after sensitivity has been established. Table III illustrates the suppression of established tuberculin hypersensitivity in the guinea pig

TABLE III

SUPPRESSION OF ACTIVITY ESTABLISHED TUBERCULIN HYPERSENSITIVITY IN GUINEA PIGS BY METHOTREXATE (MODIFIED FROM FRIEDMAN, 1964)

Experimental group	No. of days after inoculation of B.C.G.[a]			
	14	30	40	50
Control 1	15 × 12	20 × 18	20 × 17	20 × 18
2	15 × 13	20 × 20	20 × 19	20 × 20
3	15 × 14	21 × 19	20 × 20	20 × 19
Methotrexate[b] 1	15 × 14	0	0	20 × 17
2	17 × 15	0	0	20 × 19
3	18 × 15	0	0	20 × 20

[a] The figures indicate cross diameters of induration in millimeters.

[b] Each animal received 5 mg of methotrexate day 15 through day 39.

with methotrexate (Friedman, 1964), As is usually the case when immunosuppressants are used in this manner, sensitivity rapidly returns when the drug is discontinued (Aisenberg and Wilkes, 1964).

4. *Inhibition of the Inflammatory Response*

Some immunosuppressants are able to depress the banal inflammatory response to materials such as egg white and turpentine. This inhibition is an important facet of immunosuppression with adrenal corticoids (Mannick and Egdahl, 1968; Schwartz, 1968) and has been well documented with 6-mercaptopurine (Page *et al.*, 1962), where it was found that protracted treatment with high levels of antimetabolite was necessary. With other immunosuppressants (methotrexate), drug dosage that produced excellent immune inhibition was without effect on the inflammatory response (Friedman, 1964). In instances where immunosuppressants do suppress inflammation, it is difficult to assess the extent to which an inhibited delayed skin reaction reflects immune inhibition.

5. *Granulocyte Suppression and Arthus Reactivity*

The Arthus skin reaction is an immediate response caused by the combination of antigen and antibody in the skin, and is to be contrasted with the delayed cell-mediated reactions. The Arthus reaction is frequently necrotic and histologically shows polymorphonuclear leukocyte infiltration rather than the mononuclear cells of the delayed response. Many immunosuppressants, particularly the alkylating agents, profoundly depress the level of circulating polymorphonuclear leukocytes, and effectively suppress Arthus skin reactivity (Humphrey, 1955).

6. *Adaptation of the Graft*

Kidney homografts which have been in place for a protracted period of time achieve a *modus vivendi* with the host that permits survival of the graft despite the existence of potentially destructive immunological factors. The protective mechanism presumably involves either a barrier between host and graft which protects the latter from the destructive elements of the host or the coating of antigenic sites on the graft which prevents recognition by host cells. Figure 5, taken from the work of Murray *et al.* (1964), illustrates adaptation of a canine kidney homograft. In this experiment an initial kidney graft placed under the protection of immunosuppressants survived for 554 days, while skin and a second kidney from the same donor, grafted after the drugs had been tapered, were promptly rejected.

7. *Enhancement of the Immune Response*

In the course of investigating X-irradiation-induced immunosuppression, Dixon and McConahey (1963) observed that sublethal irradiation given 1 to 4 days before immunization enhanced antibody formation rather than inhibiting it. Figure 6 illustrates that very significant enhancement of antibody production can also occur with appropriately timed immunosuppressant pretreatment (Chanmougan and Schwartz, 1966). This enhancement, which should be distinguished from the enhancement of tumor immunology, has been explained by several unconvincing mechanisms. It has been suggested that the increased response is a result of increased room for proliferation in the depleted but not unsuppressed lymph node, or, alternatively, that the drug has made essential nucleic acid precursors available as a result of cell destruction (Schwartz, 1968). Regardless of the mechanism, this enhancement by immunosuppressants has important implications for the clinical worker. It indicates the potential adverse effects that may ensue from unnecessary modifications of successful immunosuppressive regimens.

C. Cellular Immunology (Immunosuppressive Mechanisms)

It is convenient to divide the immune response into an afferent or sensory side which reacts with antigen, a central mechanism which elaborates the response, and an efferent or effector side. Immunosuppressants act on the effector limb and the central mechanism; evidence for a significant inhibition of the afferent limb is not convincing (Gabrielsen and Good, 1967).

Various immunosuppressants, including alkylating agents, X-irradiation (Cronkite and Chanana, 1968), and corticosteroids (Mannick and Egdahl, 1968) are markedly destructive to effector lymphocytes. (The greater sensitivity of small lymphocytes, which mediate cellular immunity, than of plasma cells, which mediate antibody responses, explains in part why cellular reactions are more easily suppressed by these agents.) Antilymphocyte serum may also act by depletion of peripheral lymphocytes (Russell and Monaco, 1967), though an alternate explanation is that this material "blindfolds" or sterilely inactivates these effector cells (Medawar, 1968).

Quantitating effector lymphocyte depletion is difficult because of our inability to identify the several morphologically similar populations of peripheral lymphocytes (Rieke and Schwarz, 1967). At present it is believed that complete immune responsiveness requires the interaction of two populations of small lymphocytes, a long-lived thymus-derived cell and a short-lived marrow-derived cell (Davies, 1969; Miller and Mitchell, 1969; Taylor, 1969; Claman amd Chaperon, 1969). Until the exact function of the two populations is known, and until the separate populations can be enumerated, it will be impossible to evaluate lymphocyte depletion.

The second important cellular mechanism operating during immunosuppression is the induction of central inhibition or immunological tolerance.

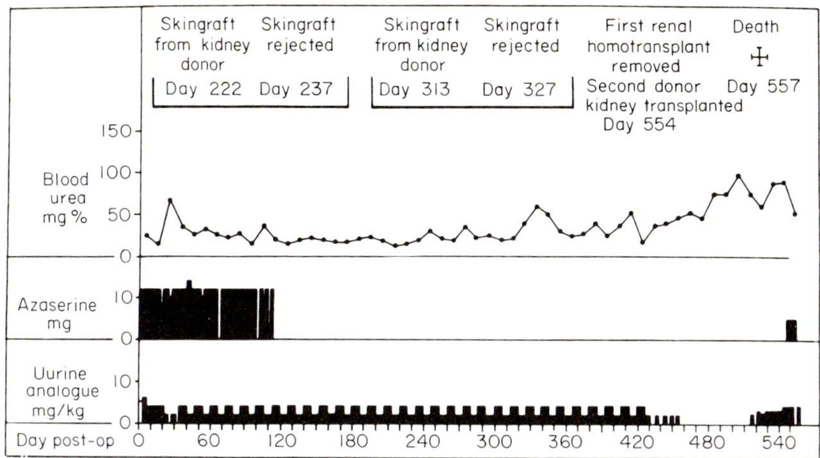

FIG. 5. Skin rejection and accelerated rejection of a second canine kidney homograft from the same donor in a dog that had tolerated an initial kidney homograft for 554 days. (Slightly modified from Murray *et al.*, 1964.)

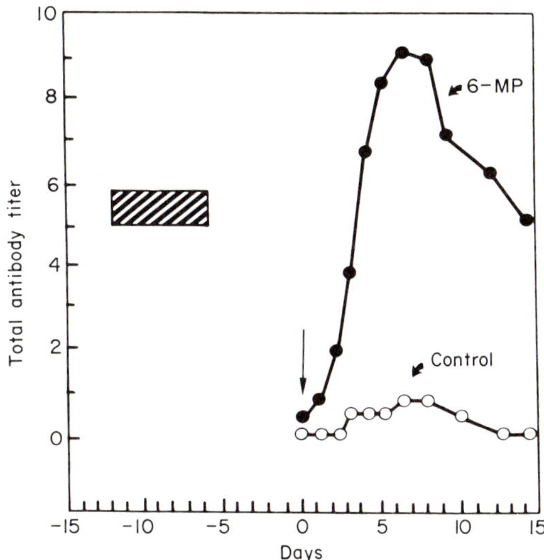

FIG. 6. Enhancement of antibody synthesis by 6-mercaptopurine (6-MP). The hatched bar indicates the timing of drug administration, and the vertical arrow the time of antigenic challenge. The amount of antigen employed (20 μg of bovine γ-globulin) was barely immunogenic in normal rabbits. (From Schwartz, 1968.)

It is well known that the immune response is accompanied by active proliferation of lymphoid cells (Humphrey, 1965; Makinodan and Albright, 1967), and it is equally well established that rapidly dividing cells are susceptible to the cytotoxic immunosuppressants (DiPalma, 1967). Thus, in the induction of drug-induced tolerance some such mechanism as the following takes place: Antigen stimulates the responsive clone of cells to divide rapidly; this rapid proliferation renders this responding clone particularly sensitive to the cytotoxic drug; and the clone responding to the particular antigen is selectively killed or inactivated. As repopulation of the lymphoid system takes place, the new lymphoid cells mature in the presence of antigen and could be expected, by conventional tolerance theory (Dresser and Mitchison, 1968), to be tolerant. The result would be a stable state of tolerance.

In actual practice there is probably a combination of partial tolerance and partial depletion of effector lymphocytes. Neither process is complete, but in successful immunosuppression the result is a satisfactory attenuation of the destructive immunological events.

V. Human Applications

A. Organ Transplantation

By far the most important human application of immunosupressants has been in the management of renal homografts. Figure 7 illustrates the results that can be achieved with current techniques in a patient who received a well-matched renal homograft from his brother (Austen and Russell, 1966). This 47-year-old man with terminal polycystic renal disease received an initial dose of azathioprine (8 mg/kg) on the evening prior to surgery, and he was subsequently maintained at a drug level (1–4 mg/kg/day) that did not significantly depress the daily determined granulocyte or platelet counts. The initial dramatic improvement in renal function was reversed on the third day (rising serum creatinine) because of the onset of a rejection crisis. Rejection was treated with prednisone, first in moderate dosage (60 mg/day) and later in large dosage (300 mg/day), and then with courses of actinomycin C (200 μg intravenously 2 successive days of each week). With this program, rejection was reversed and now, more than 5 years after grafting, he continues to do well, with satisfactory renal function.

Azathioprine is the primary immunosuppressant in almost all renal transplantation centers, though there are minor variations of timing and dose (Parker and Vavra, 1969). As would be expected from animal studies, good results are observed when the maximum immunosuppressant effect is produced shortly after grafting, and it is neither necessary nor desirable to cause severe leukopenia. Rejection occurs in many patients despite azathioprine and is best treated with a secondary drug. This is generally prednisone, which many centers now begin at the time of grafting rather than at the time of rejection, and as tertiary treatment antilymphocyte serum now frequently replaces actinomycin C or D.

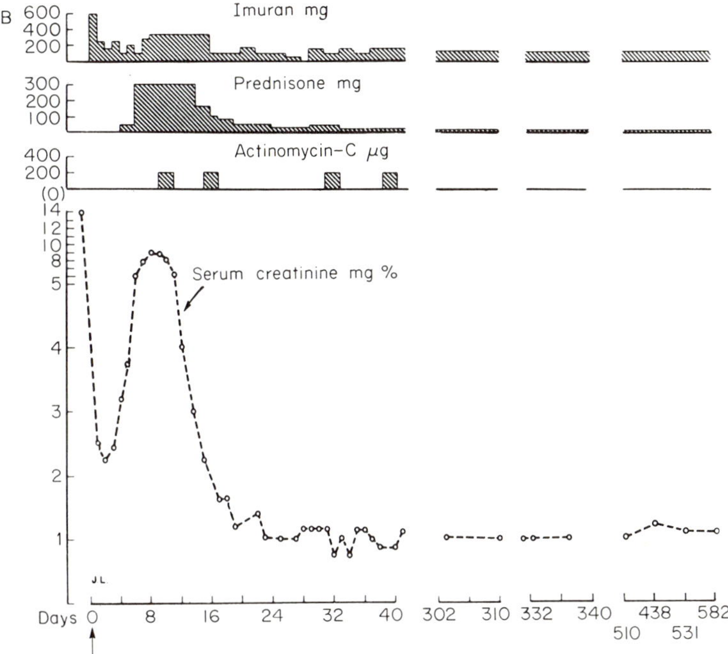

FIG. 7. Chart of a 47-year-old male with polycystic renal disease who received a kidney homograft from his 43-year-old brother on day 0. Improvement in renal function is indicated by the fall of serum creatinine from 14 to 2.3 mg per 100 ml in the first 48 hours after transplantation. The rise in serum creatinine on day 3 was caused by a rejection crisis which was successfully treated with prednisone and actinomycin C. (Modified from Austen and Russell, 1966.)

The most recent statistics of the Human Kidney Transplant Registry indicate a 1-year survival of 78% for kidneys from siblings, 71% for kidneys from parents, and 45% for grafts from unrelated cadaver donors (Advisory Committee of the Human Kidney Transplant Registry, 1968). Present evidence suggests that survival and maintenance of kidney function during the next 4 years is directly related to the histocompatibility match of the grafted kidney (Patel *et al.*, 1968). One-year survival should be capable of further improvement because many of first-year deaths are in the immediate postoperative period and are related to technical problems in surgery and organ procurement (Advisory Committee of the Human Kidney Transplant Registry, 1969). The results of transplantation of other organs (Rapaport and Dausset, 1968), such as lung (Blumenstock *et al.*, 1969), liver (Starzl *et al.*, 1969), and heart (Spencer *et al.*, 1969) are too preliminary to be evaluated at this time.

B. Autoimmune Disease

There is nc doubt that immunosuppressants can decrease the incidence, delay the onset, and ameliorate the course of autoimmune disease in experimental animals. Cyclophosphamide can completely prevent the development of autoimmune allergic encephalomyelitis in both rats and guinea pigs; other drugs will also suppress this disorder (Paterson, 1968). Therapy with 6-mercaptopurine and methotrexate will prevent the development of or completely suppress established autoimmune thyroiditis in guina pigs (Spielberg and Miescher, 1963). Very interesting results have been obtained in the fascinating and complex autoimmune disease of NZB and NZB × NZW mice which closely resembles the human disorder disseminated lupus erythematosus. To date immunosuppressive agents have been remarkably effective in influencing the development and course of lupus nephritis in NZB × NZW hybrids but have not altered the course of hemolytic disease in the NZB strain (Howie and Helyer, 1968).

When one turns to the control of human autoimmune disease, a number of difficulties arise. Perhaps the greatest problem is the uncertainty that exists as to which disorders are primarily autoimmune in causation and what criteria should be applied to establish an autoimmune pathogenesis (Miescher and Müller-Eberhard, 1968). Second, if the disease *is* autoimmune, what is the detailed mechanism? Is it abnormal distribution or structure of antigen or is the primary abnormality in the immunological responsiveness of the individual (Parker and Vavra, 1969)? A final complication arises because the remittant and prolonged course of many "autoimmune" disorders makes evaluation of therapy extraordinarily difficult.

The immunosuppressant thiopurines have found a tentative place in the clinical management of idiopathic thrombocytopenic purpura (Bouroncle and Doan, 1969; Corely, 1966; Sussman, 1967; Ogston and Fullerton, 1966) and of autoimmune hemolytic anemia (Schwartz and Dameschek, 1962; Dacie and Worlledge, 1969) after failure of corticosteroids and splenectomy (Parker and Vavra, 1969), but it is impossible to comment on the ultimate place of suppressants in the management of these two diseases. Evaluation of immunosuppressives is equally difficult in a variety of other disorders. Preliminary data suggest that recurrent renal disease (glomerulonephritis) is less frequent in immunosuppressed recipients than in *unsuppressed* individuals who receive the kidney of an identical twin (Advisory Committee of the Human

Kidney Transplant Registry, 1968). Variable results have been reported in the treatment of chronic renal disease (nephrosis, glomerulonephritis, and lupus nephritis) with immunosuppressants (Merrill, 1962; Michael *et al.*, 1967). Various other disorders (chronic hepatitis, disseminated lupus erythematosus, ulcerative colitis, regional enteritis, rheumatoid arthritis, scleraderma, dermatomyositis and periarteritis nodosa) have been treated with immunosuppressants (see Parker and Vavra, 1969). Psoriasis, a disease without immune pathogenesis, also responds to antimetabolite treatment (Demis *et al.*, 1964; Corley, 1966). Immunosuppressants are also potentially useful in controlling the adverse immune response to various biologicals of nonhuman origin, such as antihemophyllic globulin and insulin. In all these instances controlled studies with a standardized regimen in a significant number of patients are especially needed.

C. Toxicity

The immunosuppressant drugs are very toxic compounds which affect a variety of tissues and organs. Certain toxic manifestations, such as the suppression of leukocyte and platelet production, are obvious and can be minimized by careful and conservative management. Other toxicity (such as the many adverse effects of adrenal corticoids) is the inevitable but recognized result of long-term treatment, Still other toxic reactions are just coming to light, as the immunosuppressants are used for long periods of time in novel clinical situations. These include such occurrences as insidious hepatic cirrhosis developing in psoriatic patients on long-term methotrexate (Coe and Bull, 1968) and malignant lymphomas in renal transplant patients receiving antilymphocyte serum (Penn *et al.*, 1969). [In several animal systems a surprisingly high incidence of lymphomas has followed prolonged immunosuppression with antimetabolites (Casey, 1968; Armstrong *et al.*, 1968).] The varied and unpredictable toxicity of extended immunosuppression requires that it not be undertaken for trivial clinical indications.

References

Advisory Committee of the Human Kidney Transplant Registry (1968). *Transplantation* **6**, 944.

Advisory Committee of the Human Kidney Transplant Registry (1969). *Transplant. Proc.* **1**, 197.

Aisenberg, A. C. (1967). *J. Exp. Med.* **125**, 833.

Aisenberg, A. C., and Davis, C. (1968). (1968). *J. Exp. Med.* **128**, 35.

Aisenberg, A. C., and Wilkes, B. (1964). *J. Clin. Invest.* **43**, 2394.

Amiel, J. L., Brezin, C., Sekiguchi, M., Mery, A. M., Hoerni, B., Garattini, S., Daguet, G., and Mathé, G. (1964). *Rev. Fr. Etud. Clin. Biol.* **9**, 636.

Armstrong, M. Y. K., André-Schwartz, J., and Schwartz, R. S. (1968). *In* "Perspectives in Leukemia" (W. Dameshek and R. M. Dutcher, eds.), pp. 133–155. Grune & Stratton, New York.

Austen, K. F., and Russell, P. S. (1966). *Ann. N. Y. Acad. Sci.* **129**, 657.

Berenbaum, M. C. (1965). *Brit. Med. Bull.* **21**, 140.

Berenbaum, M. C., and Brown, I. N. (1964). *Immunology* **7**, 65.

Berenbaum, M. C., and Brown, I. N. (1965). *Immunology* **8**, 351.

Bertino, J. R., and Johns, D. G. (1967). *In* "Cancer Chemotherapy: Basic and Clinical Applications" (I. Brodsky and S. B. Kahn, eds.), pp. 14–25. Grune & Stratton, New York.

Billingham, R. E., Brent, L., and Medawar, P. B. (1956). *Phil. Trans. Roy. Soc. London Ser. B.* **163**, 61.

Bloom, B. R., Hamilton, L. D., and Chase, M. W. (1964). *Nature* (*London*) **201**, 689.

Blumenstock, D. A., Otte, H. P., Jean, O. B., and Mulder, M. A. (1969). *Transplant. Proc.* **1**, 223.

Borel, Y., Fauconnet, M., and Miescher, P. A. (1965). *J. Exp. Med.* **122**, 263.

Bouroncle, B. A., and Doan, C. A. (1969). *J. Amer. Med. Ass.* **207**, 2049.

Brodsky, I., and Kahn, S. B., eds. (1967). "Cancer Chemotherapy: Basic and Clinical Applications." Grune & Stratton, New York.

Bukantz, S. C., Dammin, G. J., Wilson, K. S., Johnson, M. C., and Alexander, H. L. (1949). *Proc. Soc. Exp. Biol. Med.* **72**, 21.

Burchenal, J. (1963). *Cancer Res.* **23**, 1181.

Calabresi, P., and Welch, A. D. (1965). *In* "The Pharmacological Basis of Therapeutics" (L. S. Goodman and A. Gilman, eds.), 3rd Ed., pp. 1345–1393. Macmillan, New York.

Casey, T. P. (1968). *Blood* **31**, 396.

Chanmougan, D., and Schwartz, R. S. (1966). *J. Exp. Med.* **124**, 363.

Claman, H. N., and Chaperon, E. A. (1969). *Transplant. Rev.* **1**, 92.

Coe, R. O., and Bull, F. E. (1968). *J. Amer. Med. Ass.* **206**, 1515.

Corley, C. C., Jr. (1966). *Amer. J. Med.* **41**, 404.

Cronkite, E. P., and Chanana, A. D. (1968). *In* "Human Transplantation" (F. T. Rapaport and J. Dausset, eds.). pp. 423–439. Grune & Stratton, New York.

Dacie, J. V., and Worlledge, S. M. (1969). *Progr. Hematol.* **6**, 82.

Dammin, G. J. (1968). *In* "Human Transplantation" (F. T. Rapaport and J. Dausset, eds.), pp. 170–200. Grune & Stratton, New York.

Dausset, J., and Rapaport, F. T. (1968). *In* "Human Transplantation" (F. T. Rapaport and J. Dausset, eds.), pp. 369–382. Grune & Stratton, New York.

Davies, A. J. S. (1969). *Transplant. Rev.* **1**, 43.

Demis, D. J., Brown, C. S., and Crosby, W. H. (1964). *Amer. J. Med.* **37**, 195.

Dietrich, F. M., and Dukor, P. (1967). *Pathol. Microbiol.* **30**, 909.

DiPalma, J. R. (1967). *In* "Cancer Chemotherapy: Basic and Clinical Applications" (I. Brodsky and S. B. Kahn, eds.), pp. 1–8. Grune & Stratton, New York.

Dixon, F. J., and McConahey, P. J. (1963). *J. Exp. Med.* **117**, 833.

Dresser, D. W., and Mitchison, N. A. (1968). *Advan. Immunol.* **8**, 129.

Dubois, E. L. (1954). *Arch. Intern. Med.* **94**, 667.

Dukor, P., and Dietrich, F. M. (1968). *Int. Arch. Allergy Appl. Immunol.* **34**, 32.

Dumont, A. F. (1968). *In* "Human Transplantation" (F. T. Rapaport and J. Dausset, eds.), pp. 482–488. Grune & Stratton, New York.
Dutton, R. W., and Pearce, J. D. (1962). *Immunology* **5**, 414.
Elion, G. B., Callanan, S., Bieber, S., Hitchings, G. H., and Rundles, R. W. (1961). *Cancer Chemother. Rep.* **14**, 93.
Friedman, R. M. (1964). *Proc. Soc. Exp. Biol. Med.* **116**, 471.
Friedman, R. M., and Buckler, C. E. (1963). *J. Immunol.* **91**, 846.
Friedman, R. M., Buckler, C. E., and Baron, S. (1961). *J. Exp. Med.* **114**, 173.
Gabrielsen, A. E., and Good, R. A. (1967). *Advan. Immunol.* **6**, 91.
Gale, E. F. (1963). *Pharmacol. Rev.* **15**, 481.
Goldberg, I. H., and Rabinowitz, M. (1962). *Science* **136**, 315.
Goodman, H. C., Wolff, S. M., Carpenter, R. R., Andersen, B. R., and Brandriss, M. W. (1963). *Ann. Inter. Med.* **59**, 388.
Gowans, J. L., and McGregor, D. D. (1965). *Progr. Allergy* **9**, 1.
Haas, V. H., and Stewart, S. E. (1956). *Virology* **2**, 511.
Hektoen, L., and Corper, H. J. (1921). *J. Infec. Dis.* **28**, 279.
Hersh, E. M., and Freireich, E. J. (1968). *Methods Cancer Res.* **4**, 356–454.
Hersh, E. M., Carbone, P. P., Wong, V. G., and Freireich, E. J. (1965). *Cancer Res.* **25**, 997.
Hitchings, G. H., and Elion, G. B. (1967). *In* "Cancer Chemotherapy: Basic and Clinical Applications" (I. Brodsky and S. B. Kahn, eds.), pp. 26–36. Grune & Stratton, New York.
Hotchin, J. (1962). *Cold Spring Harbor Symp. Quant. Biol.* **27**, 479.
Howie, J. B., and Helyer, B. J. (1968). *Advan. Immunol.* **9**, 215.
Humphrey, J. H. (1955). *Brit. J. Exp. Pathol.* **36**, 268.
Humphrey, J. H. (1965). *In* "Immunological Diseases" (M. Samter, ed.), pp. 100–108. Little, Brown, Boston, Massachusetts.
Karnovsky, D. A., and Clarkson, B. D. (1963). *Annu. Rev. Pharmacol.* **3**, 357.
Kligman, A. M., and Epstein, W. L. (1959). *In* "Mechanism of Hypersensitivity" (J. H. Shaffer, G. A. LoGrippo, and M. W. Chase, eds.), pp. 713–722. Little, Brown, Boston, Massachusetts.
Leskowitz, S. (1967). *Annu. Rev. Microbiol.* **21**, 157.
Levin, R. H., Landy, M., and Frei, E. (1964). *New Engl. J. Med.* **271**, 16.
Levine, B. B., and Benacerraf, B. (1965). *Science* **147**, 517.
McDevitt, H. O., and Sela, M. (1965). *J. Exp. Med.* **122**, 517.
Maguire, H. C., Jr., and Maibach, H. I. (1961). *J. Allergy* **32**, 406.
Makinodan, T., and Albright, J. F. (1967). *Progr. Allergy* **10**, 1.
Mannick, J. A., and Egdahl, R. A. (1968). *In* "Human Transplantation" (F. T. Rapaport and J. Dausset, eds.), pp. 472–481. Grune & Stratton, New York.
Medawar, P. B. (1958). *Harvey Lect.* **52**, 144.
Medawar, P. B. (1968). *In* "Human Transplantation" (F. T. Rapaport and J. Dausset, eds.), pp. 501–509. Grune & Stratton, New York.
Merrill, J. P. (1962). *Blood* **20**, 119.
Michael, A. F., Vernier, R. L., Drummond, K. N., Levitt, J. I., Herdman, R. C., Fish, A. J., and Good, R. A. (1967). *New Engl. J. Med.* **276**, 817.
Miescher, P. A., and Müller-Eberhard, H. J. (1968). "Textbook of Immunopathology," Vol. II. Grune & Stratton, New York.
Miller, J. F. A. P., and Mitchell, G. F. (1969). *Transplant. Rev.* **1**, 3.
Murray, J. E., Merrill, J. P., Harrison, J. H., Wilson, R. K., and Dammin, G. J. (1963). *New Engl. J. Med.* **268**, 1315.

Murray, J. E., Sheil, A. G. R., Moseley, R., Knight, P., McGavic, J. D., and Dammin, G. J. (1964). *Ann. Surg.* **160**, 449.

Nathans, D., and Lipmann, F. (1961). *Proc. Nat. Acad. Sci. U.S.* **47**, 497.

Ochoa, M., Jr., and Hirschberg, E. (1967). *In* "Experimental Chemotherapy" (R. J. Schnitzer and F. Hawking, eds.), Vol. 5, pp. 1–94. Academic Press, New York.

Ogston, D., and Fullerton, H. W. (1966). *Postgrad. Med.* **42**, 469.

Page, A., Condie, R. M., and Good, R. A. (1962). *Amer. J. Pathol.* **40**, 519.

Parker, C. W., and Vavra, J. D. (1969). *Progr. Hematol.* **6**, 1.

Patel, R., Mickey, M. R., and Terasaki, P. I. (1968). *New Engl. J. Med.* **279**, 501.

Paterson, P. Y. (1968). *In* "Textbook of Immunopathology" (P. A. Miescher and H. J. Müller-Eberhard, eds.), Vol. I, pp. 132–149. Grune & Stratton, New York.

Penn, I., Hammond, W., Brettschneider, L., and Starzl, T. E. (1969). *Transplant. Proc.* **1**, 106.

Philips, F. S., Sternberg, S. S., Hamilton, L. D., and Clarke, D. A. (1956). *J. Immunol.* **55**, 296.

Rapaport, F. T., and Converse, J. M. (1968). *In* "Human Transplantation" (F. T. Rapaport and J. Dausset, eds.), pp. 304–312. Grune & Stratton, New York.

Rapaport, F. T., and Dausset, J. (1968). "Human Transplantation." Grune & Stratton, New York.

Rieke, W. O., and Schwarz, M. R. (1967). *In* "The Lymphocyte in Immunology and Haemopoesis" (J. M. Yoffey, ed.), pp. 234–241. Williams & Wilkins, Baltimore, Maryland.

Russell, P. S., and Monaco, A. P. (1967). *Transplantation* **5**, 1086.

Sahier, K., and Schwartz, R. S. (1964). *Science* **145**, 395.

Schwartz, R. S. (1965). *Progr. Allergy* **9**, 246.

Schwartz, R. S. (1967). *Fed. Proc. Fed. Amer. Soc. Exp. Biol.* **26**, 879.

Schwartz, R. S. (1968). *In* "Human Transplantation" (F. T. Rapaport and J. Dausset, eds.), pp. 440–471. Grune & Stratton, New York.

Schwartz, R. S., and Dameshek, W. (1959). *Nature (London)* **183**, 1682.

Schwartz, R. S., and Dameshek, W. (1962). *Blood* **19**, 483.

Schwartz, R. S., Stack, J., and Dameshek, W. (1958). *Proc. Soc. Exp. Biol. Med.* **99**, 163.

Schwartz, R. S., Eisner, A., and Dameshek, W. (1959). *J. Clin. Invest.* **38**, 1394.

Smiley, J. O., Heard, J. G., and Ziff, M. (1964). *J. Exp. Med.* **119**, 881.

Snell, G. D., and Stimpfling, J. H. (1966). *In* "Biology of the Laboratory Mouse" (E. J. Green, ed.), 2nd Ed., pp. 457–492. McGraw-Hill, New York.

Spencer, F. C., Cooper, T., and Mitchell, S. C. (1969). *Transplant. Proc.* **1**, 691.

Spielberg, H. L., and Miescher, P. A. (1963). *J. Exp. Med.* **118**, 869.

Starzl, T. E., Brettschneider, L., Penn, F., Bell, P., Groth, C. G., Blanchard, H., Kashiwagi, N., and Putnam, C. W. (1969). *Transplant. Proc.* **1**, 216.

Sterzl, J., and Holub, M. (1957). *Csk. Biol.* **6**, 75.

Stock, J. A. (1966). *In* "Experimental Chemotherapy" (R. J. Schnitzer and F. Hawking, eds.), Vol. IV, pp. 79–377. Academic Press, New York.

Sussman, L. N. (1967). *J. Amer. Med. Ass.* **202**, 259.

Taliaferro, W. H., Taliaferro, L. G., and Jaroslow, B. N. (1964). "Radiation and Immune Mechanisms." Academic Press, New York.

Taylor, R. B. (1969). *Transplant. Rev.* **1**, 114.

Turk, J. L. (1964). *Int. Arch. Allergy Appl. Immunol.* **24**, 191.

Uhr, J. W., and Finkelstein, M. S. (1967). *Progr. Allergy* **10**, 37.

Uphoff, D. E. (1958). *Proc. Soc. Exp. Biol. Med.* **99**, 651.

Wheeler, G. P. (1967). *Fed. Proc. Fed. Amer. Soc. Exp. Biol.* **26**, 885.
Wilson, D. B., and Billingham, R. E. (1967). *Advan. Immunol.* **7**, 189.
Wolstenholme, G. E. W., and O'Connor, M. (1967). *Ciba Found. Study Group* [*Pap.*] **29**.

Glutamine Antagonists in Chemotherapy

R. B. Livingston, J. M. Venditti, D. A. Cooney, and S. K. Carter

National Cancer Institute, Bethesda, Maryland

I. Introduction

Compounds affecting the utilization of L-glutamine have a comparatively long history in the field of cancer chemotherapy. A decade ago, the "L-glutamine antagonists" azaserine and 6-diazo-5-oxo-L-nonleucine (DON) were undergoing active clinical trials. Because of their lack of effectiveness in human malignancies relative to other agents already available, interest in these compounds rapidly declined. The recent success of L-asparaginase in the therapy of certain human neoplasms has prompted a reconsideration of compounds which can alter L-glutamine metabolism, because: (1) L-glutamine is necessary, in most mammalian systems, for the synthesis of L-asparagine; (2) both azaserine and azotomycin appear to be synergistic with L-asparaginase against the L5178Y mouse leukemia (Jacobs *et al.*, 1969a,b); and (3) L-asparaginase (EC-2) of the form in clinical use in the United States has intrinsic L-glutaminase activity which may play a role in producing its therapeutic effect (Boyse *et al.*, 1967).

In the present paper an attempt has been made to summarize the information already available concerning inhibitors of enzymatic reactions which require L-glutamine. In addition, new information is presented relevant to the possible usefulness of such compounds in conjunction with L-asparaginase for the treatment of cancer (Sections VIII and IX).

II. Biological Functions and Synthesis of L-Glutamine

A. Functions

Levintow *et al.* (1957) examined the role of L-glutamine in the biosynthesis of protein by HeLa cells in tissue culture. The incorporation of ^{14}C- and ^{15}N-(amide)-labeled L-glutamine into various constituents of cell protein was measured. Labeled L-glutamine was found to be incorporated directly into cell protein without preliminary degradation. Both L-glutamine and L-glutamic acid served as the direct precursors for their corresponding residue in protein, and they did so independently of each other. Second, L-glutamine was found to furnish its carbon chain, to some extent, for the synthesis of L-aspartic acid and L-proline. In these studies, neither the amide nitrogen of L-glutamine nor ammonia served as a precursor of α-amino nitrogen in the amino acids of synthesized protein.

Ammonia and other amines, including the ϵ-amino group of protein-bound lysine (Wajda *et al.*, 1963), can be incorporated into certain proteins and polypeptides via transglutaminase-catalyzed replacement of the amido groups of L-glutamine residues. In addition, hydrolytic cleavage by transglutaminase of the amide groups of certain protein-bound L-glutamine residues produces ammonia. Evidence has been presented that the L-glutamine residues involved in both the replacement and the hydrolysis reactions are one and the same, and that specific structural requirements determine which residues may participate in these reactions (Folk and Cole, 1965). Thus protein-bound, as well as free, L-glutamine plays a metabolic role. This role may be of importance in the cross-linking of peptide chains.

Free L-glutamine furnishes its amide group in the biosynthesis of purines, pyrimidines, diphosphopyridine nucleotides (NAD, NADP), and glucosamine. The latter reaction is shown here (Ghosh *et al.*, 1960).

$$\text{Fructose-6-P} + \text{glutamine} \rightarrow \text{glucosamine-6-P} + \text{glutamic acid} \quad (1)$$

This reaction is catalyzed by the enzyme L-glutamine-D-fructose 6-phosphate transamidase. Glucosamine is an essential structural component of many glycoproteins.

The role of L-glutamine in nucleic acid and diphosphopyridine synthesis will be further examined herein as it appears relevant to the discussion of individual compounds.

Of particular interest is the function of L-glutamine in the biosynthesis of L-asparagine. In mammals, the enzyme L-asparagine synthetase catalyzes the following reaction:

$$\text{L-Aspartic acid} + \text{L-glutamine (or } NH_4^{+}) \xrightarrow[\text{ATP} \quad \text{AMP} + \text{pyrophosphate}]{(Mg^{++})} \text{L-asparagine} + \text{L-glutamic acid} \quad (2)$$

Patterson and Orr (1968) have suggested that β-aspartyladenylate is an intermediate reaction product in this equation, on the basis of (1) the stoichiometric quantities of AMP and pyrophosphate produced, and (2) the formation of β-aspartylhydroxamate when hydroxylamine was substituted for L-glutamine as a reactant.

It is now well known that certain animal tumors contain very little L-asparagine synthetase, and that it is these tumors which are, in general, most sensitive to the effects of L-asparaginase. Prager and Bachynsky (1968) found that tissues from normal and leukemic mice, as well as from normal guinea pigs, could utilize either L-glutamine or NH_4Cl as an amide donor for the synthesis of L-asparagine, but preferred L-glutamine. Inhibitors of L-asparagine synthetase could conceivably act in a number of ways, but at least one approach lies in the use of compounds which interfere with the utilization of L-glutamine. A summary of experimental work performed along these lines to date at the National Cancer Institute is given in Section IX.

B. Synthesis

L-Glutamine synthetase catalyzes the following reaction in mammalian systems:

$$\text{D- or L-glutamic acid} + NH_3 \xrightarrow[\text{ATP} \quad \text{ADP} + P_i]{} \text{D- or L-glutamine} \quad (3)$$

Meister (1968) and others have shown that γ-glutamylphosphate is an intermediate reaction product in this biosynthesis.

It has long been noted that, although L-glutamine is not an essential dietary amino acid for the intact mammal, it must be present in the medium in high concentration for the maintenance of cells in tissue culture. Levintow *et al.* (1957) suggested that the fact that L-glutamine was not nutritionally essential was a reflection of high L-glutamine synthetase activity in several mammalian organs. Under normal circumstances, they felt these organs might supply sufficient quantities of L-glutamine via the blood to meet the needs of other tissues which were low in the activity of this enzyme. In support of this reasoning, they cited the fact that blood concentrations of L-glutamine were relatively high in all mammals studied, that of human blood being one fourth the total concentration of circulating amino acids (~500–800 nmoles/ml). Eagle *et al.* (1966) later demonstrated that the requirement of mammalian cells for L-glutamine in the tissue culture medium is population dependent, given a minimal level of L-glutamine synthetase activity; under conditions of sufficiently high population density, such cells can synthesize enough L-glutamine to maintain their growth.

Levintow (1954) first compared extracts of normal tissues and those of certain neoplasms with respect to their ability to synthesize L-glutamine. (Levintow, as have other workers, actually examined the level of glutamyltransferase activity, regarding this as a measure of glutamine synthetase activity, inasmuch as the same enzyme system can catalyze both reactions.) In general, tumor extracts exhibited a low order of activity, although several mouse hepatomas had very high activity.

A number of subsequent studies have documented the inability of various neoplastic cells to synthesize L-glutamine in amounts adequate to maintain growth, even under conditions of high population density (Greenberg *et al.*, 1964). A decrease in blood and tissue levels of L-glutamine in tumor-bearing rats has also been reported by Wu *et al.* (1965), who postulated that "the decline in L-glutamine levels in tissues of tumor-bearing rats results from an inability of the host's liver to maintain or increase [sufficiently] the normal rate of L-glutamine synthesis." El-Asmar and Greenberg (1966) measured L-glutamine synthetase activity in the organs of normal mice and in selected murine tumors, with results as summarized in Table I.

A critical question with reference to L-glutamine synthetase is whether a sufficient differential exists between the activity of this enzyme in tumor cells and that in some normal cells to be therapeutically exploitable.

In summary, L-glutamine plays a vital role in protein biosynthesis, serving as a precursor not only for L-glutaminyl residues in protein but for other amino acids, notably L-asparagine, to which it donates an amido group. It also furnishes an amido group for essential reactions in nucleic acid, diphos-

TABLE I

L-GLUTAMINE SYNTHETASE ACTIVITY IN THE PRINCIPAL ORGANS OF THE MOUSE[a]

Organ or tumor	Activity (μmoles/mg of protein/15 min)
Mouse (normal)	
Brain	2.8
Bone marrow	1.0
Spleen	0.3
Liver	0.5
Lung	1.7
Intestine	0.0
Kidney	0.7
Tumor	
6C3HED	0.1
S-180 (ascites form)	0.16
L1210	0.19

[a] Data of El-Asmar and Greenberg (1966).

phopyridine, and glucosamine synthesis *de novo*. L-Glutaminyl residues in protein can, under specific conditions, undergo replacement of their amido residues through linkage with amines, and this function may be important in cross-linkage of peptide chains. [Tests of the ability of L-asparagine, in various systems, to perform the function of an amido group donor have so far yielded negative results with respect to the synthesis of diphosphopyridine (Spencer and Preiss, 1967), glucosamine (Ghosh *et al.*, 1960), guanosine monophosphate (Abrams and Bentley, 1959), and carbamylphosphate (Tatibana and Ito, 1969). However, such a role remains a possibility for L-asparagine in certain neoplastic tissues.]

The ability of cells to exist without a supply of exogenous L-glutamine depends on both the population density of the cells and on their level of L-glutamine synthetase activity. The high concentration of L-glutamine synthetase in several organs of the body presumably results in sufficient production of the amino acid to satisfy the requirements of other tissues which are less well endowed. This "exportation" explains why L-glutamine is a nutritionally nonessential amino acid for the intact animal, but cells in tissue culture may "paradoxically" require exogenous L-glutamine. Neoplastic cells in general appear to have low L-glutamine synthetase activity, but there are exceptions to this rule (Levintow, 1954).

The remainder of this paper concerns itself with antagonists and analogs of L-glutamine and their interference with the biosynthesis or metabolic roles of the parent compound, particularly as this may relate to the inhibition of tumor growth.

III. Diazo Analogs of L-Glutamine

This group of L-glutamine analogs is the only one which has received a trial against cancer in man. Structurally, these compounds exhibit a basic similarity, as is illustrated in the formulas which follow:

Structural Formulas of Diazo Antibiotics

Duazomycin A: L-norleucine, *N*-acetyl-6-diazo-5-oxo

```
                O
 -  +           ||
 N==N==CHCCH2CH2CH—COOH
                  \
                   NHC—CH3
                      ||
                      O
```

(I)

DON: 6-diazo-5-oxo-L-norleucine

```
                O
 -  +           ||
 N==N==CHCCH2CH2CHCOOH
                  \
                   NH2
```

(II)

Azotomycin (duazomycin B): *N*-(*N*-γ-glutamyl-6-diazo-5-oxonorleucinyl)-6-diazo-5-oxo-norleucine

```
          O                             O
 -  +     ||                            ||         +  -
 N==N==CHCCH2CH2          O   CH2CH2C—CH==N==N
                |         ||  |
                CH—HN—C—CH
                |             |
                COOH          NH—C—CH2CH2CHCOOH
                                 ||           \
                                 O             NH2
```

(III)

Azaserine: L-serine, diazoacetate

```
            O
 -  +       ||
 N==N==CHC—O—CH2CHCOOH
                  \
                   NH2
```

(IV)

DONV: 5-diazo-4-oxo-L-norvaline

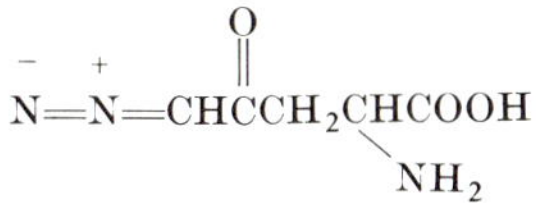

$$\overset{-}{N}=\overset{+}{N}=CH\overset{\overset{O}{\|}}{C}CH_2CH(NH_2)COOH$$

(V)

L-Glutamine

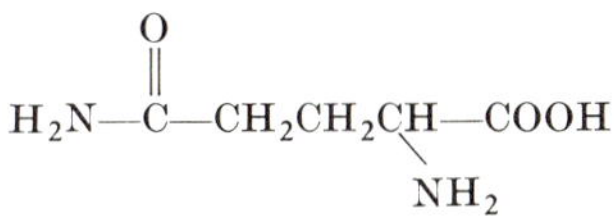

$$H_2N-\overset{\overset{O}{\|}}{C}-CH_2CH_2CH(NH_2)-COOH$$

(VI)

L-Asparagine

$$H_2N-\overset{\overset{O}{\|}}{C}-CH_2CH(NH_2)-COOH$$

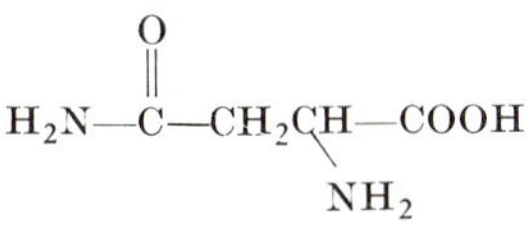

(VII)

The formulas of L-glutamine and L-asparagine are included for comparison.

Investigations of the biochemical sites of action of azaserine, DON, and duazomycin A, and their relations to antitumor activity and synergism with other drugs in animal tumor systems have been previously reviewed by Venditti and Goldin (1964). Figure 1, showing the major enzymatic steps in *de novo* purine biosynthesis, is adapted from their paper. The major steps in pyrimidine biosynthesis are shown in Fig. 2.

A. Azaserine

1. *Biochemistry and Mechanism of Action*

Azaserine has been the most thoroughly studied of this group of compounds. It has been demonstrated that azaserine interferes with several reactions in which L-glutamine participates (Venditti and Goldin, 1964), and those involving the biosynthesis of purines have been investigated most extensively. Of the latter (see Fig. 1), the reaction most sensitive to inhibition by azaserine is the conversion of FGAR (formylglycinamide ribotide) to FGAM (formylglycinamidine ribotide), which requires L-glutamine and ATP (Tomisek *et al.*, 1956, 1959; Moore and LePage, 1959; Bennett *et al.*, 1956). A representative study is that of Levenberg *et al.* (1957), who reported the effect of azaserine on several reactions leading to *de novo* inosinic acid biosynthesis

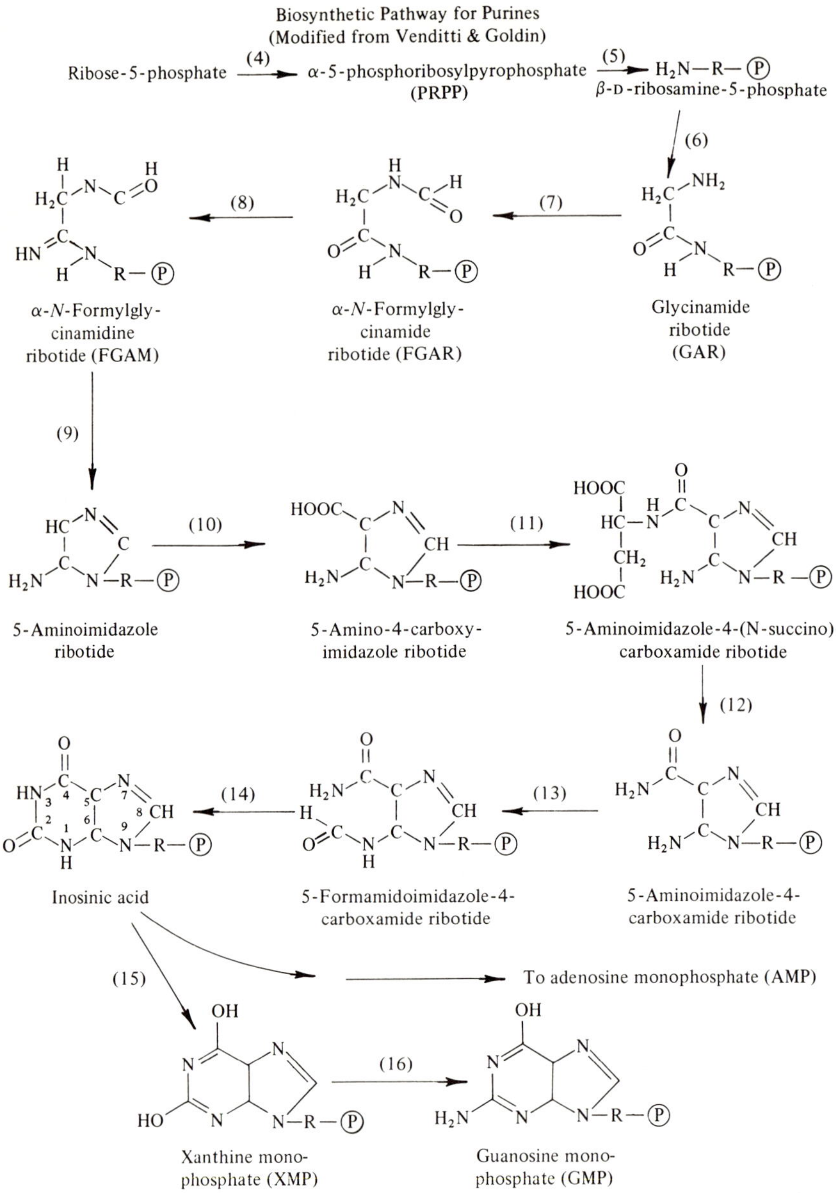

Biosynthetic Pathway for Purines
(Modified from Venditti & Goldin)

Ribose-5-phosphate —(4)→ α-5-phosphoribosylpyrophosphate (PRPP) —(5)→ $H_2N—R—Ⓟ$ β-D-ribosamine-5-phosphate

(6) → Glycinamide ribotide (GAR) —(7)→ α-*N*-Formylglycinamide ribotide (FGAR) —(8)→ α-*N*-Formylglycinamidine ribotide (FGAM)

(9) → 5-Aminoimidazole ribotide —(10)→ 5-Amino-4-carboxyimidazole ribotide —(11)→ 5-Aminoimidazole-4-(N-succino)-carboxamide ribotide

(12) → 5-Aminoimidazole-4-carboxamide ribotide —(13)→ 5-Formamidoimidazole-4-carboxamide ribotide —(14)→ Inosinic acid

Inosinic acid → To adenosine monophosphate (AMP)

Inosinic acid —(15)→ Xanthine monophosphate (XMP) —(16)→ Guanosine monophosphate (GMP)

Fig. 1. Biosynthetic pathway for purines (modified from Venditti and Goldin, 1964). In each of the following reactions, the amido group of L-glutamine serves as a nitrogen donor:

(5) catalyzed by PRPP amido transferase, (8) catalyzed by FGAR amido transferase, (16) catalyzed by GMP synthetase.

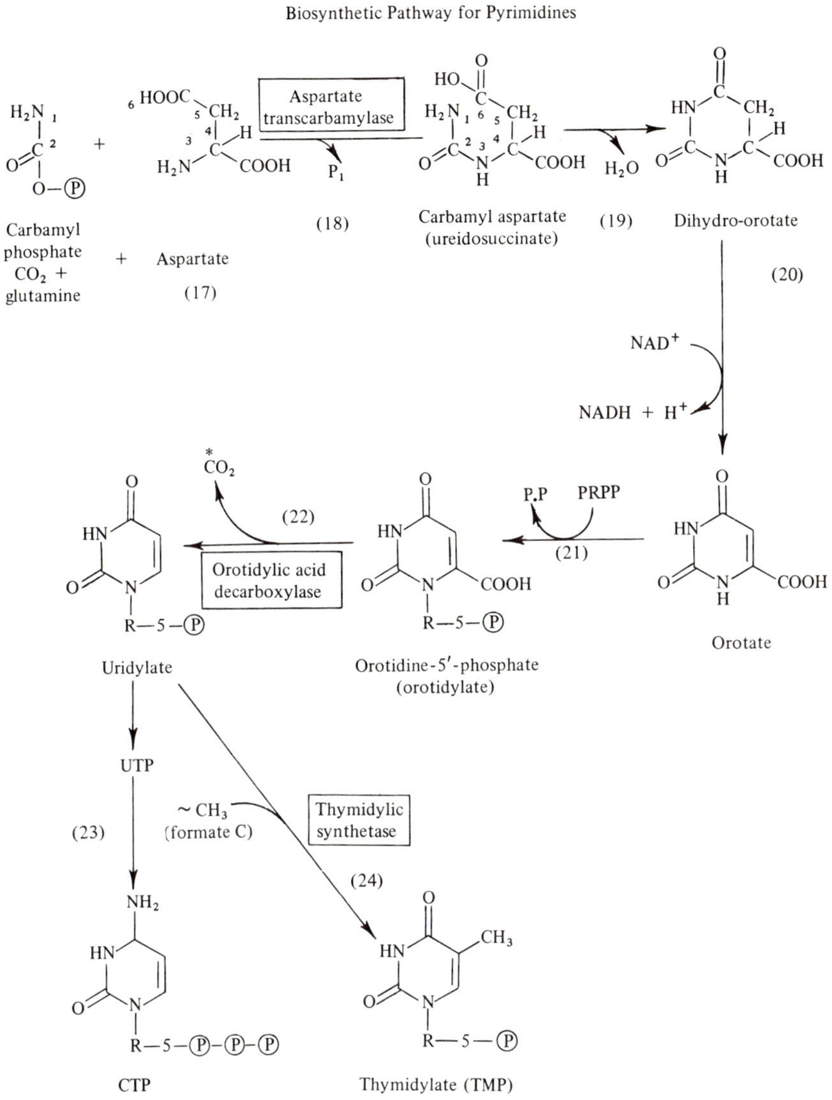

Biosynthetic Pathway for Pyrimidines

Carbamyl phosphate + Aspartate (17)
CO_2 + glutamine

Aspartate transcarbamylase (18) P_i

Carbamyl aspartate (ureidosuccinate)

(19) H_2O

Dihydro-orotate

(20) NAD^+ → $NADH + H^+$

Orotate

(21) PRPP → P.P

Orotidine-5′-phosphate (orotidylate)

(22) Orotidylic acid decarboxylase $\overset{*}{CO_2}$

Uridylate

UTP

(23)

CTP

~CH_3 (formate C)

Thymidylic synthetase (24)

Thymidylate (TMP)

Fig. 2. Biosynthetic pathway for pyrimidines. In each of the following reactions, the amido group of L-glutamine serves as a nitrogen donor:

(17) catalyzed by carbamylphosphate synthetase II,

(23) catalyzed by CTP synthetase.

in a cell-free pigeon-enzyme system. Table II summarizes their results in three reactions which were studied.

TABLE II

COMPARATIVE INHIBITORY EFFECT OF AZASERINE ON THREE DIFFERENT REACTIONS IN PURINE BIOSYNTHESIS[a]

Azaserine concentration (*M*)	L-Glutamine concentration (*M*)	% Inhibition
Reaction 1: Glutamine + PRPP → ribosylamine-5-P + glutamic acid		
2.9×10^{-3}	2.9×10^{-3}	17
2.9×10^{-2}	2.9×10^{-3}	48
Reaction 2: FGAR → FGAM		
5.7×10^{-4}	5.7×10^{-3}	61
5.7×10^{-3}	5.7×10^{-3}	95
Reaction 3: FGAM → 5-aminoimidazole carboxamide ribotide		
5.7×10^{-3}	0	40

[a] Data of Levenberg *et al.* (1957) converted from quantity/0.35 ml of incubation volume to molar concentrations. Reaction 3 is not L-glutamine dependent.

Based on an analysis of the FGAR → FGAM reaction, two mechanisms have been advanced to explain its inhibition by azaserine. Baker (1959) suggested that azaserine reacts with pyridoxal phosphate, the coenzyme essential to transfer of the amide group from L-glutamine in this and some other biological reactions, forming an inactive cofactor–azaserine complex which prevents pyridoxamine formation.

French and his co-workers (1963b) later proposed that azaserine reacts with a sulfhydryl group of the enzyme involved (FGAR amido transferase), preventing the attachment of L-glutamine to the enzyme. More recently, Mizobuchi and Buchanan (1968) also presented evidence supporting the view that the binding of L-glutamine to FGAR amido transferase initially involves a reversible reaction of the carboxamide carbon with a sulfhydryl group on the enzyme to yield a γ-glutamyl thioester and ammonia. They further showed that the azaserine–enzyme complex formed with FGAR amido transferase (derived from chicken liver) involves binding at a valylcysteine dipeptide sequence, and stated that their data "suggested that the reactive site of azaserine is the same as that of glutamine," i.e., at a specific sulfhydryl-group site on the enzyme. The weight of evidence now presented thus seems to favor French's explanation of the mechanism whereby azaserine binds to FGAR amido transferase.

Whatever the mechanism of binding to the amido transferase, both azaserine and DON do so irreversibly: L-glutamine can partially prevent but cannot reverse inhibition of purine biosynthesis by these compounds (Greenlees and LePage, 1956).

Sartorelli and Booth (1967) have shown inhibition of the synthesis of thymidine nucleotides and decreased thymidine kinase levels in sarcoma 180 ascites cells after treatment with azaserine. This effect was reversed, however, by supplying the cells with preformed adenine, suggesting a role for adenine nucleotides in regulating the activity of thymidine kinase, rather than a direct inhibitory effect of azaserine on that enzyme. Sartorelli also showed that the uptake of adenine into DNA and RNA is not inhibited by azaserine; this would seem to rule out inhibition of purine incorporation into nucleic acids as a possible mechanism of action.

Besides its effect on the purine biosynthetic pathway, azaserine also exerts an inhibitory effect on the conversion of uridine nucleotides to cytidine nucleotides (Kammen and Hurlbert, 1959), another reaction which requires donation of an amino group by L-glutamine. In a sufficiently sensitive system, such an inhibition would result not only in decreased levels of cytidine, an essential component of both DNA and RNA, but might also increase the levels of uridine nucleotides, thereby providing a mechanism for inhibition of pyrimidine synthesis itself, because increased levels of UMP are known to inhibit aspartate transcarbamylase and also orotidylic acid decarboxylase (Blair and Potter, 1961). The importance of azaserine inhibition of the conversion of UTP to CTP is, however, open to serious question for *in vivo* systems: Sartorelli and Booth (1967) have shown that azaserine, in concentrations great enough to inhibit *de novo* purine synthesis markedly in mouse sarcoma 180 cells *in vivo*, did not affect the utilization of ^{14}C-labeled orotic acid in RNA synthesis.

Simard and Bernhard (1966) have shown that azaserine at high concentrations (50 and 100 μg/ml), administered to rat embryonic cells *in vitro*, causes nucleolar segregation into three zones (granular, fibrillar, and amorphous). Other compounds which induce such nucleolar segregation, such as actinomycin D, daunorubicin and chromomycin A_3, have been shown to bind DNA and interfere with its template activity for the conduct of DNA-directed, RNA polymerase-mediated, RNA synthesis, whereas none of the "antimetabolites" do so. They concluded: "An attentive regard to [azaserine's] structure shows the existence of an unsaturated diazo grouping, capable of nucleophilic substitution. Further, azaserine possesses properties of an alkylating agent and becomes, at appropriate dose, mutagenic, antimitotic and radiomimetic."

Azaserine's ability to affect *de novo* adenine synthesis may help account for the fact that it causes a reduction in tissue levels of the diphosphopyridine nucleotides, NAD (DPN) and NADP (TPN). This effect may also be related to the role of L-glutamine's amido nitrogen as the precursor of the amido nitrogen of NAD. Narrod *et al.* (1960) first demonstrated such an effect in mouse liver, and Slater and Sawyer (1966) have shown a rapid decrease in levels of NAD and NADH in the liver of the rat after *in vivo* administration such that, 30 minutes after dosing, the sum of NAD and NADH was only 36% of the control value.

In summary, evidence has been presented that azaserine can inhibit purine biosynthesis *de novo*, that it can inhibit cytidine biosynthesis from uridine nucleotides (though, at least in one tumor system, the purine biosynthetic pathway appears much more sensitive), and that it also may bind with DNA to interfere with its template function. The inhibition of purine synthesis, mediated at the level of blocking the FGAR → FGAM reaction, has received the most attention in the literature and has been most widely accepted as azaserine's principal mechanism of antitumor action. In at least one animal tumor there is evidence to support this view. Anderson and Jacquez (1962) showed that, with intact cell suspensions of sensitive and resistant 70429 animal tumor cells, the azaserine-induced inhibition of purine synthesis was 44% for resistant cells and 85% in the sensitive cell line. They also demonstrated that there was no change in active transport of the drug in the resistant cells, which would seem to rule out a simple intracellular decrease in azaserine levels as the mechanism of resistance.

However, a number of investigators have cast doubt on blockade of *de novo* purine synthesis as the mechanism of azaserine's activity in certain tumor systems. As early as 1960, Sartorelli *et al.* (1960) showed that in hepatoma 134, chloropurine and azaserine each reduced the rate of purine formation to an extent comparable to that observed in sensitive tumors, but the hepatoma's growth was inhibited by azaserine and not by chloropurine. Hedgeaard and Roche (1966) have demonstrated, with the Ehrlich ascites tumor *in vivo*, that treatment with azaserine combined with the addition of various purine precursors (formylglycinamide, FGAR, 5-aminoimidazole carboxamide, and/or purines) did not alter the antitumor effect of azaserine. McFall and Magasanik (1960) added guanosine and observed a "tremendous increase in adenine and guanine pools" but no reversal of growth inhibition in the tumor system which they studied. One might argue that in these tumor systems, purine produced by *de novo* synthesis is utilized in preference to preformed purines, and that, therefore, failure of preformed purines to reverse azaserine inhibition of tumor growth does not *a priori* vitiate the blockade-of-purine-synthesis theory. However, Vandevoorde *et al.* (1964) demonstrated that the Osgood J-128 cell line (a tissue culture line derived from a patient with chronic granulocytic leukemia) utilized hypoxanthine, adenine, or aminoimidazole carboxamide (AICA) in preference to formation of purine by *de novo* synthesis. The cell line's growth was inhibited by azaserine, and the inhibition could not be reversed by adding any of these preformed purines to the culture medium. Thus it appeared clear that the drug interfered with biochemical reactions other than those leading to synthesis of the purines utilized by the tumor. The same investigators (Hansen and Vandevoorde, 1966) later duplicated these results and demonstrated a new finding: J-128 cells exposed to azaserine increased markedly in size and DNA content. During attempted cell division, a lesion appeared in the "central sphere of attraction" in azaserine-treated cells, increased in size, and "apparently caused death of the cell." This marked increase in size of the J-128 cells was observed in medium without AICA or preformed purine added, suggesting that *de novo* purine synthesis was not seriously inhibited.

This apparent disruption in the process of cell replication itself would seem to be compatible with the Simard thesis that azaserine acts by interference with the DNA template mechanism.

There is some evidence that azaserine, unlike most "antimetabolites," can kill cells which are not actively replicating. Only it and bischloroethyl nitrosourea (BCNU) were found to produce significant kill of nondividing L1210 cells in a study by Schabel *et al.* (1965). This, too, might be taken as evidence in support of the Simard and Bernhard thesis (1966).

The antitumor mechanism of action of azaserine is, therefore, not at all clear. However, it does inhibit *de novo* purine biosynthesis in all systems where this has been measured, and this inhibition is probably related to its ability to compete successfully with L-glutamine at a specific sulfhydryl site for the enzyme in the L-glutamine-dependent reaction, FGAR → FGAM.

2. *Clinical Studies*

Clinical experience with azaserine was first reported by Ellison *et al.* (1954). In this study a number of adults and children with a variety of malignancies received both oral and intravenous preparations of the drug, first in crude form, then as a crystalline preparation. An adequate trial was defined as "that producing definite signs of toxicity." The toxic effects encountered with the crystalline or synthetic preparation are summarized in Table III.

Mouth lesions were usually the earliest sign of toxicity after both oral and intravenous administration. "The oral lesions first appeared, after five or more days of treatment, as reddening and hypertrophy of the papillae on the tip of the tongue." Soreness of the tongue then developed, and then "erythema usually developed inside the vermilion border of the lip and on the buccal mucosa. The erythema was accompanied by a burning sensation and some soreness of the mouth. If the drug was continued, the diffuse reaction then proceeded to mucosal ulcerations."

TABLE III

TOXIC EFFECTS OF AZASERINE IN A CLINICAL TRIAL[a]

		% Adequate trials developing abnormality						
		Digestive tract				Hematologic		
Group and route	No. of adequate trials	Oral lesions	Nausea and vomiting	Anorexia	Epigastric pain	Platelets	WBC	Pyrogenic
Adults								
IV	8	87	62	87	12	12	25	25
PO	26	69	69	73	23	0	8	0
Children (all acute leukemia)								
IV	3	100	0	0	0	—	—	0
PO	6	83	0	0	0	—	—	0

[a] After Ellison *et al.* (1954).

TABLE IV

DOSES OF CRYSTALLINE AND SYNTHETIC AZASERINE TOLERATED BY INTRAVENOUS AND ORAL ADMINISTRATION[a]

	Daily dose (mg/kg)		Mean duration of treatment (days)	Total dose (mg/kg)	
	Range	Average		Range	Average
Intravenous					
Adults	1–10	8.1	9	21–125	69
Children	12	—	10	120	—
Oral					
Adults	3.3–20	8.1	13	46–245	108
Children	7.1–10	8.1	16	50–368	156

[a] Data of Ellison *et al.* (1954).

The smallest dose producing signs of toxicity was also determined by these investigators, and their findings are shown in Table IV.

Ellison *et al.* concluded that "about 60–70% more azaserine may be required to produce toxicity by the oral as compared to the intravenous route, suggesting that the drug is either incompletely absorbed or is inactivated in the stomach.

. . . On the basis of our experience, an effective dosage schedule for azaserine is 8 to 10 mg/kg (400–800 mg in the adult) given daily PO or IV and continued to the first signs of toxicity." Such toxicity was seen usually after 5 to 20 days of a single daily dose at this level.

Therapeutic effects were seen in both Hodgkin's disease and in acute leukemia. Five of nineteen patients with Hodgkin's disease had brief partial remissions (0.5–3.5 months); of these five, three received parenteral drug and two received it only by the oral route. Three of fourteen children with acute leukemia had brief partial remissions (3–10 weeks); at least one of these achieving remission received only oral drug.

Although the report of Ellison's group seemed to demonstrate significant oral absorption of drug, at least in some patients, it also pointed up the erratic nature of absorption by this route. It has been shown that the half-life of intact azaserine at a pH of 2 is only 7 minutes (Lim, 1968), which supports this clinical observation and casts some doubt on the validity of other studies which have been performed only with the oral preparation, such as the largest clinical study of the drug reported by Heyn *et al.* (1960). This study failed to show any significant difference between the therapeutic results of oral therapy with 6-mercaptopurine (6-MP) alone and therapy with 6-MP plus oral azaserine, in 125 cases of acute childhood leukemia. Comparative toxicity was not reported between the two regimens. Sherman (1963) criticized the conclusions of this report (which were that azaserine added nothing to 6-MP therapy), stating, "It is doubtful that orally administered azaserine survives exposure to gastric secretion."

In support of this contention, he cited the successful use of parenteral azaserine plus oral 6-MP in two cases of 6-MP-resistant acute lymphocytic leukemia. In one, a partial remission was reportedly obtained and maintained for 4.5 months. A subsequent remission was obtained by replacing 6-MP with 9-butyl-6-MP and continuing parenteral azaserine. No details were furnished on the other case.

Schroeder *et al.* (1964) published the results of their studies of the combination of azaserine and thioguanine in advanced solid malignant neoplasms. Ten patients participated in the Phase I studies. Each drug was given intravenously twice a day at equal doses, varying from 0.4 to 1.7 mg/kg per dose, for 5 to 9 days. "Because of leukopenia, thrombocytopenia, and the less significant side reactions [primarily stomatitis and alopecia], it became evident that a dosage level of 3.4 mg/kg/day of each drug . . . for five to nine days was the maximum that could be conveniently tolerated." Interestingly, only two instances of nausea and one of diarrhea were observed in 27 separate courses of therapy. A repeat course of therapy was instituted 1 month after the last dose of the previous course, and evaluations were made 1 month after the last dose of the second course. Six patients were then enrolled in a Phase II study at 3.4 mg/kg/per day of each agent given intravenously 5 or more days, divided into two daily doses. Of the total of 16 patients treated, five showed improvement, including four of seven patients with breast carcinoma. One patient died from leukopenia secondary to the therapy, with complicating infection. Four patients developed marked thrombocytopenia, each after more than three courses of the combination for 6 days or more. The authors felt this was a common enough complication to warrant the abandonment of therapy at this dose level for more than 5 days per course. They stated: "It appears that if successive courses of therapy are given at intervals of 28 days between the last dose of one course and the beginning of the next, thrombocytopenia will supervene in almost all patients in three months." The authors concluded that the effectiveness in carcinoma of the breast was "very encouraging," but that "another dose schedule should be employed in an attempt to circumnavigate the serious thrombocytopenia while preserving therapeutic effectiveness."

Holland *et al.* (1961) reported a comparative study of "optimal medical care" with and without azaserine in 20 patients with multiple myeloma. The schedule of drug dose was 3 mg/kg per day for 28 days, 6 mg/kg per day for the next 7 days, and 12 mg/kg per day for the last 7 days, unless dose-limiting toxicity appeared first. The drug was given orally with sodium bicarbonate in an attempt to prevent its destruction by gastric juice. The nine azaserine-treated patients sustained more toxicity than the 11 placebo-treated patients, but showed no therapeutic benefit from the drug.

Hayes *et al.* (1967) reported on combination therapy with thioguanine and azaserine in multiple myeloma. Fifteen patients received 0.2 mg/kg of azaserine orally twice daily, and 1 mg/kg of thioguanine orally per day. The mean duration of treatment was 122.3 days. Twelve of the cases were evaluable, of whom two had subjective pain relief, two had a significant decrease in marrow plasma cells, and one had a significant decrease in Bence-Jones proteinuria. Myelosuppression was seen in five patients, jaundice in one, and pharyngitis and GI disturbances in three, with one death possibly related to the treatment. The group's conclusion was that the combination "does not warrant further study as primary therapy."

The effect of azaserine as an inhibitor of L-asparagine synthetase is presented in Section IX. Section VIII presents evidence for its synergism with L-asparaginase in the L5178Y tumor system and reviews its activity against leukemia L1210.

B. DON

1. *Biochemistry and Mechanism of Action*

DON has been evaluated almost as extensively as azaserine. In reference to presumed mechanisms of action, it has been shown that DON inhibits the biosynthesis of D-glucosamine (Ghosh *et al.*, 1960), purines, diphosphopyridine nucleotides, and pyrimidine nucleotides, with the FGAR → FGAM reaction, of those examined, again most sensitive to this inhibition (Moore and LePage, 1957). At higher doses DON effectively inhibits purine biosynthesis at a point prior to FGAR formation (Moore and LePage, 1957). DON is much more effective on an equimolar basis as an inhibitor of purine synthesis, both in isolated reaction systems and *in vivo*, than is azaserine (Buchanan, 1957). Moore and LePage (1957) have measured the *in vivo* sensitivity of normal and neoplastic mouse tissues to azaserine and DON, and their results are summarized in Table V. They found that FGAR accumulated in the treated tumor tissues.

TABLE V

INTRAPERITONEAL DOSES OF AZASERINE AND DON CALCULATED TO INHIBIT *in vivo* GLYCINE-^{14}C INCORPORATION INTO ACID-SOLUBLE PURINES by 90%[a]

Tissue (normal mice)	Azaserine (mg/kg)	DON (mg/kg)
Spleen	7.2	0.36
Intestine	14.0	0.72
Kidney	57.0	3.6
Lung	110.0	11.0
Liver	180.0	18.0
Ehrlich carcinoma (solid)	2.9	0.14

[a] Date of Moore and LePage (1957).

As in the case of azaserine, synthesis of the pyrimidine nucleotide cytidine is inhibited by DON, and the mechanism in both cases is thought to be inactivation of the L-glutamine-requiring enzyme system which catalyzes the conversion of uridine to cytidine nucleotides. Moore and Hurlbert (1961) have shown, however, that the concentrations of DON required to inhibit completely this amination step in the biosynthesis of cytidine nucleotides were at least ten times the concentrations required to inhibit completely *de novo* biosynthesis of purine nucleotides. Furthermore, the lowest concentration (1×10^{-4} M in the presence of 30×10^{-6} M of exogenous L-glutamine) of DON which was effective in inhibiting purine formation actually stimulated pyrimidine formation from labeled orotic acid in the *in vitro* suspension of Novikoff tumor cells which Moore and Hurlbert used. They explained this apparent anomaly as follows: inactivation of the more sensitive of two enzymes competing for L-glutamine permits an increased availability of intracellular L-glutamine for the other enzyme, in this case that which catalyzes the amination of uridine nucleotides. Moore and Hurlbert found that 4.5×10^{-3} *M* of DON in the presence of 30×10^{-6} *M* exogenous L-glutamine completely inhibited *de novo* formation of purine and cytidine nucleotides by the Novikoff tumor cell suspension, yet the cells were able to maintain synthesis (or turnover) of RNA at 60% of their usual rate. The investigators concluded: "It may be judged that the relative effectiveness of DON in inhibition of growth of tissues and cells may be diminished by the availability of pre-existing nucleotides or of nucleotides from sources other than the *de novo* pathways."

DON has more recently been shown to have another site of action in pyrimidine synthesis, at least in some systems. This was demonstrated in studies whose primary aim was the characterization of a possible new form of carbamylphosphate synthetase. A form of this enzyme which uses ammonia as a nitrogen source for the synthesis of carbamylphosphate, the first intermediate in the pathway of pyrimidine biosynthesis, has long been known. The reaction it catalyzes is shown below:

$$CO_2 + NH_3 \xrightarrow[\text{ATP} \curvearrowright \text{ADP}]{Mg^{++},\ N\text{-acetylglutamate}} H_2N{-}\overset{\overset{O}{\|}}{C}{-}O{-}\underset{\underset{OH}{|}}{\overset{\overset{O}{\|}}{P}}{-}OH \qquad (25)$$

This reaction requires *N*-acetylglutamic acid and Mg^{++}. Carbamylphosphate then reacts with L-aspartate in the presence of transcarbamylase to form carbamylaspartic (ureidosuccinic) acid, a precursor of orotic acid.

The ammonia-utilizing form of carbamylphosphate synthetase, however, is limited in its distribution, appearing principally in mammalian liver (Brown and Cohen, 1960), although it has also been demonstrated in the intestinal mucosa, salivary gland, and kidney of the normal rat (Jones *et al.*, 1961; Hager and Jones, 1965). Furthermore, carbamylphosphate which is synthesized in the liver is apparently not available to other tissues, since no significant amount of it can be found in blood (Hager and Jones, 1965). Hager and Jones (1965) chose the Ehrlich ascites carcinoma as a convenient example of a nonhepatic tissue with a high pyrimidine requirement which apparently lacked carbamylphosphate synthetase but contained high levels of other enzymes of the orotic acid pathway. They incubated intact Ehrlich ascites cells *in vitro* for a short time with bicarbonate-^{14}C and found that the ^{14}C was incorporated into carbon atom two of the uracil ring in the cell's uridine nucleotides. The incorporation was increased by L-glutamine, with 0.1 m*M* extracellular L-glutamine saturating the system. It was also increased by ammonium chloride, but 5 m*M* of the latter compound was required to obtain nearly full activity in the system. Ammonia and L-glutamine did not give an additive increase in UMP biosynthesis when they were present simultaneously, indicating that they function as alternative substrates for a single enzyme system, with L-glutamine clearly the preferred nitrogen donor. DON, azaserine, and *O*-carbamyl-L-serine, another antagonist of L-glutamine which has never been used clinically, were then each added to the system. It was known that these compounds do not inhibit enzymes specific for ammonia. However, when used as competitive inhibitors of the enzymes which catalyze amido nitrogen transfer from L-glutamine, they will inhibit whether L-glutamine or the less efficient substrate, ammonia, is used. In the experience of Hager and Jones, the addition of 10 m*M* of DON or of 10 m*M* of *O*-carbamyl-L-serine gave 44% and 78% inhibition of carbamylphosphate formation, respectively, when only ammonium chloride served as the nitrogen source. Azaserine at the same concentration caused no inhibition. When 8 m*M* L-glutamine was added to the system, the degree of inhibition by 10 m*M* of DON and *O*-carbamyl-L-serine was reduced to 29% and 24% respectively. The authors concluded that their data suggested "synthesis of carbamylphosphate in the Ehrlich ascites cell by an enzyme requiring bicarbonate and L-glutamine and the subsequent incorporation of this carbamylphosphate into uridine nucleotides by the orotic acid pathway." They also stated, "An important extension of these results is the possibility that, in mammals and other vertebrates, the L-glutamine-dependent carbamyl-P-synthetase [since called carbamyl-P-synthetase II] provides carbamyl-P solely or mainly for pyrimidine biosynthesis while the ammonia-specific carbamyl-P-synthetase provides carbamyl-P solely or mainly for biosynthesis of arginine and urea."

Since their report was published, it has been shown by Mayfield *et al.* (1967) that the Novikoff ascites tumor also utilizes L-glutamine rather than ammonia as the chief nitrogen donor for the synthesis of carbamylaspartate. DON is 1×10^{-5} *M*, in the presence of 5×10^{-6} *M* of added L-glutamine, inhibited by nearly 50% the amount of incorporation of ^{14}C-labeled bicarbonate into carbamylaspartate which otherwise would take place with that amount of L-glutamine present. It may be noted that Moore and Hulbert (1961), working also with the Novikoff tumor, found that DON, at 1×10^{-4} *M*, in the presence of 30×10^{-6} *M* of added L-glutamine, was necessary to achieve 90% inhibition of purine formation, and that this concentration of DON stimulated pyrimidine biosynthesis. This apparent paradox is explained when one remembers that Moore and Hulbert furnished the cells with preformed orotic acid.

In subsequent experiments, Hager and Jones (1967), working with fetal rat liver, and Tatibana and Ito (1967) working with hematopoietic mouse spleen, have demonstrated the presence of the L-glutamine-dependent carbamylphosphate synthetase II in both systems, residing in the supernatant fraction of tissue homogenates. It was apparently a rate-limiting enzyme for pyrimidine synthesis in these systems, inasmuch as it was inhibited by pyrimidine nucleotides. Activity of the ammonia-dependent synthetase was also present in the fetal rat liver and increased with maturation of the organism. The ammonia-dependent synthetase is now thought to reside in mitochondria and to catalyze the initial steps in arginine and urea synthesis (Kerson and Appel, 1968).

Kerson and Appel (1968) have confirmed the inhibition of carbamylphosphate synthetase in the supernatant fraction of adult rat liver by pyrimidine nucleotides. Cytidine triphosphate was the most potent of these, cytosine derivatives being more potent than uracil derivatives. This would seem to confirm the function of carbamylphosphate synthetase as a rate-limiting enzyme in pyrimidine biosynthesis. However, these workers found the enzyme which they isolated to be synthetase I (dependent on NH_3), and L-glutamine did not serve as a nitrogen source for it. They felt that during purification the affinity of the *in vivo* enzyme for L-glutamine may have been lost, as has been shown to occur with the L-glutamine-dependent carbamylphosphate synthetase in *E. coli* (Kalman *et al.*, 1965).

The relevance of these experiments to a discussion of DON is at least twofold: (1) they demonstrate that L-glutamine antagonists can serve as powerful confirmatory tools in the investigation of whether a biosynthetic enzyme is dependent on L-glutamine and (2) they demonstrate another site of L-glutamine-dependent enzyme inhibition by antagonists of L-glutamine, with *O*-carbamyl-L-serine appearing, in the work of Hager and Jones, to be more powerful than DON, and azaserine almost without effect. This is in contrast to the order of effectiveness of the three in other L-glutamine-dependent reactions which they inhibit, in which DON is more effective than azaserine, and the latter is more effective than *O*-carbamyl-L-serine (Hager and Jones, 1965).

2. *Clinical Studies*

Clinical experience with DON prior to 1960 has been summarized in a previous review by Duvall (1960): In a study comparing DON with nitrogen mustard, 41 adults were placed on DON in an oral dose regimen at 0.2 mg/kg per day for 30 days. Thirty-eight percent required temporary withdrawal because of toxicity. Diagnoses among the 41 patients were bronchogenic carcinoma, 18; Hodgkin's disease, 11; lymphosarcoma, 7; and malignant melanoma, 5. Some of the patients with lymphomas showed transient reductions in lesion size, but no significant objective changes were noted in any of the other patients. Nitrogen mustard was concluded to be the superior agent. In another preliminary study, 32 evaluable patients with advanced solid tumors were treated for from 9 to 67 days with DON at oral doses of 0.3–1 mg/kg per day or parenteral doses of 0.06–0.4 mg/kg per day. Transient benefit was seen in two cases of metastatic carcinoma, one of malignant melanoma, and one of lymphoma. A later study of 47 patients considered to have had "acceptable" trials of DON (therapy for 2 weeks or longer at doses of 0.2–1.1 mg/kg per day, either IV, IM, or orally, showed seven cases with transient evidence of disease regression. These included two of 14 cases of breast carcinoma (two others had reversal of hypercalcemia), two of nine cases of bronchogenic carcinoma, one of six cases of gastrointestinal carcinoma, one of five cases of endometrial or cervical cancer, and one of four lymphomas. Four patients with melanoma and four with "miscellaneous carcinomas" were treated without response.

Also cited by Duvall, and largely compiled from the preliminary clinical studies just discussed, were "marked reversals of hypercalcemia and hypercalciuria . . . effected in 11 patients on DON or DON–6-MP combination therapy." Calcium changes were not paralleled by X-ray evidence of bone healing or regression in soft tissue calcifications present in some patients, and all patients succumbed to progression of their disease. Transient clinical improvement noted in some of the patients was considered largely attributable to correction of hypercalcemia. The patients, all with radiographically demonstrable osteolysis, had the following types of carcinoma: breast (6 cases), bronchogenic (2 cases), adrenocortical (1 case), and metastatic carcinoma of unknown origin (2 cases). DON was given intravenously or intramuscularly in single daily doses ranging from 0.1 to 0.6 mg/kg, generally starting with high initial doses and then tapering to 0.2 mg/kg per day. Treatment periods ranged from 9 to 69 days. Calcium intake was restricted in all patients to 200 mg/day or less. "6-MP was administered orally in doses of 2.5 mg/kg/day for 12–40 days. . . . The periods of treatment and total dosages of DON and 6-MP were approximately the same in each patient." Treatment of four patients with hypercalcemia and/or hypercalciuria with 6-MP alone effected no substantial change in calcium metabolism.

Toxic reactions in the series compiled by Duvall were analyzed in 63 adult patients who received DON orally or parenterally, generally in doses ranging from 0.2 1.1 mg/kg once daily, and usually continued as long as tolerated. Ulceration of tongue and mucous membranes occurred in 83% of patients and appeared to be selectively blocked by adenine in daily oral doses of 400–500 mg. Forty-eight percent had diarrhea and 30% had nausea and vomiting. Twenty-four percent of patients developed moderate leukopenia and 11% developed thrombocytopenia of mild degree—no drug-related deaths attributable to myelosuppression occurred. No hepatic dysfunction related to DON was seen.

M. C. Li (1960) cited its use in eight patients with metastatic testicular carcinomas, in combination with 6-MP. Drug dose schedules were not mentioned. One patient had a response, in that a persistently elevated HCG titer returned to normal and remained negative for more than 39 months. In a later paper (1961), Li mentions the use of DON in the following manner: 10 to 15 mg/day orally for 3–5 weeks or to toxicity, then no drug until toxicity subsides, then back on drug again in cyclic maintenance fashion; this was used in patients with trophoblastic tumors. Of four who received DON, three had favorable responses. However, the one patient with metastatic disease did not respond to the drug.

Masterson and Nelson (1965) have reported on the treatment of three women with choriocarcinoma who received DON as primary treatment: two of the three were in remission after 6 and 8 years.

Sullivan *et al.* (1962) reported on the use of 6-MP plus DON in a large cooperative study in acute leukemias of childhood, carried out by Children's Cancer Study Group A. They treated 259 evaluable cases of previously untreated acute leukemia (basic study) and 44 evaluable cases of children with acute leukemia who had relapsed from a steroid-induced remission or failed to achieve remission on steroids (steroid substudy). The children in the basic study group were randomized among three treatment regimens with dosage schedules as follows: (a) standard dose 6-MP, 2.5 mg/kg body weight, by mouth, daily; (b) 6-MP standard dose plus DON, 0.25 mg/kg body weight, by mouth, daily; and (c) high-loading dose 6-MP, 6.6 mg/kg per day, by mouth, daily for 21 days, followed by standard dose therapy. Children in the steroid substudy were randomized between a standard dose regimen of 6-MP and a DON-supplemented regimen as above. The results obtained in the basic study (only 194 received adequate drug trial) are shown in Table VI.

TABLE VI

6-MP + DON vs. 6-MP in Acute Childhood Leukemia[a]

Regimen	CR (complete remission)	PR (partial remission)	No. response and failure
6-MP (59 patients)	21 (35.6%)	29 (49.1%)	9 (15.3%)
6-MP + DON (71 patients)	30 (42.3%)	35 (49.4%)	6 (8.3%)
High-load 6-MP (64 patients)	22 (34.4%)	35 (54.7%)	7 (10.9%)

[a] Data of Sullivan *et al.* (1962).

M_1 marrows were attained by 50/71 (70.4%) patients on 6-MP plus DON, by 31/59 (52.5%) patients on 6-MP "standard dose," and by 37/64 (57.8%) on "high-loading" 6-MP.

There was no statistically significant difference among the three with regard to rapidity of response, duration of control, or survival time.

The number and percentage of adequate trials in the basic study, and drug toxicity observed, are shown in Table VII.

TABLE VII

TOXICITY OF 6-MP VS. 6-MP + DON IN ACUTE CHILDHOOD LEUKEMIA[a]

	6-MP (59 patients)	6-MP + DON (71 patients)	High-loading 6-MP (64 patients)
Leukopenia	42 (71.2%)	43 (60.6%)	40 (62.5%)
Mouth ulcers	5 (10.2%)	61 (85.9%)	21 (32.8%)
GI signs	6 (10.2%)	20 (28.2%)	7 (10.9%)
Skin rash	2 (3.4%)	6 (8.5%)	3 (4.7%)
Marrow aplasia	9 (15.3%)	14 (19.7%)	8 (12.5%)

[a] Data of Sullivan *et al.* (1962).

The major difference, as seen from this table, was an increased incidence of mouth ulcers and GI symptoms in the 6-MP plus DON group.

The percentage of inadequate trials was 31.4% for 6-MP, 14.5% for 6-MP plus DON, and 28.9% for high-loading dose 6-MP regimens.

The investigators' conclusion about the basic study was that DON added to 6-MP gave a greater complete remission and M_1 marrow rate which was statistically significant at the expense of increased, but not trial-limiting, toxicity. The number of children on DON-supplement in the inadequate trial group was significantly less than the number of children on the other two regimens. No "striking difference" in age distribution, duration of untreated disease, toxicity, or complications during study was noted which could account for this difference. They stated: "It would appear that the combined drug regimen was more effective than either of the single drug regimens in controlling the early course of the disease, thereby permitting a longer period of therapy." In the steroid substudy, no statistically significant difference was seen, in response or in other parameters, between the group treated with 6-MP alone and that treated with the combination of 6-MP and DON.

C. Azotomycin

1. *Biochemistry and Mechanism of Action*

Azotomycin, because of its structural similarity, has been supposed to have a similar mechanism of action to DON and azaserine. Studies on this subject have not yet been published.

2. *Clinical Studies*

Ansfield (1965) reported results of a Phase I clinical study of azotomycin in 112 patients with far-advanced solid tumors. The patients received single daily intravenous injections, and "moderate leukopenia, thrombocytopenia, and vomiting appeared consistently when a dose of 5 mg/kg per day for 5 days was reached." There were no deaths from drug toxicity and no responses were observed in these patients, all of whom had very far-advanced disease.

A Phase II study of azotomycin was subsequently reported by Weiss *et al.* (1968). The drug was given to 252 adult patients with a variety of solid tumors at a dose schedule of 2.0 mg/kg per day for 10 days or to dose-limiting toxicity. Nausea and vomiting were the principal toxicities classed as "severe" in 87 patients (35%), most of whom were unable to complete the 10-day course of therapy because of it. Forty patients (17%) developed "severe" marrow suppression, but there was no evidence of prolonged hematopoietic toxicity. Fourteen patients (5%) developed oral toxicity classed as "severe." Objective responses were reported in 11/64 patients with cancer of the colon and rectum, 2/21 with bronchogenic cancer, 1/15 with breast carcinoma, 3/21 with melanoma, 2/7 with lymphomas, 1/21 with head and neck tumors, 1/4 with carcinoma of the pancreas, and 4/14 patients with soft tissue sarcomas. The response in pancreatic carcinoma and one of the responses in melanoma were classed as "complete." Further studies of azotomycin, both alone and in combination with 5-FU (Central Drug Evaluation Program) and with L-asparaginase (National Cancer Institute; Southwest Cancer Chemotherapy Study Group) are now in progress.

The effect of azotomycin as an inhibitor of L-asparagine synthetase is shown in Section IX. Section VIII presents evidence for its synergism with L-asparaginase in the L5178Y tumor system and reviews its antitumor activity against the L1210 leukemia.

D. Duazomycin A

1. *Biochemistry and Mechanism of Action*

Duazomycin A (*N*-acetyl-DON) has been studied less than azaserine and DON with regard to possible mechanisms of antitumor action. Anderson and Brockman (1963) have shown, however, that sublines of the mouse plasma cell neoplasm 70429 which have been made resistant to duazomycin A are also resistant to azaserine and DON. As with the latter two compounds, they found that duazomycin A inhibited incorporation of formate into soluble purine nucleotides and into nucleic acids in growing 70429 cells and produced large accumulations of FGAR in the soluble fraction of these cells. The accumulations of FGAR were much reduced at higher levels of duazomycin A, although purine nucleotide synthesis continued to be blocked: "... this would be consistent with an effective secondary inhibition earlier in the *de novo* pathway of purine biosynthesis in the L-glutamine-requiring synthesis of phosphoribosylamine. In this respect duazomycin A resembled DON, but azaserine did not show this effect." Duazomycin A was also shown by Anderson and Brockman to be an effective inhibitor of the conversion of uridine to cytidine nucleotides in these cells, but not so potent as DON. Acylase activity in the 70429 cells was weak and had no detectable effect on duazomycin, although it was readily deacetylated to DON by mammalian acylase I purified from hog kidney.

2. *Clinical Trials*

Duazomycin A has received limited clinical trial. Lefkowitz *et al.* (1965) reported on their experience with the drug in combination with thioguanine in the treatment of 15 patients with solid neoplasms of the head and neck: The patients were treated intravenously with a combination of 6-thioguanine and duazomycin A at daily dosages of 3.0 and 0.6 mg/kg, respectively, in two divided doses. In general, the patients who were selected for this study had received and had become resistant to conventional therapy. Nine of the 15 patients showed some objective improvement, defined as a 50% or greater regression of tumor, but in no case was there complete eradication of the tumor clinically. "Toxicity to the drug combination appeared between the 11th and the 20th day following treatment, with leukopenia and thrombocytopenia as the major toxic manifestations. Seven patients developed leukopenia, and thrombocytopenia was noted in five; four patients developed a significant eosinophilia. Seven patients exhibited some loss of hair, but no stomatitis, gastrointestinal toxicity, or evidence of hemorrhage were noted." The objective tumor regressions obtained were all "of short duration."

Colsky *et al.* (1966) reported on the use of duazomycin A by the Eastern Solid Tumor Group in patients with metastatic malignancy. One hundred and four patients received the drug on a daily intravenous schedule. After initial trials at much lower levels had established lack of significant toxicity, the daily dose was established at 3 mg/kg for 6 to 14 days (until limiting toxicity developed). Anorexia and nausea occurred in almost all patients at this dose level, but were not usually severe enough to warrant discontinuation of treatment. Stomatitis occurred in one half of the patients and mild nonbloody diarrhea in one fourth at the 3 mg/kg per day level. "Although stomatitis generally did not become severe enough to force cessation of therapy, its appearance usually heralded or occurred concomitantly with hematopoietic depression."

A white blood count of $<5000/mm^3$ occurred in 64 of the 104 patients on daily drug dose, but was usually mild and reversible. Thrombocytopenia (defined as <100,000 platelets/mm^3) was noted in 26 of the 104 patients treated daily, and was again usually mild and reversible.

Thirty-nine patients in the study of Colsky *et al.* received duazomycin A as intermittent treatment by the following regimens: (1) intravenous infusion over a 4-hour period once weekly at 10–20 mg/kg (7 patients); (2) direct intravenous "push" once weekly at 4–14 mg/kg (17 patients); (3) intramuscular injection twice weekly at 6–16 mg/kg (13 patients); and (4) direct intravenous "push" three times per week at 4 or 6 mg/kg (2 patients). Only one of the patients on intermittent dosage developed leukopenia and none developed thrombocytopenia.

Six patients in the total of 143 had objective, measurable tumor regression; five of the six had bronchogenic carcinoma and one had an anaplastic carcinoma of unknown primary site. All six tumor regressions were observed in patients on the initial daily intravenous study.

Foley *et al.* (1966) reported on the treatment of 23 patients with carcinoma of the lung who were randomized as follows: nine received radiation therapy alone; seven received radiation plus duazomycin A at 0.75 or 1 mg/kg per day intravenously with the drug being started 4 days prior to the onset of radiation therapy, and thereafter given only on days that radiation therapy was given (usually 5 days per week). The third group of seven patients received radiation therapy plus methotrexate, 1.2 mg/kg IM two times per week. There were no responses in the duazomycin plus radiation group, two in the group treated with radiation alone, and three in the methotrexate plus radiation groups, although there was no increase in survival time for responders. Toxicity specific to duazomycin A included four out of seven with "mild bone marrow suppression."

The effect of duazomycin A as an inhibitor of L-asparagine synthetase is presented in Section IX. Data on its activity against leukemia L1210 are shown in Section VIII.

E. Duazomycin C

Duazomycin C, a fourth diazo compound, received limited clinical trials by Colsky's group (Dr. J. J. Oleson, personal communication), before the drug became unavailable. Twelve patients were treated with up to 2 mg/kg per day IV for 10 days. No dose-limiting toxicity and no therapeutic responses were seen. Duazomycin C was without activity against L1210 leukemia using daily IP treatment, in contrast to the other diazo compounds previously discussed (see Section VIII). No work on its structure or mechanism of action has been published.

F. DONV

DONV (5-diazo-4-oxo-L-norvaline) is the next lower homolog of DON. It is classed by Handschumacher *et al.* (1967) as an analog of L-asparagine; they have shown that preincubation of guinea pig serum or a purified preparation of L-asparaginase from *E. coli* with 1.2×10^{-4} *M* DONV causes inactivation of the amidase activity of L-asparaginase. This is not restored by passage through Sephadex. The apparent successful competition of DONV with L-asparagine for binding sites on L-asparaginase at physiological pH is reversed if L-asparagine or L-aspartic acid are provided and the pH is below 5.5. In the same experiment, "DONV had no effect on L-glutaminase or other L-glutamine-dependent reactions." This is in contrast to the findings of French *et al.* (1963a), who found that DONV, as the DL-compound in micromolar concentration, caused 50% inhibition of FGAR → FGAM conversion in an enzyme system derived from *Salmonella typhimurium*, and referred to it as an "L-glutamine antagonist."

Handschumacher *et al.* (1967) found that incubation of L5178Y cells, which require L-asparagine for growth, for 1 to 4 hours with 6×10^{-4} DONV in the absence of exogenous L-asparagine caused a logarithmic rate of cell death (80% cell kill at 4 hours). An identical study with P815Y cells, which do not require L-asparagine for growth, showed 30% cell kill in 4 hours. The total growth of L5178Y cells in culture for 4 days in the presence of 8×10^{-5} *M* L-asparagine was 87% inhibited by 9×10^{-4} *M* DONV. Preincubation of cells with DONV at 6×10^{-4} *M* did not affect the cells' ability to concentrate L-asparagine from the medium. They also retained the ability to incorporate ^{14}C-labeled L-asparagine into protein. He concluded that these findings suggest "a more subtle mechanism of action [in tumor growth inhibition] than a gross effect on protein synthesis. . . ." It would appear that DONV has at least two separate properties: (1) inactivation of L-asparaginase at physiological pH and (2) inhibition of the L-asparagine-dependent aspect of growth in tumors which have such dependence. The latter effect does not appear to be mediated through blocking L-asparagine's entrance into the cell or through inhibiting its incorporation into protein. It would therefore seem reasonable to assume that DONV mediates its latter effect by interaction with an L-asparagine-requiring enzyme system, as the L-glutamine antagonists do with L-glutamine-requiring enzyme systems. No such systems have so far been demonstrated. It is, however, tempting to speculate that they exist, and that some of the reactions involved may be those which rely on L-glutamine for donation of an amido group in the biosynthetic pathways of normal tissues.

Becker and Broome (1967) have confirmed the L-asparaginase-inactivating activity of DONV. They showed that L-asparaginase in untreated agouti serum inhibits the first wave of mitosis occurring in rat liver after partial hepatectomy, whereas DONV-treated serum does not inhibit mitosis.

It is of particular interest that DONV inactivates L-asparaginase when cells are preincubated with the enzyme, whereas azaserine, a very similar compound, potentiates the effect of L-asparaginase in the L5178Y system and DON itself has no ability to inactivate L-asparaginase, although there is evidence it can inactivate L-glutaminase (Ghosh *et al.*, 1960) derived from *E. coli*. It should be noted also, however, that the possible effects of sequential use of L-asparaginase and DONV have not been determined.

The effects of DONV as an asparagine synthetase inhibitor are presented in Section IX. Section VIII summarizes screening data for this compound against leukemia L1210.

IV. Inhibitors of L-Glutamine Synthetase

A. L-Methionine DL-Sulfoximine

L-Methionine DL-sulfoximine is an antagonist of L-glutamine with this structure:

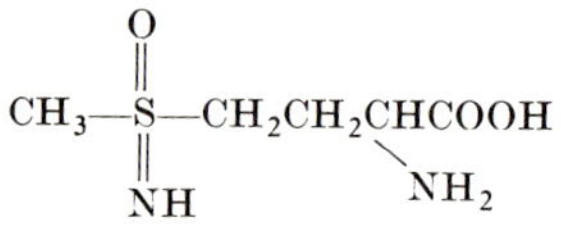

$$CH_3{-}\overset{\overset{\displaystyle O}{\|}}{\underset{\underset{\displaystyle NH}{\|}}{S}}{-}CH_2CH_2\underset{\underset{\displaystyle NH_2}{\diagdown}}{C}HCOOH$$

(VIII)

It is the active toxic material in flour bleached with nitrogen trichloride (agene), and as such is the cause of convulsions in dogs, cats, monkeys, and rats fed "agenized" flour (Misani and Reiner, 1950). Because of its structural resemblance to other amino acid analogs with animal antitumor activity, Clarke *et al.* (1957) studied its effect on the growth of sarcoma 180 in mice. They found L-methionine DL-sulfoximine to be ineffective by itself as a tumor inhibitor, but it appeared to potentiate the antitumor effects of azaserine and DON. Sloan-Kettering then carried out pharmacological studies of L-methionine DL-sulfoximine and DON in combination in rats, mice, and dogs (Krakoff, 1961). They found pathological, biochemical, and hematological changes similar to those produced by DON alone; the only toxic effect of L-methionine DL-sulfoximine appeared to be on the central nervous system.

Greenlees and LePage (1956) found that L-methionine DL-sulfoximine appeared to be an effective inhibitor of *de novo* purine formation, reducing the accumulation of GAR in Ehrlich ascites cells to 14% of control; they proceeded to test L-methionine DL-sulfoximine in combination with azaserine against the Ehrlich ascites carcinoma *in vivo*. Combination treatment led to shorter survival times than were obtained with azaserine alone, which led the authors to the conclusion that "methionine sulfoximine must be more harmful to the host tissues than to the tumor's." The doses used were azaserine 0.2 mg/kg per day plus methionine sulfoximine 20 mg/kg per day for 6 days.

Krakoff (1961) has reported on the effects of L-methionine DL-sulfoximine in man. It was given orally to seven patients with far-advanced malignancies, in divided doses totaling from 10 to 400 mg per day. No antitumor effects were seen, and the toxic effects of the drug were limited to the central nervous system. Four patients developed toxic psychoses, with frank hallucinations, disorientation, and marked agitation which continued for from 1 to 3 days after administration of the compound was discontinued. The onset of these abnormalities was related to the size of the daily dose rather than the cumulative dose received: "Thus, a dose of 200 to 400 mg daily produced toxic psychoses in three to five days, whereas smaller doses could be given for much longer periods of time without evidence of toxicity." One to 2 days of restlessness and apprehension usually preceded the onset of frank psychosis. The mental state returned to the pretreatment level without the addition of L-methionine. However, L-methionine, administered at the same time as L-methionine DL-sulfoximine, appeared to exert a protective effect: a patient with carcinoma of the cervix received 400 mg/day for 5 days of L-methionine DL-sulfoximine, and concurrently, 6–7.5 gm/day of L-methionine. No neurological or psychological abnormalities were seen, and the EEG was normal during this period. When L-methionine DL-sulfoximine was readministered alone in smaller doses, however, it produced hallucinations, disorientation, and agitation.

One patient in Krakoff's study received DON at 2.5 mg/day and L-methionine DL-sulfoximine at 100 mg/day for 3 days. In this individual, mental aberrrations appeared which regressed only partially after administration of the two compounds was stopped, and subsequently peripheral neuropathy developed. He died of metastatic bronchogenic carcinoma, and postmortem examination of the central nervous system failed to reveal a cause for the mental and neurological abnormalities. Krakoff stated: "In this single instance, the possibility cannot be excluded that L-methionine DL-sulfoximine together with DON produced irreversible functional changes in the central nervous system."

L-Methionine DL-sulfoximine is a powerful inhibitor of the biosynthesis of L-glutamine from L-glutamate. It exerts this effect through irreversible binding to the enzyme L-glutamine synthetase, which phosphorylates it so that the enzyme's usual production from L-glutamate of the intermediate, γ-glutamyl phosphate, is prevented (Ronzio and Meister, 1968).

The efficacy of L-methionine DL-sulfoximine as an inhibitor of L-asparagine synthetase is shown in Section IX.

B. δ-HYDROXYLYSINE

A second compound which probably acts as an inhibitor of L-glutamine synthetase is δ-allohydroxy-L-lysine (HL), which has the structural formula IX:

$$\begin{array}{l} H_2N\text{—}CH_2\underset{\displaystyle OH}{CH}\text{—}CH_2CH_2\underset{\displaystyle NH_2}{CH}\text{—}COOH \end{array}$$

(IX)

Rabinowitz *et al.* (1957) found HL to be a noncompetitive inhibitor of radioactive leucine incorporation into the protein of Ehrlich ascites carcinoma cells *in vitro*. A concentration of 2×10^{-3} *M* HL produced 30 to 40% inhibition, which could be prevented by the addition of L-glutamine to the medium at concentrations as low as 5×10^{-4} *M*. Similar results were obtained with the study of lysine, valine, phenylalanine, and methionine incorporation. Although the antagonism produced by HL closely resembled that produced by L-methionine DL-sulfoximine and the two compounds were almost equally potent at the same concentrations, twice the concentration of L-glutamine was required to prevent inhibition of protein synthesis by L-methionine DL-sulfoximine as was required to prevent the inhibition due to HL.

In addition to preventing HL-induced inhibition of protein synthesis, Rabinowitz *et al.* found that L-glutamine could also reverse such inhibition after it has occurred. Furthermore, these authors showed that a single low concentration ($\sim 2 \times 10^{-5}$ *M*) of L-glutamine could prevent HL-induced inhibition of L-valine incorporation into protein, despite concentrations of the inhibitor which ranged as high as 1×10^{-2} *M*. They concluded that the absence of a competitive relationship between HL and L-glutamine indicated that HL did not interfere with the utilization of L-glutamine for protein synthesis. To support this conclusion, they demonstrated that HL failed to inhibit L-glutamine incorporation into protein, even at concentrations of L-glutamine which were too low to prevent the inhibitory effect of HL on valine incorporation. They felt these data were all "consistent with the postulation that HL interferes with synthesis of L-glutamine rather than its utilization," and that the partial inhibition of incorporation of various amino acids seen with HL was due to the requirements of the tumor cells for L-glutamine to carry out *de novo* protein synthesis. If insufficient exogenous L-glutamine were available, HL could largely block new protein synthesis by blocking endogenous L-glutamine synthesis.

A major difference noted by Rabinowitz *et al.* between HL and L-methionine DL-sulfoximine was the relative absence of toxicity due to the former. The LD_{50} of L-methionine DL-sulfoximine was found to be 100 mg/kg when given to mice intraperitoneally. HL was apparently nontoxic and could be injected in doses up to 5 gm/kg.

In the only reported attempt to assay animal antitumor activity, Rabinowitz *et al.* administered HL at 500 mg/kg per day for 7 days to mice with the Ehrlich ascites tumor; no inhibition was observed.

In a later study (Rabinowitz *et al.*, 1959), the same authors, examined the effect of L-methionine DL-sulfoximine, HL, *O*-carbamyl-DL-serine, and azaserine on amino acid incorporation into protein. The incorporation of valine-^{14}C and isoleucine-^{14}C was measured to determine the overall effect of the analogs on protein synthesis, and the results obtained are summarized in Table VIII.

TABLE VIII

In Vitro PROTEIN SYNTHESIS AFTER EXPOSURE TO L-GLUTAMINE ANALOGS IN NORMAL AND ASCITES TUMOR CELLS OF RATS[a]

		Incorporation (as % of control) after exposure to:					
		L-Methionine DL-sulfoximine		δ-Hydroxylysine		*O*-Carbamyl-DL-serine	
Tissue	Amino acid	0.002 *M*	0.005 *M*	0.002 *M*	0.005 *M*	0.002 *M*	0.005 *M*
Liver (normal)	L-Isoleucine	92	70	80	84	51	81
Spleen (normal)	L-Isoleucine	91	91	92	93	71	70
	L-Valine	88	86	94	88	87	76
Ehrlich ascites carcinoma cells	L-Isoleucine	57	57	62	62	98	106
	L-Valine	65	60	66	63	103	108
6C3HED	L-Isoleucine	84	88	84	90	119	123
Lymphoma cells	L-Valine	89	90	99	103	104	128

[a] Data of Rabinowitz *et al.* (1959).

The investigators concluded that Ehrlich ascites carcinoma cells (and those of sarcoma S-180, hepatoma 134, and leukemia L4946, which also had significant inhibition of protein synthesis) "carry out a trace synthesis of L-glutamine which . . . determines the incorporation of other amino acids by supplying L-glutamine as the limiting amino acid." The 6C3HED cells, on the other hand, were not affected by L-methionine DL-sulfoximine or HL; they were "markedly stimulated" in their incorporation of L-isoleucine and L-valine into protein by addition of γ-glutamyl hydrazide (GH) to the medium. "The results suggest," they continued, "that these two lymphomas [6C3HED and C3HSX] have a high requirement for L-glutamine and that, in the absence of any synthetic capacity for supplying this amino acid, they incorporated GH (or a metabolic by-product of it) to support their incorporation of the other amino acids." This correlates well with the observation of El-Asmar and Greenberg (see Table I) that the 6C3HED lymphoma has a relatively small amount of L-glutamine synthetase activity.

V. L-Glutaminase

Several investigators have, as previously noted, documented the inability or only slight capacity of various neoplastic cells to synthesize L-glutamine. Greenberg *et al.* (1964) attempted to capitalize on this apparent difference between such cells and normal tissues by administering the enzyme L-glutaminase to rats with a variety of tumors (6C3HED, ascites form; S-180, ascites form; L-4946 leukemia; Ehrlich ascites carcinoma; and CA-755). The enzyme used was isolated from a strain of *Pseudomonas* (GG 13) and contained both L-glutaminase and L-asparaginase activity, with its optimum at pH 6.6 and a range of high activity from pH 5 to 8. One enzyme unit (EU) was defined as the amount of enzyme which catalyzed the liberation of 1 μmole of NH_3 in 15 minutes at 37°C. (One enzyme unit, or IU, of EC-2 asparaginase is defined as that amount necessary to liberate 1 μmole of NH_3 in 1 minute at 37°C.) These investigators succeeded in lowering measurable blood L-glutamine levels to virtually zero in both normal and tumor-bearing mice by the administration of 15 EU on days 1, 3, and 5 after inoculation of the tumor-bearing mice. In the 6C3HED lymphoma, they obtained the following results with respect to effect on tumor growth: 92% (average) tumor growth inhibition in the ascites form with daily dosage at 30 EU for 5 days, intraperitoneally or subcutaneously; and 58% tumor inhibition in the solid form with the same treatment daily for 8 days. In all these groups, blood L-glutamine in treated animals was undetectable. Interestingly, with a lower dose (15 EU) given over a longer period (daily for 12 days), there was 72% tumor growth inhibition although blood L-glutamine was only slightly reduced. In no instance did enzyme administration extend the survival time of tumor-bearing hosts, although the tumor growth was markedly inhibited during treatment in both the 6C3HED tumor and the Ehrlich carcinoma, with about 80% inhibition observed in the latter.

With regard to toxicity of the L-glutaminase preparation, treatment of a group of normal mice with 15 EU daily for 7 days did not result in any deaths over a 3-month period of observation. However, weight gain was inhibited. In regard to the tumor-bearing mice, Greenberg and his co-workers concluded: "It . . . seems improbable that in enzyme-treated mice death is due merely to proliferation of tumor [since marked inhibition of tumor growth did not cause an increased survival time]. Pathologic exam, both gross and microscopic, of the organs and carcasses of treated mice bearing the Gardner [6C3HED] lymphosarcoma showed no changes other than an enlargement and spotting of the liver . . . certain cells of the body may be nearly as sensitive to a deficiency of L-glutamine as are a variety of neoplastic cells."

In a later report, El-Asmar and Greenberg (1966) investigated the mechanism of inhibition of tumor growth by L-glutaminase. They injected two groups of mice with 2×10^6 cells of 6C3HED and 1×10^6 cells of the L1210 leukemia, respectively. One EU of L-glutaminase (at least 50 EU/kg) was injected on days 1, 3, and 5 after tumor implantation. The growth of 6C3HED was 66% inhibited, and that of L1210 about 70%. However, again there was no increase in overall survival time.

Administration of three doses of 1 EU or more of L-glutaminase reduced the L-glutamine content of the blood to an undetectable level. After a single injection of 1 EU, L-glutamine content was zero for the first 24 hours and only 1.75 mg % (112 nmoles/ml) at 48 hours, and it had returned to normal levels by 72 hours.

In the same report, the effect of L-glutaminase on nucleic acid metabolism of tumor cells *in vivo* was determined. Glycine-^{14}C was used to measure *de novo* purine synthesis. The incorporation of glycine was 50 to 60% inhibited in the 6C3HED cells and was 100% inhibited in L1210 cells.

El-Asmar and Greenberg also attempted combination chemotherapy with L-glutaminase and azaserine against the 6C3HED tumor. The results of optimal tested single-drug and optimal tested combination treatment are shown in Table IX.

TABLE IX
COMBINED EFFECT OF L-GLUTAMINASE AND AZASERINE ON THE 6C3HED LYMPHOMA[a,b]

Treatment	Dose schedule	Mean concentration of L-glutamine in blood: Treated (mg/100 ml)	Mean concentration of L-glutamine in blood: Control	% Growth inhibition	Mean survival time (days): Treated	Mean survival time (days): Control
1 EU enzyme	× 3, alternate days	0	5	68	10.5	10.5
Azaserine, 0.2 mg/kg	× 5, daily	7.4	5	67	11.3	10.5
1 EU enzyme + azaserine, 0.2 mg/kg	× 3, alternate days × 5, daily	0	5	95	12.0	10.5

[a] Data of El-Asmar and Greenberg (1966).
[b] No significant increase was seen in lifespan.

Again in these experiments, El-Asmar and Greenberg used an enzyme prepared from *Bacillus coagulans* (*Pseudomonas*); their results may be compared with those of Mashburn and Wriston, who found an L-asparaginase prepared from *Bacillus coagulans* to be ineffective in inhibiting tumor growth (Mashburn and Wriston, 1964).

As noted in the introduction, the L-asparaginase derived from *E. coli* which is active at a physiological pH also has intrinsic L-glutaminase activity. L-Asparaginase derived from guinea pig or agouti serum, on the other hand, lacks such activity. Both EC-2 and the preparations with only L-asparagine-hydrolyzing capacity have marked antitumor activity against a number of animal neoplasms. However, the EC-2 preparation appears to be more active, at least against the 6C3HED tumor, on a basis of equivalent L-asparaginase activity (Boyse *et al.*, 1967). Whether this is due to its additional L-glutaminase activity remains to be proven. Clearly, L-glutaminase deserves further evaluation with regard to possible usefulness as an antineoplastic agent, especially in combination chemotherapy.

VI. Competitive Inhibitors of L-Glutaminyl t-RNA Synthesis

γ-Aminobutyramide

Yellin (1968) has reported on the compound γ-aminobutyramide (GABM) as an inhibitor of protein synthesis in cell suspensions of the Ehrlich ascites cell carcinoma. He used the incorporation of leucine-^{14}C, uridine-^{3}H, and methylthymidine-^{3}H into acid-insoluble material as a measure of protein, RNA, and DNA synthesis, respectively. Increasing concentrations of GABM

TABLE X

GABM Inhibition of Protein Synthesis[a]

Additions	Relative activity (as % of control incorporation of leucine-^{14}C into protein)	P (significance value)
None	100	
GABM (1×10^{-3} M)	52	0.001
GABM (2×10^{-3} M)	42	
GABM (3×10^{-3} M)	38	
GABM (5×10^{-3} M)	32	
GABA[b] (1×10^{-3} M)	108	Not significant
NH_4Cl (1×10^{-3} M)	144	0.001

[a] Data of Yellin (1968).
[b] γ-Aminobutyric acid.

caused a progressive decrease in protein synthesis, as shown in Table X.

The inhibition of protein synthesis by GABM was largely reversed by an extracellular concentration of 0.1 m*M* L-glutamine (a ratio of amino acid to analog of 1:10). Concentrations of L-glutamine greater than this completely prevented the inhibitory effect of GABM.

Yellin pointed out that "the high concentration of GABM necessary to demonstrate inhibition intracellularly is not unreasonable if we allow that the inhibition is probably of the competitive type and that L-glutamine synthesis continues at a normal rate."

While protein synthesis was markedly inhibited, RNA and DNA synthesis remained unaffected for at least 20 minutes under similar conditions.

As shown in Table X, protein synthesis was not inhibited by GABA (γ-aminobutyric acid), a hydrolysis product of GABM, in concentrations as high as 1×10^{-3} *M*. NH_4Cl, on the contrary, stimulated incorporation of leucine. Yellin states, "This effect may be due, in part, to the role of NH_3 as amide nitrogen donor in L-glutamine synthesis. NH_4Cl did not stimulate in cell suspensions to which L-glutamine (0.1 m*M*) had been added."

GABM-induced, L-glutamine-reversed inhibition of protein synthesis of similar degree was obtained also in cell suspensions from the 6C3HED and L1578Y animal tumors. Again quoting Yellin, "the striking fact in each case is that of all the essential factors in Eagle's medium [in which the cells were suspended], L-glutamine alone antagonizes the inhibitory effect of GABM."

The author felt his data suggested that GABM acts by competitively inhibiting the binding of L-glutamine to glutaminyl-t-RNA synthetase. A compound with such activity would be expected to produce similar effects, namely, selective inhibition of protein synthesis without immediately affecting nucleic acid synthesis; in addition, its effects should be reversed by adding L-glutamine. Yellin cited recent evidence that the carboxyl group of an amino acid may not be necessary for binding of an amino acid to its "specific" aminoacyl-t-RNA synthetase. GABM is the decarboxylation product of L-glutamine. In conclusion, he reported that, in preliminary experiments, GABM (10^{-6} to 10^{-4} *M*) inhibited the activation of glutamine-^{14}C but not leucine-^{14}C by the S_{100} enzyme system of *E. coli*: "It is possible that potent, reversible inhibitors of aminoacyl-t-RNA synthetases would be useful against tumors which are deficient in one or more amino acids such as L-glutamine or L-asparagine."

VII. Other Analogs

A. *O*-Carbamyl-L-Serine

O-Carbamyl-L-serine has been mentioned herein as an effective inhibitor of the L-glutamine-dependent form of carbamylphosphate synthetase; its potency against other L-glutamine-dependent enzymes in nucleic acid synthesis appears to be much less than that of DON or azaserine. Rabinowitz *et al.* (1959) determined the effect of *O*-carbamyl-L-serine and of azaserine on incorporation of 2-^{14}C-labeled L-glutamine into protein, using a trace concentration of 2×10^{-5} *M* DL-glutamine in media containing both normal mammalian cells and cells from ascites tumors. Both compounds inhibited the incorporation of L-glutamine into protein of normal tissues, while markedly stimulating such incorporation into the protein of Ehrlich ascites, L4946, and 6C3HED tumor cells. The inhibitors were added at a molar ratio of analog to L-glutamine of 100:1. Table XI summarizes their results.

TABLE XI

DIFFERENTIAL INHIBITION OF L-GLUTAMINE INCORPORATION INTO PROTEINS OF NORMAL AND TUMOR TISSUES[a]

Tissue (*in vitro*)	L-Glutamine incorporation in presence of inhibitor (as % of control): *O*-Carbamyl-DL-serine, 0.002 *M*	Azaserine, 0.001 *M*
Normal		
Spleen, mouse	33	63
Bone marrow, rabbit	31	69
Liver, mouse (tumor)	71	44
Ehrlich ascites carcinoma	130	133
Leukemia L4946	145	140
Lymphoma 6C3HED	198	168

[a] Data of Rabinowitz *et al.* (1959).

The authors concluded that "the striking variation of inhibitions and stimulations . . . can best be explained by inhibition of multiple pathways for L-glutamine utilization." They suggested that in normal tissues the analogs principally blocked incorporation of L-glutamine into protein, while their primary effect in tumors seemed to be blocking the utilization of the trace amount of L-glutamine by other pathways (e.g., nucleic acid synthesis), thus conserving L-glutamine for incorporation into protein. Supporting this was their observation that *O*-carbamyl-L-serine-induced stimulation of L-glutamine incorporation into protein occurred only when the L-glutamine was present in trace concentrations. When equimolar amounts of L-glutamine and *O*-carbamyl-L-serine were incubated with 6C3HED cells, no stimulation occurred. There was, then, no direct stimulation by the inhibitors of L-glutamine incorporation into protein of the tumor cells; the stimulation seen apparently resulted from greater sensitivity of nucleic acid synthesis to their L-glutamine-antagonist effects, and when enough L-glutamine was provided to overcome these effects, protein synthesis was unaffected.

B. γ-Glutamylhydrazide

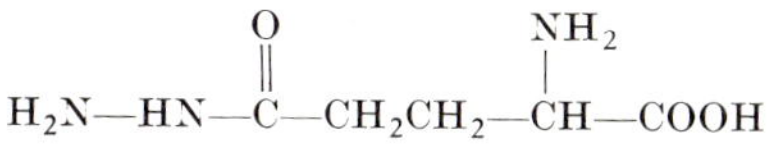

$$H_2N{-}HN{-}\overset{\overset{\displaystyle O}{\|}}{C}{-}CH_2CH_2{-}\overset{\overset{\displaystyle NH_2}{|}}{CH}{-}COOH$$

(X)

γ-Glutamylhydrazide (GH), with the structure shown in (X), is a compound which has been mentioned as a stimulator of protein synthesis in the 6C3HED system, but not in the Ehrlich ascites system. Smulson and Neal (1965) investigated this different effect, confirmed its existence, and showed that labeled GH was incorporated into the primary structure of protein. At the same time, it proved to be a moderately effective inhibitor of incorporation of formate-^{14}C into RNA in both tumor systems. DON was found to be an even more effective stimulator of protein synthesis than GH, with azaserine somewhat less so, and L-glutamine itself the most effective (each at a concentration of 5×10^{-3} M). There was no stimulation by any of the compounds of protein synthesis by the Ehrlich ascites cells, in whom significant L-glutamine synthesis takes place. These observations would also tend to support the hypothesis that enhancement of protein synthesis in L-glutamine-dependent tumor systems by various analogs of L-glutamine is a consequence of sparing of L-glutamine for protein synthesis by the inhibitory action of the analogs on more sensitive amido transfer reactions. Smulson and Neal's demonstration that GH can apparently substitute for L-glutamine in proteins (*in vitro*) also would help explain its stimulating activity. Whether the protein synthesized is biologically functional has not been determined.

VIII. Possible Future Therapeutic Use of Analogs of L-Glutamine

The future therapeutic role of any of these compounds is uncertain. The compounds which have received clinical trials are primarily the diazo group of analogs (DON, azaserine, azotomycin, and duazomycin A). These have not proven effective enough as sole therapy to make any of them the treatment of choice for any type of malignancy. Theoretically, it would seem that an L-glutamine antagonist might be of value in conjunction with L-asparaginase; the results to be presented in this section (Part B) of combination therapy in animal tumors with azaserine plus L-asparaginase and azotomycin plus L-asparaginase support this contention. Clinical trials will be necessary to judge the possible usefulness of either combination; these are under way. Combination therapy with azotomycin, a drug of some effectiveness in at least colon cancer and soft tissue sarcomas, and other agents of established effectiveness like 5-FU, may also prove to be of clinical value.

A number of compounds discussed in this view have received little or no clinical trial, including the inhibitors of L-glutamine synthetase, L-glutaminase, γ-aminobutyramide, and *O*-carbamyl-L-serine. It would seem that at least further preclinical investigation of the mode of action and therapeutic effectiveness of these compounds is warranted, and it would be of special interest to know whether any of these demonstrates synergism with L-asparaginase.

The effectiveness of the compounds discussed herein as inhibitors of L-asparagine synthetase is presented in the last section. L-Asparaginase is an agent of definite clinical usefulness in acute lymphocytic leukemia, whose effectiveness is, however, limited by the rapid development of resistance. Such resistance may be on the basis of development of an efficient system for synthesizing the amino acid, in tumors which were previously deficient in L-asparagine synthetase. A really effective inhibitor of the latter enzyme might thus prevent or delay the development of the resistant state, both enhancing and prolonging remissions induced by L-asparaginase. Clearly the ideal compound has yet to be found, but some of these may be worthy of trial on this basis.

A. Effectiveness of Glutamine Analogs and Related Materials Against Mouse Leukemia L1210

A number of glutamine analogs and related materials have been examined by the Cancer Chemotheraphy National Service Center (CCNSC) for their ability to prolong the lifetime of mice with leukemia L1210. The general experimental design for such testing has been published (Cancer Chemotherapy National Service Center, 1962; Goldin and Venditti, 1970; Venditti and Abbott, 1967) and is described in the legend for Figs. 3 and 4.

The profound influence of the treatment schedule on the effectiveness of azaserine against L1210 is shown by the data summarized in Table XII and Figs. 3 and 4. When the drug was given intraperitoneally (IP), daily treatment or one treatment every second or fourth day produced increases in median survival time over controls of 40–60%. When IP treatment was limited to one injection per treatment day, there was a decrease in activity as the interval (days) between treatments was increased. One treatment on day 1 only or on days 1 and 9 was ineffective. However, IP treatment administered every

TABLE XII

Azaserine (NSC-742). Influence of Treatment Schedule on Antileukemic (L1210) Effectiveness[a]

Treatment route	Treatment schedule	Doses (mg/kg/day)[b] Range	Doses (mg/kg/day)[b] Optimal	% Increase in mean survival time over controls[c]
		(Experiment 01–1647)		
IP	qd; Days 1–9	4.0–3.2	8.0	51
IP	q4d; Days 1,5,9	8.0–64	32	57
IP	E3hr; q4d; Days 1,5,9	16/8–128/8	32/8	74
PO	qd; Days 1–9	8.0–64	32	39
PO	q4d; Days 1,5,9	16–128	32	28
PO	E3hr; q4d; Days 1,5,9	32/8–256/8	128/8	64
		(Experiment 08–2968)		
IP	Once; Day 2	27–135	—	Neg.
IP	qd; Days 2–16	5.3–27	12	60
IP	q2d; Days 2–16	6.2–31	31	56
IP	q4d; Days 2–14	18–94	42	44
IP	E3hr; q4d; Days 2–14	10/8–72/8	32/8	140
		(Experiment 08–3403)[d]		
IP	Once; Day 1	16–128	—	Neg.
IP	E3hr; Day 1	16/8–128/8	128/8	56
IP	qd; Days 1–9	1.0–32	8.0	60
IP	q8d; Days 1,9	8.0–128	—	Neg.
IP	E3hr; q8d; Days 1,9	8.0/8–128/8	128/8	74
IP	q4d; Days, 1,5,9	8.0–64	64	50
IP	E3hr; q4d; Days, 1,5,9	8.0/8–64/8	64/8	160
SC	Once; Day 1	16–128	—	Neg.
SC	qd; Days 1–9	4.0–32	16	56
PO	Once; Day 1	32–256	32	36
PO	qd; Days 1–9	8.0–64	32	42
		(Experiment 08–3550)[d]		
IP	q6d; Days 1,7,13	4.0–128	64	33
IP	E3hr; q6d; Days 1,7,13	4.0/8–128/8	64/8	120
PO	q6d; Days 1,7,13	8.0–128	—	Neg.
PO	E3hr; q6d; Days 1,7,13	8.0/8–128/8	128/8	74
PO	q4d; Days 1,5,9	8.0–128	—	Neg.
PO	E3hr; q4d; Days 1,5,9	8.0/8–128/8	128/8	90

[a] Data obtained from Microbiological Associates, Inc. (Expt. 01–1647) and Southern Research Institute (Expts. 08–2968, 3403, 3550) under contract to CCNSC.

[b] Where more than one injection per day was given, doses are expressed as total daily dose per number of injections per day.

[c] Neg. = increase <25%.

[d] Results of treatment with selected dosage levels are graphically illustrated in Figs. 3 and 4.

AZASERINE (NSC 742) vs L1210 LEUKEMIA
IP TREATMENT SCHEDULE
1/day, Days 1—5
1/day, Days 1—9
1/day, Day 1 only
8/day, Day 1 only
1/day, Days 1,5,9
8/day, Days 1,5,9
1/day, Days 1,9
8/day, Days 1,9
(60)
(60)
(56)
(11)
(160)
(50)
(74)
(20)
Controls
( ) = Maximum increase in survival time over controls, %
Expt. - 08-LE-3403
MEAN SURVIVAL TIME (days)
INCREASE OVER CONTROLS (%)
TOTAL DAILY DOSE (mg/kg)

FIG. 3.

AZASERINE (NSC 742) vs L1210 LEUKEMIA
TREATMENT ROUTE AND SCHEDULE
PO; 1/day, Days 1,5,9
PO; 8/day, Days 1,5,9
PO; 1/day, Days 1,7,13
PO; 8/day, Days 1,7,13
IP; 1/day, Days 1,7,13
IP; 8/day, Days 1,7,13
(90)
(19)
(74)
(20)
(120)
(33)
Controls
( ) = Maximum increase in survival time over controls, %
Expt. - 08-LE - 3550
MEAN SURVIVAL TIME (days)
INCREASE OVER CONTROLS (%)
TOTAL DAILY DOSE (mg/kg)

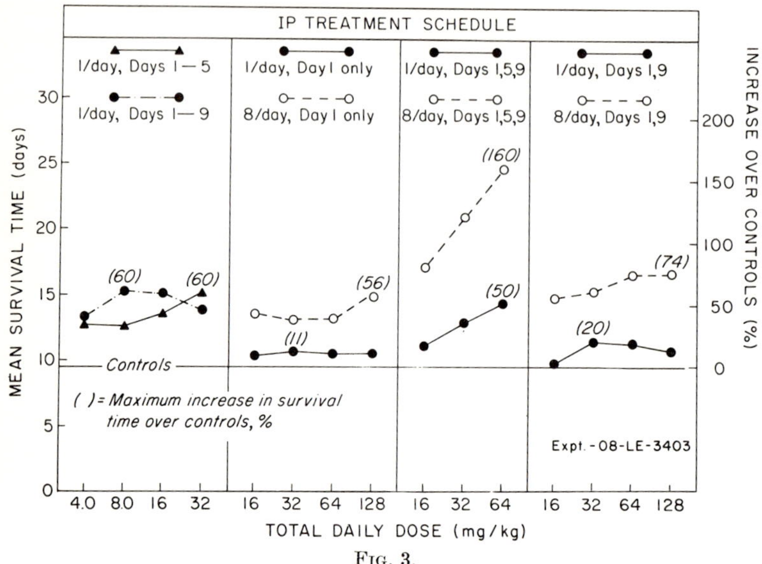

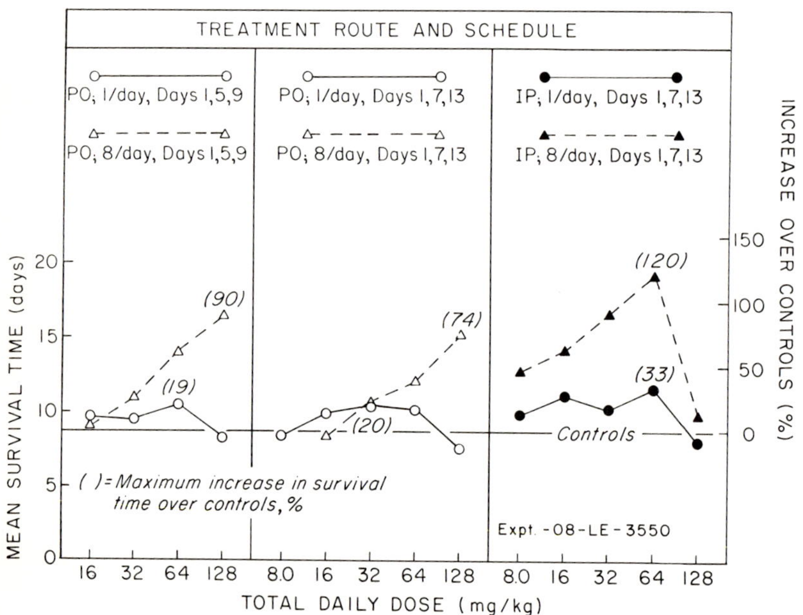

FIG. 4.

3 hours for a 24-hour period on day 1 or on every fourth, sixth, or eighth day, resulted in marked increases in efficacy. For example, in experiment 08-3403 (Fig. 3), IP treatment every 3 hours on day 1 only; days 1,5, and 9; or days 1 and 9 ellicited maximum increases in mean survival time of 56, 160, and 74%, respectively. In general (Table XII), azaserine was most effective when given IP every 3 hours on every fourth day. The advantage of such divided, intermittent therapy with azaserine is illustrated further in experiment 08-3550 (Table XII, Fig. 4) where the total duration of treatment was extended to 13 days. In this case, IP treatment given eight times per day on days 1,7, and 13 was approximately four times more effective than a single treatment on those days. The data summarized in Table XII and Fig. 4 show also that the advantage of divided, intermittent therapy with azaserine was retained when the drug was given orally, although oral treatment was somewhat less effective than IP treatment.

The pattern of schedule dependency against L1210 seen with azaserine contrasts with those observed with duazomycin A (Table XIII), DON (Table XIV), and azotomycin (Table XV). With duazomycin A, single treatments given every fourth or eighth day were about as effective as daily treatment and appeared to be more effective than a single treatment on day 1 only (Table XIII). The data suggest that there was some advantage to divided, intermittent therapy with duazomycin A, but not to the extent observed with azaserine (Table XII). In limited testing, orally administered duazomycin A was moderately effective when given daily and ineffective as a single treatment (Table XIII).

FIGS. 3 and 4. Influence of treatment schedule and route on activity of azaserine against mouse leukemia L1210 (Data of Schabel *et al.*, Southern Research Institute). In each experiment summarized in these figures and in Tables XII–XVII, BDF_1 or CDF_1 mice (18–22 gm) were implanted IP with 10^5 L1210 ascites cells/mouse on Day 0 and distributed 8–10 per group and 30 controls. In the L1210 assay, thereapeutic efficacy is based on the increase in survival time of treated mice over controls. Typically, an effective treatment produces an increase in survival time with increasing dosage until toxicity for the host becomes limiting. Further increase in dosage results in a diminished efficacy. Results of these and other experiments with azaserine are summarized in table XII which lists each route and treatment schedule; the range of doses used, the most effective dose (optimal dose), and the maximum percentage increase in mean survival time over controls achieved. Experiments conducted similarly with duazomycin A, DON, and azotomycin are summarized in Tables XIII–XV, respectively. In the present experiments, there were a number of instances in which the highest dose given was optimal for the leukemic mice. For each therapy regimen, parallel groups of mice without tumor were included. The mean survival times for normal mice are not shown, but the results indicated that there would be no advantage to the treatment of the leukemic mice at still higher doses.

TABLE XIII

DUAZOMYCIN A (NSC-51097). INFLUENCE OF TREATMENT SCHEDULE ON ANTILEUKEMIC (L1210) EFFECTIVENESS[a]

Treatment route and schedule	No. of expts.	Doses (mg/kg/day)[b] Range	Doses (mg/kg/day)[b] Optimal	% Increase in mean survival time over controls[c]
IP–Once; Day 1	2	0.25–16	16	25
IP–E3hr; Day 1	2	0.24/8 –16/8	8.0/8	39
IP–q8d; Days 1,9	2	0.13–16	16	37
IP–E6hr; q8d; Days 1,9	1	2.0/4–16/4	8.0/4	56
IP–E3hr; q8d; Days 1,9	2	0.08/8–16/8	16/8	52
IP–q4d; Days 1,5,9	2	0.13–16	16	54
IP–E6hr; q4d; Days 1,5,9	1	2.0/4–16/4	4.0/4	58
IP–E3hr; q4d; Days 1,5,9	2	0.08/8–16/8	8.0/8	81
IP–qd; Days 1–5	1	1.0–16	1.0	30
IP–qd; Days 1–9	6	0.1–8.0	0.8	50
IP–qd; Days 1–15	1	0.2–1.0	0.6	23
PO–Once; Day 1	1	1.0–8.0	—	Neg.
PO–qd; Days 1–9	1	0.13–1.0	0.50	37

[a] Compiled data obtained from A. D. Little, Inc., Battelle Memorial Institute, and Charles Pfizer and Co., Inc., under contract to CCNSC.

[b] See footnote [b], Table XII.

[c] Neg. = increase <25%.

The extent of schedule dependency of DON against L1210 is unclear from the experiments summarized in Table XIV. In experiments 10-1117–1177, daily IP treatment increased the survival time of the mice by more than 100% and was considerably more effective than a single IP treatment. Treatment IP or orally every second day was as effective as daily IP treatment. In experiments 08-3639 and 3696, IP daily treatment with DON was less effective and there appeared to be a tendency toward greater activity when treatment was given every fourth or eighth day. It is possible that the differences in total duration of daily treatment could account for the observed differences in response in the two studies. However, it is clear that with DON, divided, intermittent treatment failed to provide an "azaserine-like" therapeutic advantage.

With azotomycin, maximum therapeutic efficacy against L1210 was achieved when IP treatments were given on every second or fourth day, and

TABLE XIV

DON (NSC-7365). INFLUENCE OF TREATMENT SCHEDULE ON ANTILEUKEMIC (L1210) EFFECTIVENESS[a]

Treatment route and schedule	Doses (mg/kg/day)[b]		% Increase in mean survival time over controls
	Range	Optimal	
(Expts. 10–1117, 1118, 1135, 1136, 1177)			
IP-qd; Days 1–15	0.05–0.80	0.20,0.40	114
IP-q2d; Days 1–15	1.25–15	5.0	116
PO-q2d; Days 1–15	1.25–20	10	105
IP-Once; Day 2	25–300	150	52
(Expts. 08–3639, 3696)			
IP-Once; Day 1	50–400	100	56
IP-E3hr; Day 1	3.1/8–400/8	12.5/8	38
IP-q8d; Days 1,9	3.1–400	100	68
IP-E3hr; q8d; Days 1,9	3.1/8–25/8	6.2/8	65
IP-q4d; Days 1,5,9	1.56–200	12.5	81
IP-E3hr; q4d; Days 1,5,9	3.1/8–25/8	6.2/8	94
IP-qd; Days 1–9	0.05–0.4	0.1	36
PO-Once; Day 1	100–800	100	47
PO-qd; Days 1–9	0.06–0.8	0.25	64
PO-q2d; Days 1–9	0.2–26	26	87

[a] Data obtained from Charles Pfizer and Co., Inc. (Expts. 10–1117–1177) and Southern Research Institute (Expts. 08–3639, 3696) under contract to CCNSC.
[b] See footnote [b], Table XII.

there was no advantage in dividing the injections on the days of therapy (Table XV). Orally, azotomycin was more effective when given every second day than when given daily or as a single treatment.

Analysis of the influence of treatment schedule on the optimal antileukemic (L1210) dose of azaserine, duazomycin A, DON, and azotomycin (Table XVI) provides a further basis for assessing the degree to which toxicity for the host limited therapeutic efficacy. This, in turn, provides a possible explanation for the observed patterns of schedule dependency against L1210. For azaserine, the maximally tolerated dose (MTD) given once on day 1 was 64 mg/kg and was without antileukemic effectiveness. This dose could be repeated every fourth day for a total of three treatments and under the latter circumstances, it was moderately effective. Widening of the interval between treatments to 8 days resulted in inactivity. Of significance is the observation

TABLE XV

AZOTOMYCIN (NSC-56654). INFLUENCE OF TREATMENT SCHEDULE ON ANTILEUKEMIC (L1210) EFFECTIVENESS[a]

Treatment route and schedule	No. of expts.	Doses (mg/kg/day)[b]		% Increase mean survival time over controls
		Range	Optimal	
IP–Once; Day 1 or 2	9	12.5–500	100–200	40–58
IP–E3hr; Day 1	1	6.2/8–50/8	25/8	41
IP–qd; Days 1–9	5	0.05–2.0	0.07–0.10	37–56
IP–qd; Days 1–15	1	0.09–0.80	0.30	61
IP–qd; Days 1–17	2	0.05–0.50	0.20	57,58
IP–q2d; Days 1–9	1	1.0–8.0	6.0	97
IP–q2d; Days 1–15	1	1.25–10	10	80
IP–q4d; Days 1,5,9	5	7.5–80	15–40	91–109
IP–E12hr; q4d; Days 1,5,9	1	20/2–80/2	40/2	88
IP–E3hr; q4d; Days 1,5,9	1	6.2/8–50/8	6.2/8	93
IP–q7d; Days 1,8	3	10–500	100–150	71–94
PO–Once; Day 1	1	50–400	200	55
PO–qd; Days 1–15	1	0.20–1.0	0.6	37
PO–q2d; Days 1–9	1	1.0–8.0	6.0	104
PO–q2d; Days 1–15	3	1.25–20	5.0–10	98–118
SC–Once; Day 1	1	50–400	100	42
SC–qd; Days 1,9	1	0.05–0.20	0.10	49
SC–qd; Days 1–15	1	0.09–0.30	0.30	56

[a] Compiled data obtained from Microbiological Associates, Inc., Hazleton Laboratories, and Charles Pfizer and Co. under contract to CCNSC.

[b] See footnote [b], Table XII.

that division of the dose per day into eight injections on day 1 only, every fourth day, or every eighth day did not reduce the total amount of drug tolerated compared with the corresponding schedules involving one injection per treatment day. Indeed, when treatment was restricted to day 1 only or days 1 and 8, dividing the doses permitted the administration of a greater total amount of drug before toxicity became limiting. This relative lack of cumulative toxicity with azaserine could possibly explain its remarkable effectiveness when given on the divided, intermittent schedules. In terms of the total amount of drug administered, the optimal daily dose of azaserine (8.0 mg/kg for 9 days) was close to the MTD for a single treatment (64 mg/kg).

TABLE XVI

INFLUENCE OF TREATMENT SCHEDULE ON OPTIMAL ANTILEUKEMIC (L1210) DOSE[a]

IP Treatment schedule	Azaserine, optimal dose (mg/kg)				Duazomycin A, optimal dose (mg/kg)				DON, optimal dose (mg/kg)				Azotomycin, optimal dose (mg/kg)			
	Per dose	Per day	Total D1–9	Max. ILS[b] (%)	Per dose	Per day	Total D1–9	Max. ILS[b] (%)	Per dose	Per day	Total D1–9	Max. ILS[b] (%)	Per dose	Per day	Total D1–9	Max. ILS[b] (%)
Once Day I only	(64)	(64)	(64)	Neg.	16	16	16	25	100	100	100	56	150	150	150	50
E3hr Day 1 only	16	128	128	56	8.0	8.0	8.0	39	1.56	12.5	12.5	38	3.1	25	25	41
Once/day Days 1–9	8.0	8.0	72	60	0.8	0.8	7.2	50	0.1	0.1	0.9	36	0.1	0.1	0.9	50
q4d Days 1,5,9	64	64	192	50	16	16	48	54	12.5	12.5	37.5	81	30	30	90	100
E3hr; q4d Days 1,5,9	8.0	64	192	160	1.0	8.0	24	81	0.78	6.2	18.6	94	0.78	6.2	18.6	93
q8d Days 1,9	(64)	(64)	(128)	Neg.	16	16	32	37	100	100	200	68	100[c]	100[c]	200[c]	83[c]
E3hr; q8d Days 1,9	16	128	256	74	2.0	16	32	56	0.78	6.2	18.6	65	—	—	—	—

[a] Where more than one test was conducted using a treatment schedule, the doses and activities shown were selected on the basis of reproducibility among tests or represent the average values from a number of tests. Since doses higher than the optimal dose were less effective because of toxicity, the optimal dose is regarded as approximating the maximally tolerated dose in leukemic mice. Where therapy was ineffective (Neg.), the highest nonlethal dose (LD_{10} or less) in normal mice is shown in parentheses.

[b] The maximum increase in mean survival time over controls.

[c] Treatment schedule: q7d; Days 1,8.

Duazomycin A, DON, and azotomycin, in sharp contrast to azaserine, exhibited very low optimal daily doses relative to the dose tolerated as a single treatment or on intermittent treatment schedules. The marked difference in the MTD of azotomycin given daily compared with a single treatment or treatments spaced 2 or 3 days apart have been previously reported (Venditti and Abbott, 1967). Also with duazomycin A, DON, and azotomycin, multiple injections on day 1 only or on every fourth or eighth day resulted in a decrease in the total amount of tolerated drug relative to the amount tolerated when the mice were given one injection per treatment day.

The data indicate that, in the L1210 assay, the optimal conditions for usage of duazomycin A, DON, and azotomycin contrast sharply to those for azaserine, and suggest that caution be used in planning protocols for toxicological or clinical evaluation of these drugs on the basis of experiences with azaserine. Despite evidence suggesting similar biochemical sites of action for

TABLE XVII

Activity of Miscellaneous Glutamine Analogs and Inhibitors of L-Glutamine Synthetase Against Leukemia L1210[a]

NSC No.	Name	Treatment route and schedule	Dose or dose range tested (mg/kg/day)	% Increase in mean survival time over controls[b]
132938	D-Hydroxy-L-lysine	IP–Once; Day 1	400	Neg.
		IP–qd; Days 1–9	400	Neg.
128373	*O*-Carbamyl-L-serine	IP–Once; Day 1	400	Neg.
		IP–qd; Days 1–9	400	Neg.
7786	Glutamylhydrazine	IP–qd; Day 1–death	34–86	Neg.
			(100 mg/kg/day, lethal)	
7891	DL-Asparagine	IP–qd; Day 1–death	500	Neg.
82391	L-Asparagine	IP–Once; Day 1	100–400	Neg.
		IP–qd; Days 1–15	400	Neg.
117613	DONV	IP–Once; Day 1	50–400	Neg.
		IP–qd; Days 1–9	400	29
53397	Duazomycin C	IP–qd; Day 1–death	0.5	50

[a] CCNSC Screening Data.

[b] Neg. = increase <25%.

azaserine and these related agents, they elicit distinctly different responses *in vivo* with respect to the influence of treatment schedule on antileukemic activity and toxicity.

CCNSC screening results with a series of other glutamine analogs and inhibitors of L-glutamine synthetase against L1210 are summarized in Table XVII. Of these, only duazomycin C provided important increases in the mean survival time of the mice.

B. Combination Chemotherapy of Mouse Leukemias L1210 and L5178Y Using Glutamine Analogs and L-Asparaginase

The role of glutamine analogs as inhibitors of glutamine utilization was discusssed earlier in this chapter. Historically, most workers have pointed to the inhibition of glutamine utilization of nucleic acid biosynthesis as a likely mechanism leading to antitumor specificity. More recently, the role of L-glutamine as a precursor in L-asparagine biosynthesis has received considerable attention (Adamson and Fabro, 1968; Horowitz *et al.*, 1968; Prager and Bachynsky, 1968). A number of studies (Adamson and Fabro, 1968; Jacobs *et al.*, 1969a,b; Haskell and Canellos, 1969) have shown that tumors with low asparagine synthetase activity generally require an extracellular source of L-asparagine and are sensitive to L-asparaginase treatment (e.g., leukemia L5178Y). In contrast, tumors with relatively high levels of asparagine synthetase activity are generally not dependent on circulating L-asparagine and are insensitive to L-asparaginase (e.g., leukemia L1210).

In studies of the effectiveness of combination chemotherapy against L1578Y, Jacobs *et al.* (1969a,b; and personal communication) confirmed the activity of L-asparaginase alone and found that azaserine or azotomycin alone were about as effective against L5178Y as against L1210; they showed that combinations of L-asparaginase plus azaserine or azotomycin provided a therapeutic effect that was markedly superior to that produced by the individual drugs. It would appear from these studies that depletion of circulating L-asparagine by the dual process of inhibiting a precursor for its extracellular synthesis and enhancing its deamidation can lead to a synergistic response against a tumor with little or no asparagine synthetase activity. It is also possible that the synergistic action of glutamine analogs and L-asparaginase against L5178Y resulted from L-asparagine depletion and concurrent block of *de novo* purine biosynthesis.

Combination chemotherapy of L1210 with azaserine or azotomycin plus L-asparaginase failed to provide a therapeutic effect greater than that achieved with azaserine or azotomycin alone, and L-asparaginase alone was ineffective (Jacobs *et al.*, 1969a,b; and personal communication). The failure of L-asparaginase to provide a therapeutic advantage when combined with azaserine or azotomycin against L1210 suggests that any inhibition of glutamine utilization for L-asparagine biosynthesis intracellularly or extracellularly was insufficient to create dependence on circulating L-asparagine.

IX. Glutamine Analogs and Other Compounds as Inhibitors of L-Asparagine Synthetase

Since L-asparagine is the next lower homolog of L-glutamine, analogs of the latter amino acid are, by definition, analogs of the former. On this basis and despite the consistently different chemical properties of the two amino acids (Steward and Thompson, 1952), it was felt worthwhile to reexamine, in enzymatic systems having L-asparagine as their principal substrate or product, the analogs and antagonists of L-glutamine whose biological activity has been recapitulated in the preceding sections of this paper.

The Gardner lymphosarcoma resistant to L-asparaginase has been used as the source of the crude L-asparagine synthetase examined in these studies; L-asparagine α-ketoacid transaminase, and murine L-asparaginase were studied in extracts of mouse liver. Bacterial L-asparaginase was a clinical formulation of EC-2, purified by Merck to a specific activity of 340 IU/mg of protein. Other details of the methods and materials used are given in the legends to the appropriate tables.

A. Analogs and Antagonists of L-Glutamine as Inhibitors of L-Asparaginase from *E. coli* (EC-2)

1. *Amido Hydrolysis of L-Asparagine*

In Table XVIII the interaction of analogs and antagonists of L-glutamine with L-asparaginase, EC-2, is described.

Out of the panel of 13 candidate compounds, two inhibitors emerged: DONV and carbamyl-L-serine. DONV at a concentration of 2×10^{-3} *M* proved to be a moderate inhibitor, yielding 50–82% inhibition depending on the concentration of L-asparagine. That the inhibitory effect of DONV, a known titrant of the active site of EC-2 is not total, may be explained by the observations of Handschumacher *et al.* (1968) and Jackson *et al.* (1969) that L-asparaginase from *E. coli* catalytically decomposes DONV to gaseous nitrogen and 5-hydroxy-4-oxonorvaline (HONV). If the enzyme is preincubated with the diazo-ketone in the absence of its natural substrate, more efficient alkylation transpires and stronger inhibition results (Handschumacher *et al.*, 1967). Aqueous environments also appear to favor hydrolysis of DONV by L-asparaginase; conversely, when the ordinary high molarity of water is lowered, as, for example, in 50% aqueous DMSO, DONV becomes a far more

TABLE XVIII

INTERACTION OF ANALOGS AND ANTAGONISTS OF L-GLUTAMINE WITH L-ASPARAGINASE (EC-2)[a]

$$\text{L-asparagine or L-glutamine} \xrightarrow{\text{EC-2}} \text{L-aspartic acid} + NH_3 \text{ or L-glutamic acid} + NH_3 \quad (26)$$

Inhibitor (2×10^{-3} *M*)	NSC No.	% Inhibition, L-glutamine at: 1×10^{-3} *M*	% Inhibition, L-glutamine at: 1×10^{-4} *M*	% Inhibition, L-asparagine at: 1×10^{-3} *M*	% Inhibition, L-asparagine at: 1×10^{-4} *M*
Control		—	—	—	—
Serine, diazoacetate (ester), L- (azaserine)	742	0	0	0	0
Norleucine, 6-diazo-5-oxo-, L- (DON)	7,365	0	0	0	0
Glutamine, *N*-{1-[(1-carboxy-5-diazo-4-oxopentyl) carbamyl]-5-diazo-4-oxopentyl}-, sodium salt (azotomycin)	56,654	0	0	0	0
Norleucine, *N*-acetyl-6-diazo-5-oxo, L- (duazomycin A)	51,097	0	0	0	0
Norvaline, 5-diazo-4-oxo-, L- (DONV)	117,613	50	90	50	82
Sulfoximine, *S*-(L-3-amino-3-carboxypropyl) *S*-methyl- (L-methionine-DL-sulfoximine)		0	0	0	0
Lysine, 5-hydroxy-, monohydrochloride, DL- *allo*-(+)- (δ-OH-lysine	132,938	0	0	0	0
Butyramide, 4-amino- (γ-aminobutyramide)		0	0	0	0
Serine, carbamate (ester), L- (carbamyl-L-serine)	128,373	40	56	20	56
Glutaminic acid, 5-hydrazide, L- (γ-glutamylhydrazide)	7,786	0	0	0	0
Levulinic acid, 2-amino-5-chlorohydrochloride, L- (CONV)	124,412	27	50	20	64

[a] Inhibitors were dissolved in deionized water and neutralized. The substrates, L-asparagine and L-glutamine, were prepared at the requisite concentrations in 0.1 *M* Tris pH 8.0. With L-asparagine, 0.02 IU of enzyme was added to 5 ml of substrate solution; after 30 minutes at 37°C, any L-aspartic acid produced was measured spectrophotometrically in a coupled enzymatic assay utilizing glutamic oxalacetic transaminase and malic dehydrogenase (Cooney and Handschumacher, 1968). With L-glutamine, 20 IU of enzyme was added to 5 ml of substrate solution; after 30 minutes at 37°C, ammonia was measured enzymatically as follows: to an appropriate aliquot of the reaction mixture were added 200 nmoles of DPNH in 50 μliter of 0.04 *M* Tris; and 50 μliter of commercial L-glutamic dehydrogenase in glycerin. After 10 minutes of incubation at room temperature *A* was measured at 340 nm; 600 nmoles of α-ketoglutaric acid were added in 10 μliters of water and the $-\Delta A$ measured 15 minutes later. Then 20 nmoles of NH_4Cl were added in 10 μliters of H_2O and a second $-\Delta A$ recorded. The addition of NH_4Cl served to check the viability of the assay system in the presence of inhibitors. All reactions with L-asparagine were terminated by immersion of the glass reaction vessels in a bath of boiling water for 15 minutes. All reactions with L-glutamine were terminated with PCA which was then neutralized with KOH. The percent inhibition of the hydrolysis of L-glutamine by DONV is a minimal value inasmuch as significant enzymatic decomposition of the diazoketone certainly took place during these incubations.

efficient inhibitor, inasmuch as its catalytic decomposition by the target enzyme L-asparaginase is strongly curtailed (Jackson *et al.*, 1969).

Carbamyl-L-serine also inhibited amido hydrolysis by EC-2, yielding 20% inhibition when the molar concentration of L-asparagine was 1×10^{-3} *M*, and 56% inhibition when the concentration of L-asparagine was lowered to 1×10^{-4} *M*. These data are suggestive of a competitive inhibiton.

2. *Amido hydrolysis of* L-*glutamine*

In keeping with the consensus that hydrolysis of both L-asparagine and L-glutamine is accomplished on one and the same active site of EC-2 (Campbell and Mashburn, 1969) are the present experimental results showing that both DONV and carbamyl-L-serine inhibit the activities toward both amino acids to a roughly comparable degree (Table XVIII). While it was observed that carbamyl-L-serine was more inhibitory to the L-glutamine amido hydrolase activity than to the L-asparagine amido hydrolase activity of EC-2, the magnitude of this differential effect was not great. Moreover, of the other 13 candidate compounds studied, no agent was found which selectively repressed the hydrolysis of only one of the two major substrates of L-asparaginase from *E. coli*.

TABLE XIX

LACK OF INHIBITION BY DON OF THE L-GLUTAMINASE ACTIVITY OF L-ASPARAGINASE (EC-2) AT pH 5.0[a]

Concentration of L-glutamine	Concentration of DON	L-Asparaginase added (IU)	NH_3 generated (μmoles/min)
1×10^{-2} *M*	0	100	0.5182 ± 0.02
1×10^{-2} *M*	1×10^{-3} *M*	100	0.4852 ± 0.02

[a] To 10 ml of 0.01 *M* L-glutamine in 0.1 *M* acetate buffer was added 100 IU of L-asparaginase in 50 μliters of H_2O; in the case of the blank, 50 μliters of water only was added. DON was prepared in ice-cold distilled water and the iced solution brought to pH 5 immediately before its addition to the reaction vessel. (Spectrophotometric monitoring did reveal a very slow acid hydrolysis of the diazo function. No molar corrections have been made for this decomposition inasmuch as >95% of the inhibitor was intact after 1 hour at 37°C. Moreover, L-asparaginase did not catalyze any detectable hydrolysis of the diazo group of DON at pH 5.) After 1 hour at 37°C, the capped glass reaction vessels were immersed in a bath of boiling water for 10 minutes. Ammonia was measured enzymatically. The low final concentration of DON was noninhibitory in this spectrophotometric assay which uses L-glutamic dehydrogenase to aminate α-ketoglutaric acid reductively in the presence of ammonia (cf. Table XVIII).

Miller and Balis (1969) have demonstrated that DON, a powerful inhibitor of the L-glutaminase from *E. coli* (pH optimum ~ 5.0), only marginally depressed L-glutaminase activity of L-asparaginase (EC-2) from *E. coli*. These authors used a concentration of about 3 m*M*. In the present experiments with somewhat lower concentrations of DON no inhibition was detectable. It is possible that, at the markedly different pH optima of these two enzymes, the inhibitors themselves exist in a sufficiently distinct ionic configuration, that a molecule which is strongly inhibitory at pH 5 (such as DON versus L-glutaminase from *E. coli*) could become ineffective at pH 8 (such as DON versus L-asparaginase from *E. coli*). In order to explore this possibility, the inhibition of EC-2 by DON was studied at pH 5.0 (Table XIX). At this hydrogen-ion concentration, coliform L-asparaginase exhibits ~80% of its maximal activity toward L-asparagine, but only ~16% of its activity toward L-glutamine. Despite the shift of pH, no significant inhibition of the amido hydrolysis of L-glutamine by EC-2 could be detected.

Because clinical toxicity due to coliform L-asparaginase is not uncommon and because inhibitors of the enzyme may be able to function as antidotes to this toxicity, the search for antagonists to EC-2 ought to continue. Nevertheless, the present results would suggest that the most fruitful field for that search is probably not among the five-carbon (L-glutamine-like) compounds.

B. Analogs and Antagonists of L-Glutamine as Inhibitors of L-Asparaginase from Mouse Liver

While their catalytic roles are isologous, the L-asparaginases of mammalian and bacterial origins are distinct enzymes with distinctive properties. The former enzyme is thermolabile (Errera and Greenstein, 1947), often stereospecific, and largely restricted to the hydrolysis of four-carbon dicarboxylic acids bearing ω-nitrogen functions; the latter enzymes can be remarkably thermostable (as is EC-2) (Whelan and Wriston, 1969; Cooney and Davis, 1970), nonstereospecific, and capable of hydrolyzing L-glutamine with fair, moderate, or excellent catalytic efficiency. Thus, under saturating conditions L-asparaginase from *E. coli*, *E. carotovora*, and a *Pseudomonas* species hydrolyze L-glutamine at about 3% (Campbell and Mashburn, 1969), 10%, and 90% (Ramadan and Greenberg, 1963), respectively, the rate of their hydrolysis of L-asparagine. With such individuating notes in mind, and despite the generally negative effects found when the analogs of L-glutamine were studied as inhibitors of L-asparaginase from *E. coli*, crude L-asparaginase from mouse liver was assayed in the presence and absence of the analogs and antagonists of L-glutamine.

Azaserine, one of the most generally effective antagonists of L-glutamine significantly inhibited the murine hepatic L-asparaginase. This finding is superficially surprising because most mammalian L-asparagine amido hydrolases will not attack L-glutamine; it is therefore unlikely that L-glutamine gains access to their active site. In keeping with such a suggestion is the finding that L-glutamine itself does not materially inhibit the L-asparagine amido hydrolase of mouse liver (Table XX). Because, however, azaserine is capable

TABLE XX

INTERACTION OF ANALOGS AND ANTAGONISTS OF L-GLUTAMINE WITH L-ASPARAGINASE OF MOUSE LIVER[a]

$$\text{L-Asparagine} \xrightarrow{\text{L-asparaginase}} \text{L-aspartic acid} + NH_3 \qquad (27)$$

Inhibitor	NSC No.	L-Asparagine hydrolyzed 37°C (nm/gm wet wt/min)	Percent of control
None		455	—
Serine, diazoacetate (ester), L- (azaserine)	742	350	77
Norleucine, 6-diazo-5-oxo-, L- (DON)	7,365	520	114
Glutamine, *N*-{1-[(1-carboxy-5-diazo-4-oxopentyl)carbamyl]-5-diazo-4-oxopentyl}-, sodium salt (azotomycin)	56,654	660	145
Norleucine, *N*-acetyl-6-diazo-5-oxo-, L- (duazomycin A)	51,097	514	113
Norvaline, 5-diazo-4-oxo-, L- (DONV)	117,613	388	85
Sulfoximine, *S*-(L-3-amino-3-carboxypropyl)-*S*-methyl- (L-methionine-DL-sulfoximine)		493	108
Lysine, 5-hydroxy-, monohydrochloride, DL-*allo*-(+)- (δ-OH-lysine)	132,938	368	81
Butyramide, 4-amino- (γ-aminobutyramide)		418	92
Serine, carbamate (ester), L- (carbamyl-L-serine)	128,373	436	96
Glutamic acid, 5-hydrazide, L- (γ-glutamylhydrazide)	7,786	375	82
Levulinic acid, 2-amino-5-chlorohydrochloride, L- (CONV)	124,412	174	38
L-Glutamine		455	100

[a] Mouse liver was homogenized with 0.1 *M* Tris, pH 8.0, and centrifuged at 17,000 *g* for 20 minutes at 4°C. The supernatant was dialyzed against 4 liters of 0.05 *M* Tris, pH 8.0, and the dialysate used as such. For the measurement of L-asperaginase, each reaction vessel contained, in a net volume of 550 μliters, 500 μliters of dialyzed liver, 10 μmoles of L-asparagine, and, where indicated, inhibitor at 8×10^{-3} *M*. After 30 minutes at 37°C, the reaction was terminated with heat, and L-aspartic acid was measured in 100-μliter aliquots of the centrifuged reaction mixture, by an enzymatic, spectrophotometric technique (Cooney and Handschumacher, 1968).

of alkylating sulfhydryl groups (Section III, A, 1), quite possibly the agent is inhibiting hepatic L-asparaginase, a sulfhydryl enzyme, by nonspecifically alkylating some essential sulfhydryl function. To explore this hypothesis, the inhibitory action of *N*-ethyl maleimide was studied. This sulfhydryl reagent virtually abolished the action of hepatic L-asparaginase when used at concentrations above 5×10^{-4} *M*.

γ-Glutamylhydrazide also inhibited murine L-asparaginase to a moderate degree. Because this hydrazide bears a strong resemblance to L-glutamine, but is even bulkier at the site of hydrolysis, it is not easy to suppose that it can enter the catalytic site on L-asparaginase when L-glutamine is probably unable to do so. Nevertheless, as Gass and Meister (1970) have abundantly demonstrated in the case of L-glutamine synthetase, seemingly small substitutions can confer substrate potential on otherwise inert analogs. Similarly, in the present situation, the hydrazino grouping may so alter topography as to permit γ-glutamylhydrazide to behave as an inhibitor.

DONV, and to a far greater degree CONV, inhibited the hydrolysis of L-asparagine by hepatic L-asparaginase. While high concentrations only were used, this finding nevertheless confirms the role of these agents as reactive analogs of L-asparagine.

One paradox emerged from these studies with murine L-asparaginase: Azotomycin stimulated, rather than inhibited, the enzyme. This effect was repeatedly observed in liver extracts of Swiss as well as BALB/c mice. Azotomycin itself did not stimulate the synthesis of L-aspartic acid, the product of amido hydrolysis which was measured in these studies; only in the presence of L-asparagine was the effect demonstrable. However, while the stimulation was most often modest (~145%, as shown in Table XX), in some preparations 200% stimulation of L-asparaginase was observed. DON and *N*-acetyl-DON also consistently yielded marginal stimulation. Whether the greater stimulative potency of azotomycin derives from the fact that each mole of it bears two diazo functions for every one such function on DON or *N*-acetyl-DON, is a matter of conjecture. It is also possible that the labile diazo functions of DON and *N*-acetyl-DON are susceptible to enzymatic cleavage while those of azotomycin—a bulky tripeptide—are more resistant to such cleavage and thus available for stimulation of the enzyme.

C. Analogs and Antagonists of L-Glutamine as Inhibitors of L-asparaginase from Agouti Serum

The L-asparaginase which circulates in the bloodstream of rodents from the superfamily Caviodea probably arises in the liver. The same general pattern of inhibition which was seen when the antagonists of L-glutamine were incubated with murine hepatic L-asparaginase might, accordingly, have been anticipated when a similar series of incubations were undertaken with the agouti enzyme. Nevertheless, the experiments were carried out for the following reasons. Most of the L-asparagine-utilizing enzymes of liver are absent from serum; inhibitory effects, when seen with the L-asparaginase of serum are therefore susceptible of more straightforward interpretation. Also, the agouti is sufficiently removed from the mouse phylogenetically that interesting variations of the structure and function of homologous enzymes are likely. The results of this study are given in Table XXI. Of the agents studied, DONV was clearly the most powerful inhibitor of amido hydrolysis, significantly more powerful in this system, in fact, than CONV. This order of efficacy is the reverse of that seen with L-asparaginase of liver, toward which CONV was a stronger inhibitor than DONV. γ-Aminobutyramide, which is an α-decarboxylated glutamine, exerted a minimal inhibitory action on the agouti enzyme comparable in magnitude to its effect on the hepatic hydrolase. At a concentration of 2×10^{-3} M, the other agents of the panel of candidate inhibitors examined were without influence on the L-asparaginase of agouti serum. Thus, both L-glutamine and the diazo compounds, azotomycin, DON, and duazomycin A, failed to stimulate or inhibit amido hydrolysis. However, when the molarity of these analogs was raised to 8×10^{-3} M, azotomycin did marginally accelerate the hydrolysis of L-asparagine to 110% of controls. Even at this higher molarity, L-glutamine produced no inhibitory effects on the agouti L-asparaginase, a finding which suggests that this amino acid cannot enter the active site of the enzyme.

D. Analogs and Antagonists of L-Glutamine as Inhibitors of L-Asparagine Transaminase of Mouse Liver

The interaction of the analogs of L-glutamine with the L-asparagine α-ketoacid transaminase of murine liver was also explored. Dialyzed supernatants of homogenized mouse liver furnished the enzyme for these experiments. L-Asparagine transaminase, a little-studied enzyme, is of interest for several reasons. It is known to be capable of catalyzing the synthesis of L-asparagine from α-ketosuccinamic acid and an amido donor (Meister, 1953) provided only that α-ketosuccinamic acid is present in high enough (but probably nonphysiological) concentrations to drive the reaction to the left or that L-asparagine is drained off rapidly. Efflux into plasma could provide such a drain. When the meagre synthetic rate of mouse liver L-asparagine synthetase (~10–100 μmoles/gm wet weight/hr) is contrasted with the rapid rate of L-asparagine transaminase from the same source (~12 μmoles/gm wet weight/hr), the potential importance of this transaminase is emphasized. Several agents of those studied yielded significant inhibition of the enzyme

TABLE XXI

INTERACTION OF ANALOGS AND ANTAGONISTS OF L-GLUTAMINE WITH THE L-ASPARAGINASE OF AGOUTI SERUM[a]

$$\text{L-Asparagine} \xrightarrow{\text{L-asparaginase}} \text{L-aspartic acid} + NH_3 \qquad (28)$$

Inhibitor	NSC No.	% Inhibition, L-asparagine at: $1 \times 10^{-3}\ M$	$1 \times 10^{-4}\ M$
Serine, diazoacetate (ester), L- (azaserine)	742	0	0
Norleucine, 6-diazo-5-oxo-, L- (DON)	7,365	0	0
Glutamine, *N*-{1-[(1-carboxy-5-diazo-4-oxopentyl) carbamyl]-5-diazo-4-oxopentyl}-, sodium salt (azotomycin)	56,564	0	0
Norleucine, *N*-acetyl-6-diazo-5-oxo-, L- (duazomycin A)	51,097	0	0
Norvaline, 5-diazo-4-oxo-, L- (DONV)	117,613	74	78
Sulfoximine, *S*-(L-3-amino-3-carboxypropyl)-*S*-methyl- (L-methionine-DL-sulfoximine)	—	0	0
Lysine, 5-hydroxy-, monohydrochloride, DL-*allo*-(+)- (δ-OH-lysine)	132,938	7	10
Butyramide, 4-amino- (γ-aminobutyramide)	—	0	0
Serine, carbamate (ester), L- (Carbamyl-L-serine)	128,373	0	0
Glutamic acid, 5-hydrazide, L- (γ-glutamylhydrazide)	7,786	60	33
Levulinic acid, 2-amino-5-chlorohydrochloride, L- (CONV)	124,412	37	44
L-Glutamine	—	0	0

[a] Agouti serum (10 IU/ml) was procured by cardiac puncture and kindly provided by Dr. Florence White, NCI, NIH. L-Asparagine, $1 \times 10^{-3}\ M$, and $1 \times 10^{-4}\ M$ was prepared in 0.05 *M* Tris, pH 8.2. Five-ml aliquots of substrate were dispensed, in duplicate, into screw-capped glass tubes. Inhibitors were added to a final concentration of $2 \times 10^{-3} M$. At timed intervals of 0.1 IU of agouti enzyme was added to the paired reaction vessels. After 30 minutes at 37°C, the tubes were immersed in a bath of boiling water for 10 minutes, and cooled. Any L-aspartic acid released by the hydrolysis of L-asparagine was quantitated, by an enzymatic spectrophotometric method in 1-ml aliquots of the reaction mixture. CONV and γ-glutamylhydrazide materially retarded the velocity of the coupling enzymes used in this assay; however, quantitative measurements were possible by doubling the reaction time.

(Table XXII). Azaserine and CONV reduced the reaction rate more than 75%; carbamyl-L-serine virtually abolished transamination of pyruvic acid and L-asparagine.

Several ancillary observations of interest emerged from these studies. Azaserine itself was found to stimulate the production of L-alanine in the

TABLE XXII

INTERACTION OF ANALOGS AND ANTAGONISTS OF L-GLUTAMINE WITH L-ASPARAGINE TRANSAMINASE FROM MOUSE LIVER[a]

L-Asparagine + pyruvic acid ⟶ α-ketosuccinamic + alanine (29)

Inhibitor	NSC No.	L-Asparagine transaminated at 37°C (mean nm/gm wet wt/min)
None (control)		200
Serine, diazoacetate (ester), L- (azaserine)	742	60
Norleucine, 6-diazo-5-oxo-, L- (DON)	7,365	200
Glutamine, *N*-{1-[(1-carboxy-5-diazo-4-oxopentyl)carbamyl]-5-diazo-4-oxopentyl}-, sodium salt (azotomycin)	56,654	170
Norleucine, *N*-acetyl-6-diazo-5-oxo-, L- (duazomycin A)	51,907	200
Norvaline, 5-diazo-4-oxo-, L- (DONV)	117,613	190
Sulfoximine, *S*-(L-3-amino-3-carboxypropyl)-*S*-methyl- (L-methionine-DL-sulfoximine)	—	190
Lysine, 5-hydroxy-, monohydrochloride, DL-*allo*-(+)- (δ-OH-lysine)	132,938	170
Butyramide, 4-amino- (γ-aminobutyramide)	—	200
Serine, carbamate (ester), L- (carbamyl-L-serine)	128,373	25
Glutamic acid, 5-hydrazide, L- (γ-glutamylhydrazide)	7,786	160
Levulinic acid, 2-amino-5-chlorohydrochloride, L- (CONV)	124,412	60
L-Glutamine		200

[a] Mouse liver was homogenized with 3 volumes of iced 0.05 *M* Tris buffer, pH 8.0. The homogenate was centrifuged at 17,000 *g* for 20 minutes at 4°C, and the resulting supernatant was dialyzed against 4 liters of 0.05 *M* Tris, pH 8.0; a 10% dilution of homogenate took place during dialysis. For the measurement of L-asparagine transaminase, in a net reaction volume of 650 μliters were admixed: 500 μliters of dialyzed liver supernatant, 10 μmoles of L-asparagine, and 10 μmoles of pyruvic acid, both of the latter two compounds brought to neutrality before addition. Inhibitors were dissolved in water, neutralized, and used immediately at a concentration of 8×10^{-3} *M*. After 30 minutes at 37°C, the reaction vessels were heated at 95°C for 20 minutes and centrifuged at 12,000 rpm for 3 minutes. Ten μliters of 30% H_2O_2 was added to decarboxylate pyruvic acid quantitatively. After an additional 1 hour at 37°C, the H_2O_2 was decomposed with 10 μliters of crystalline catalase. Twenty minutes after all effervescence ceased, the concentration of L-alanine in 20-μliter aliquots of supernatant fluid was measured spectrophotometrically as follows: in a net volume of 1.1 ml, in individual glass cuvettes were admixed 200 nmoles of DPNH, 1 μmole of α-ketoglutaric acid, 50 μmoles of Tris, pH 7.4, and one IU of lactic dehydrogenase. Ten minutes after admixture of the ingredients, *A* at 340 was recorded. Twenty μliters of glutamic pyruvic transaminase (Boehringer) were added, and the cuvettes incubated at 37°C for 45 minutes. At this time $-\Delta A$ was complete, *A* was recorded again

presence of L-asparagine and in the absence of pyruvate. Thus, at 37°C, 100 nmoles of L-alanine were generated per minute per gram wet weight of liver when azaserine was incubated together with L-asparagine and the crude enzyme. Very likely the following conjoint reactions are producing this effect:

$$\text{Azaserine} \xrightarrow[\text{dehydratase}]{\text{serine}} \text{pyruvate} + \text{ammonia} + \text{diazo compound X}$$

$$\text{Pyruvate} + \text{L-asparagine} \xrightarrow[\text{transaminase}]{\text{L-asparagine}} \text{L-alanine} + \alpha\text{-ketosuccinamic acid} \quad (30)$$

Under the conditions of these measurements, azotomycin also stimulated the production of L-alanine, but only in the presence of pyruvate. Thus 1.5 μmoles of L-alanine were generated per minute per gram wet weight of liver when azotomycin and pyruvic acid were incubated together. It is very likely that azotomycin was entering into transamination with pyruvic acid. On the other hand, it is possible that ammoniagenesis in the thoroughly dialyzed extracts of liver used in these studies along with traces of DPNH provided enough ammonia and coenzyme for the reaction:

$$\text{Pyruvic acid} + \text{DPNH} + NH_3 \xrightarrow{\text{L-glutamic dehydrogenase}} \text{L-alanine} + \text{DPN} + H_2O \quad (31)$$

This sequence of events seems unlikely for the following two reasons: The reductive amination of pyruvate in the presence of low concentrations of ammonia is an exceedingly sluggish reaction, and azotomycin was found to inhibit, *not stimulate* the reductive amination of pyruvate, by purified bovine L-glutamic dehydrogenase.

DON, L-methionine-DL-sulfoximine and γ-glutamylhydrazide all stimulated the generation of L-alanine to a minor degree (61, 54, and 21 nmoles, respectively, of L-alanine/gm wet weight/minute at 37°C were the rates observed). Whether these small effects stem from transamination or reductive amination of pyruvate is not known.

E. The Interaction of Analogs and Antagonists of L-Glutamine with L-Asparagine Synthetase

Because L-asparagine synthetase can utilize both L-glutamine and ammonia in the synthesis of the amido group of L-asparagine, it might be anticipated

---

and the net $-\Delta A$ calculated. Under these conditions 20 nmoles of L-alanine yielded a $-\Delta A$ at 340 nmeters of 0.110–0.115. Corrections have been made in all cases for L-alanine generated in the absence of pyruvic acid or in the absence of L-asparagine. The results of a single experiment are given. The results of three similar experiments while not quantitatively identical yielded entirely comparable percentages of inhibition.

that the panel of known antagonists of L-glutamine would inhibit the reaction with L-glutamine to a greater degree than the reaction with ammonia. There is ample precedent for this kind of selective effect in other enzymatic systems using either amido donor (Khedouri *et al.*, 1966). Thus CONV will selectively inactivate the L-glutamine binding site of *Escherichia coli* carbamylphosphate synthetase. In the present series of experiments, using an L-asparagine synthetase from the Gardner lymphosarcoma resistant to L-asparaginase the action of antagonists of L-glutamine on amido donation by both L-glutamine and by ammonia was studied. A new radiometric assay was developed for these measurements which permitted an examination of the interaction of each of the several inhibitors with both amido donors and the same crude enzyme preparation. L-Aspartic acid-4-^{14}C was used as labeled precursor, along with saturating amounts of ATP, magnesium, and either L-glutamine or ammonium chloride. Any L-asparagine synthesized was separated completely from L-aspartic acid on miniature columns of Dowex 1×8 in the formate form. The effluent, containing L-asparagine-4-^{14}C was incubated with α-ketoglutaric acid, zinc ions, and glutamic oxalacetic transaminase in acetate buffer, at pH 5.0. After any entrained CO_2 had been driven off by agitation, L-asparaginase was added to hydrolyze L-asparagine back to L-aspartic acid. The L-aspartic acid was then transaminated to oxalacetic acid and that latter compound was catalytically β-decarboxylated by the zinc ions. $^{14}CO_2$ was trapped in center wells and its radioactivity quantitated in a liquid scintillation counter.

Marked differential effects on amido donation by L-glutamine as opposed to ammonia were, in fact, observed in the case of DON and its bulkier congener, azotomycin. These effects are given in Table XXIII and conform closely in magnitude to those described by Haskell and Canellos (1970) with a synthetase from KB cells using L-glutamine as the amido donor.

Both DONV and its chloroketone analog (CONV) also inhibited L-asparagine synthetase to a significant degree. In the case of the former agent, a diazo compound, homologous in the descent of the series to DON, differential inhibition of amido donation by L-glutamine as contrasted with ammonia was marked. The chloroketone, CONV, also exhibited effects that were marked and strikingly differential; amido donation by L-glutamine was 80% inhibited at an inhibitor concentration of $8 \times 10^{-3}\ M$, whereas use of ammonia continued to a significant, albeit depressed, degree. The residual synthesis of L-asparagine under these conditions of inhibition of the L-glutamine site may proceed through the ammonia site, with ammonia present or generated in the extracts.

An examination of Table XXIII shows that several other agents depressed the enzymatic synthesis of L-asparagine. But azaserine, the classic antagonist of L-glutamine only marginally inhibited the amido donation by both ammonia and L-glutamine.

TABLE XXIII

INHIBITION OF THE L-ASPARAGINE SYNTHETASE OF THE L-ASPARAGINASE-RESISTANT GARDNER LYMPHOSARCOMA BY ANALOGS AND ANTAGONISTS OF L-GLUTAMINE[a]

$$\text{L-Aspartic acid} + NH_3 \text{ or L-glutamine} + \text{ATP·magnesium} \xrightarrow[\text{Synthetase}]{\text{L-asparagine}} \text{L-asparagine} + \text{AMP} + \text{pyrophosphate} + \text{L-glutamic acid or } H_2O \text{ (32)}$$

Inhibitor	NSC No.	% Inhibition			
		With NH_3 as amido donor, and inhibitor at:		With L-glutamine as amido donor, and inhibitor at:	
		2×10^{-3} M	8×10^{-3} M	2×10^{-3} M	8×10^{-3} M
Serine, diazoacetate (ester), L- (azaserine)	742	8	10	15	17
Norleucine, 6-diazo-5-oxo-, L- (DON)	7,365	8	10	75	76
Glutamine, *N*-{1-[(1-carboxy-5-diazo-4-oxopentyl) carbamyl]-5-diazo-4-oxopentyl}-, sodium salt (azotomycin)	56,654	8	12	78	78
Norleucine, *N*-acetyl-6-diazo-5-oxo-, L- (duazomycin A)	51,097	20	24	20	24
Norvaline, 5-diazo-4-oxo-, L- (DONV)	117,613	22	33	55	59
Sulfoximine, *S*-(L-3-amino-3-carboxypropyl)-*S*-methyl- (L-methionine-DL-sulfoxime)		0	18	8	20
Lysine, 5-hydroxy-, monohydrochloride, DL-*allo*-(+)- (δ-OH-lysine)	132,938	0	20	0	16
Butyramide, 4-amino- (γ-aminobutyramide)		0	12	0	18
Serine, carbamate (ester), L- (carbamyl-L-serine)	128,373	0	8	8	8
Glutamic acid, 5-hydrazide, L- (γ-glutamyl hydrazide)	7,786	0	0	0	0
Levulinic acid, 2-amino-5-chlorohydrochloride, L- (CONV)	124,412	4	25	80	84

[a] Freshly excised or deep-frozen (liquid N_2) tumor nodules of the 6C3HED lymphosarcoma resistant to L-asparaginase were homogenized in 3 volumes (w/v) of 0.05 M Tris buffer, pH 7.4. A clear supernatant was procured by centrifugation of the homogenates at 17,000 g for 20 minutes at 4°C. In conical Eppendorf reaction vessels, in a net volume of 240 μliters were admixed: 200 μliters of tumor extract; 5 μmoles of L-glutamine or 12.5 μmoles of NH_4Cl; 2.5 μmoles of ATP and MgCl; and 0.25 μmoles of L-aspartic acid-4-^{14}C 250,000 cpm (Calbiochem). Inhibitors were neutralized and added to a final concentration of 2×10^{-3} M and 8×10^{-3} M. The reaction mixtures were incubated at 37°C for 1 hour, heated at 96°C for 5 minutes and centrifuged at 19,000 g for 3 minutes. One hundred μliters of the supernatant was applied to a miniature column of Dowex 1 × 8 in the formate form and rinsed through with three 500-μliter aliquots of 0.001 M L-asparagine in 0.005 M Tris, pH 8.45. The effluent (2 ml) was collected in a scintillation vial; to it was added 1 ml of 0.66 M acetate buffer, pH 5.0, containing 500 μg of α-ketoglutaric acid and 5 mg of $ZnSO_4$. After incubation at 40°C for 1 hour, 10 μliters, containing 10 IU of EC-2 L-asparaginase was added and center wells containing 200 μliters of 10% KOH were screwed into place. Three hours later the caps were removed and immersed in a scintillator-solution containing toluene, ethanol, POPOP, PPO, and Cabosil; a thixotropic gel formed instantly and served to entrap $^{14}CO_2$ in minimally volatile form. The vials were counted with ~45% efficiency in a scintillation spectrometer. At the concentrations used, L-glutamine was a 25% more efficient amido donor than ammonia.

It is well to point out that in all of these studies with enzymatic systems having L-asparagine as their ordinary substrate or product, high concentrations of antagonists were used, in order unequivocally to characterize any inhibitory effect. However, it is unlikely that such concentrations could be reached in the *melieu interieur* unless concentrative phenomena or affinity effects were to come into play. Thus, although striking inhibitory effects were detected *in vitro*, they are probably not extrapolatable *in vivo*. Moreover, on a molar basis these inhibitions, where observed, should not be termed powerful. In keeping with this viewpoint are the negative findings given in Section VIII. No agent, in this series, even those presently shown to be inhibitors of L-asparagine synthetase was able to confer sensitivity to L-asparaginase on a tumor resistant to the enzyme. Since there is strong evidence that resistance to L-asparaginase emerges via induction (or at least augmentation) of L-asparagine synthetase, this failure must mean that the agents in question cannot be given in large enough doses to inhibit the enzyme to a significant degree or for a significant duration *in vivo*. The search for truly powerful inhibitors of L-asparagine synthetase should continue then inasmuch as, in theory at least, such agents could render whole classes of resistant tumors sensitive to the chemotherapeutic action of L-asparaginase.

In summary, several analogs and antagonists of L-glutamine were found to exert the following effects on enzymatic reactions utilizing or producing L-asparagine; proceeding seriatim those effects were:

1. Azaserine did not inhibit coliform or agouti L-asparaginases but was minimally inhibitory toward the L-asparaginase of mouse liver and strongly inhibitory toward the L-asparagine transaminase from the same source. Only marginal inhibition of L-asparagine synthetase was detectable at concentrations of azaserine up to 8×10^{-3} *M*.

2. DON did not inhibit the L-glutamine or the L-asparagine amido hydrolytic activity of EC-2 either at an acid or alkaline pH. The compound was also without effect on agouti L-asparaginase but did marginally stimulate the L-asparaginase of mouse liver. DON was without influence on the murine L-asparagine transaminase and profoundly depressed the utilization of L-glutamine but not of NH_3 by murine L-asparagine synthetase.

3. Azotomycin also was inert toward EC-2 and stimulated both agouti and hepatic L-asparaginases. This tripeptide was marginally inhibitory toward hepatic L-asparagine transaminase but strongly inhibitory towards L-asparagine synthetase when L-glutamine was acting as the amido donor.

4. Duazomycin A (*N*-acetyl-DON) exerted only marginal effects on all the L-asparagine enzymes studied.

5. DONV, a five-carbon diazo ketone, inhibited the bacterial and both mammalian L-asparagine amido hydrolases as well as L-asparagine synthetase, especially when L-glutamine was used as the amido donor in the

latter reaction. L-Asparagine transaminase, on the other hand was not significantly inhibited by DONV.

6. L-Methionine-DL-sulfoximine, a powerful inhibitor of ovine cerebral glutamine synthetase, produced only marginal inhibition of murine L-asparagine synthetase at the concentrations studied, and no inhibition either of the three L-asparaginases studied or of L-asparagine transaminase.

7. δ-OH-Lysine inhibited both mammalian L-asparaginases, but the effect was not a powerful one.

8. γ-Aminobutyramide did not significantly inhibit any enzyme utilizing or producing L-asparagine. However, it should be stressed that the amino acid activating enzymes and L-asparaginyl t-RNA synthetase(s) were not examined.

9. Carbamyl-L-serine significantly inhibited amido hydrolysis of L-asparagine and of L-glutamine by EC-2; however, hepatic and agouti L-asparaginases were unaffected by the compound. Since hepatic L-asparagine transaminase was exceptionally susceptible to the inhibitory effects of this carbamate ester, it promises to be useful as a tool for studying the role of this transaminase in the homeostasis of L-asparagine by higher organisms.

10. γ-Glutamylhydrazide did not inhibit the L-asparaginase of *E. coli* or agouti serum but did exert a modest inhibitory action on murine hepatic L-asparaginase. Moreover, despite the presence of a reactive and potentially labile γ-hydrazino function, this agent was only marginally inhibitory toward L-asparagine transaminase of mouse liver and appeared to be transaminated itself to a minor but measurable degree. Lastly, although γ-glutamylhydrazide closely resembles L-glutamine, it did not significantly inhibit L-asparagine synthetase even when L-glutamine was being tested as the amido donor.

11. CONV, a reactive chloroketone, strongly inhibited L-asparaginase from *E. coli* and agouti serum, strongly inhibited L-asparaginase and L-asparagine transaminase from the liver of *Mus musculus*, and strongly inhibited L-asparagine synthetase of lymphosarcomatous origin when L-glutamine was the amido donor. Of all the candidate compounds studied then, and despite the fact that on the face of it, CONV, being a 5-C compound is formally and functionally (Khedouri *et al.*, 1966) similar to L-glutamine, this agent is also a most reactive antagonist of L-asparagine.

ACKNOWLEDGMENTS

We would like to express our appreciation to Mrs. Martha Harshman for her work in preparing the manuscript and to Mrs. Ruth Davis for her critical review and suggestions.

REFERENCES

Abrams, R., and Bentley, M. (1959). *Arch. Biochem. Biophys.* **79**, 91.
Adamson, R., and Fabro, S. (1968). *Cancer Chemother. Rep.* **52**, 617.

Anderson, E., and Brockman, R. (1963). *Biochem. Pharmacol.* **12**, 1335.
Anderson, E., and Jacquez, J. (1962). *Cancer Res.* **22**, 27.
Ansfield, F. (1965). *Cancer Chemother. Rep.* **46**, 37.
Baker, B. (1959). *Biochem. Pharmacol.* **2**, 161.
Becker, F., and Broome, J. (1967). *Science* **156**, 1602.
Bennett, L., Schabel, F., and Skipper, H. (1956). *Arch. Biochem. Biophys.* **64**, 423.
Blair, D., and Potter, V. (1961). *J. Biol. Chem.* **236**, 2503.
Boyse, E., Old, L., Campbell, H., and Mashburn, L. (1967). *J. Exp. Med.* **125**, 17.
Brown, G., Jr., and Cohen, P. (1960). *Comp. Biochem.* **2**, 227–250.
Buchanan, J. (1957a). *Tex. Rep. Biol. Med.* **15**, 148.
Buchanan, J. (1957b). *Tex. Rep. Biol. Med.* **15**, 169.
Campbell, H., and Mashburn, L. (1969). *Biochemistry* **8**, 3768.
Cancer Chemotherapy National Service Center (1962). *Cancer Chemother. Rep.* **25**, 1–66.
Clarke, D., Reilly, H., and Stock, C. (1957). *Antibiot. Chemother.* **7**, 653.
Colsky, J., Shnider, B., and Franzino, A. (1966). *Clin. Pharmacol. Ther.* **1**, 353.
Cooney, D., and Davis, R. (1970). *Biochim. Biophys. Acta* **212**, 134.
Cooney, D., and Handschumacher, R. (1968). *Proc. Amer. Ass. Cancer Res.* **9**, 15.
Duvall, L. (1960). *Cancer Chemother. Rep.* **7**, 86.
Eagle, H., Washington, D., Levy, M., and Cohen, L. (1966). *J. Biol. Chem.* **241**, 4994.
El-Asmar, F., and Greenberg, D. (1966). *Cancer Res.* **26**, 116.
Ellison, R., Karnofsky, D., Sternberg, S., Murphy, L., and Burchenal, J. (1954). *Cancer* **7**, 801.
Errera, M., and Greenstein, J. (1947). *J. Nat. Cancer Inst.* **7**, 437.
Foley, H., Shnider, B., and Gold, G. (1966). *J. New Drugs* **6**, 105.
Folk, J., and Cole, P. (1965). *J. Biol. Chem.* **240**, 2951.
French, T., Dawid, I., Day, R. A., and Buchanan, J. (1963a). *J. Biol. Chem.* **238**, 2171.
French, T., Dawid, I., Day, R. A., and Buchanan, J. (1963b). *J. Biol. Chem.* **238**, 2186.
Gass, J., and Meister, A. (1970). *Biochemistry* **9**, 842.
Ghosh, S., Blumenthal, H., Davidson, E., and Roseman, S. (1960). *J. Biol. Chem.* **235**, 1265.
Goldin, A., and Venditti, J. (1970). *Proc. 6th Int. Cancer Congr., Tokyo* (in press).
Greenberg, E., Blumenthal, G., and Ramadan, M. (1964). *Cancer Res.* **24**, 957.
Greenlees, J., and LePage, G. (1956). *Cancer Res.* **16**, 808.
Hager, S., and Jones, M. (1965). *J. Biol. Chem.* **240**, 4556.
Hager, S., and Jones, M. (1967). *J. Biol. Chem.* **242**, 5667.
Handschumacher, R., Bates, C., Chang, P., Andrews, A., and Fischer, G. (1967). *Proc. Amer. Ass. Cancer Res.* **8**, 25.
Handschumacher, R., Bates, C., Chang, P., Andrews, A., and Fischer, G. (1968). *Science* **161**, 62.
Hansen, H., and Vandevoorde, J. (1966). *Proc. Soc. Exp. Biol. Med.* **123**, 209.
Haskell, C., and Canellos, G. (1969). *Proc. Amer. Ass. Cancer Res.* **10**, 36.
Haskell, C., and Canellos, G. (1970). *Cancer Res.* **30**, 1081.
Hayes, D., Costa, J., Moon, J., Hoogstraten, B., and Harley, J. (1967). *Cancer Chemother. Rep.* **51**, 235.
Hedegaard, J., and Roche, J. (1966). *C. R. Soc. Biol.* **160**, 539.
Heyn, R., Brubaker, C., Burchenal, J., Cramblett, H., and Wolff, J. (1960). *Blood* **15**, 350.
Holland, J., Gehan, E., Brindley, C., Dederick, M., Owens, A., Jr., Shnider, B., Taylor, R., Frei, E., III, Selawry, O., Regelson, W., and Hall, T. (1961). *Clin. Pharmacol. Ther.* **2**, 22.

Horowitz, B., Madras, B., Meister, A., Old, L., Boyse, E., and Stockert, E. (1968). *Science* **160**, 533.

Jackson, R., Cooney, D., and Handschumacher, R. (1969). *Fed. Amer. Soc. Exp. Biol.* **28**, 601.

Jacobs, S., Wodinsky, I., Kensler, C., and Venditti, J. (1969a). *Proc. Amer. Ass. Cancer Res.* **10**, 43.

Jacobs, S., Wodinsky, I., Venditti, J., and Kensler, C. (1969b). *Pharmacologist* **11**, 234.

Jones, M., Anderson, A., Anderson, C., and Hodes, S. (1961). *Arch. Biochem. Biophys.* **95**, 499.

Kalman, S., Duffield, P., and Brzozowski, T. (1965). *Biochem. Biophys. Res. Commun.* **18**, 530.

Kammen, H., and Hurlbert, R. (1959). *Cancer Res.* **19**, 654.

Kerson, L., and Appel, S. (1968). *J. Biol. Chem.* **243**, 4279.

Khedouri, E., Anderson, P., and Meister, A. (1966). *Biochemistry* **5**, 3552.

Krakoff, I. (1961). *Clin. Pharmacol. Ther.* **2**, 599.

Lefkowitz, E., Creasey, W., and Calabresi, P. (1965). *Cancer Res.* **25**, 1207.

Levenberg, B., Melnick, I., and Buchanan, J. (1957). *J. Biol. Chem.* **225**, 163.

Levintow, L. (1954). *J. Nat. Cancer Inst.* **15**, 347.

Levintow, L., Eagle, H., and Piez, K. (1957). *J. Biol. Chem.* **227**, 929.

Li, M. C. (1960). *J. Amer. Med. Ass.* **174**, 1291.

Li, M. C. (1961). *Med. Clin. N. Amer.* **45**, 661.

Lim, P. (1968). Personal communication. (Report to Drug Development Branch, Cancer Chemotherapy National Service Center.)

McFall, E., and Magasanik, B. (1960). *J. Biol. Chem.* **235**, 2103.

Mashburn, L., and Wriston, J. J., Jr. (1964). *Arch. Biochem. Biophys.* **105**, 450.

Masterson, J., and Nelson, J., Jr. (1965). *Amer. J. Obstet. Gynecol.* **93**, 1102.

Mayfield, E., Jr., Lyman, K., and Bresnick, E. (1967). *Cancer Res.* **27**, 476.

Meister, A. (1953). *J. Biol. Chem.* **200**, 571.

Meister, A. (1968). *Advan. Enzymol. Relat. Areas Mol. Biol.* **31**, 183–218.

Miller, H., and Balis, M. (1969). *Biochem. Pharmacol.* **18**, 2225.

Misani, F., and Reiner, L. (1950). *Arch. Biochem.* **27**, 234.

Mizobuchi, K., and Buchanan, J. (1968). *J. Biol. Chem.* **243**, 4853.

Moore, E., and Hurlbert, R. (1961). *Cancer Res.* **21**, 257.

Moore, E., and LePage, G. (1957). *Cancer Res.* **17**, 804.

Narrod, S., Bonavita, V., and Kaplan, N. (1960). *Proc. Amer. Ass. Cancer Res.* **3**, 137.

Oleson, J. (1969). Personal communication.

Patterson, M., Jr., and Orr, G. (1968). *J. Biol. Chem.* **243**, 376.

Prager, M., and Bachynsky, N. (1968). *Arch. Biochem. Biophys.* **127**, 645.

Rabinowitz, M., Olson, M., and Greenberg, D. (1957). *Cancer Res.* **17**, 885.

Rabinowitz, M., Olson, M., and Greenberg, D. (1959). *Cancer Res.* **19**, 388.

Ramadan, M., and Greenberg, D. (1963). *Anal. Biochem.* **6**, 144.

Ronzio, R., and Meister, A. (1968). *Proc. Nat. Acad. Sci. U.S.* **59**, 164.

Sartorelli, A., and Booth, B. (1967). *Mol. Pharmacol.* **3**, 71.

Sartorelli, A., Akers, C., Jr., and Booth, B. (1960). *Biochem. Pharmacol.* **5**, 238.

Schabel, F., Skipper, H., Trader, M., and Wilcox, W. (1965). *Cancer Chemother. Rep.* **48**, 17.

Schroeder, J., Ansfield, F., Curreri, A., and LePage, G. (1964). *Brit. J. Cancer* **18**, 449.

Sherman, H. (1963). *Bull. Tulane Univ. Med. Fac.* **22**, 275.

Simard, R., and Bernhard, W. (1966). *Int. J. Cancer* **1**, 463.

Slater, T., and Sawyer, B. (1966). *Biochem. Pharmacol.* **15**, 1267.
Smulson, M., and Neal, A. (1965). *Arch. Biochem. Biophys.* **112**, 25.
Spencer, R., and Preiss, J. (1967). *J. Biol. Chem.* **242**, 385.
Steward, F., and Thompson, J. (1952). *Nature (London)* **169**, 739.
Sullivan, M., Beatty, E., Hyman, C., Murphy, M., Pierce, M., and Severo, N. (1962). *Cancer Chemother. Rep.* **18**, 83.
Tatibana, M., and Ito, K. (1967). *Biochem. Biophys. Res. Commun.* **26**, 221.
Tatibana, M., and Ito, K. (1969). *J. Biol. Chem.* **244**, 5403.
Tomisek, A., Kelly, H., and Skipper, H. (1956). *Arch. Biochem. Biophys.* **64**, 437.
Vandevoorde, J., Hansen, H., and Nadler, S. (1964). *Proc. Soc. Exp. Biol. Med.* **115**, 55.
Venditti, J., and Abbott, B. (1967). *Lloydia* **30**, 332.
Venditti, J., and Goldin, A. (1964). *Advan. Chemother.* **1**, 397–484.
Wajda, I., Acs, G., Clarke, D., and Waelsch, H. (1963). *Biochem. Pharmacol.* **12**, 241.
Weiss, A., Ramirez, G., Grage, T., Stawitz, J., Goldman, L., and Downing, V. (1968). *Cancer Chemother. Rep.* **52**, 611.
Whelan, H., and Wriston, J. J., Jr. (1969). *Biochemistry* **8**, 2386.
Wu, C., Roberts, E., and Bauer, J. (1965). *Cancer Res.* **25**, 677.
Yellin, T. (1968). *Biochem. Biophys. Res. Commun.* **32**, 307.

The Combined Action of Pyrimidines and Sulfonamides or Sulfones in the Chemotherapy of Malaria and Other Protozoal Infections

W. H. G. RICHARDS

Wellcome Laboratories of Tropical Medicine
Langley Court
Beckenham, Kent, England

I. Introduction

Research into the problems of controlling malaria has been notable for the intermittent attention it has received. All too frequently there have been periods when the rapid accumulation of vital knowledge has lulled workers in this field into a state of false security where further research appears to be unnecessary. The discovery and proven use of prophylactic drugs such as paludrine and pyrimethamine, and the use of primaquine and chloroquine in the treatment of malaria, appeared to have the problem solved. These coupled with the widespread use of insecticides and their dramatic effect on the insect vector led to the general impression that the threat of malaria was at last conquered. It was Hackett (1937) who said, "the simplicity of the theory of malaria control is surpassed only by the difficulties involved in its application."

In spite of the widespread control and eradication campaigns malaria still constitutes one of the leading causes of mortality and morbidity in the tropics today. Sadun (1964) reported that in 1957 nearly one billion or one-third of the world's population were exposed to malarial infections.

By the early 1960's resistance of the malaria parasites to treatment with all the major antimalarial drugs had been reported. With the renewed threat of malaria now apparent, research was once again intensified in this field.

The major advances in chemotherapy during the first half of the present century can, without doubt, be attributed to an empirical approach to the subject. This approach has provided a wealth of information relating the structure of compounds to their biological activity, but it has yielded little or no information about the mechanism of their action. The aim of chemotherapy is the selective toxicity of the chemotherapeutic agent between host and parasite producing a differential effect, beneficial to the host. A knowledge of the biochemistry of a parasite facilitates a more rational approach to drug design and chemotherapy.

This scientific approach has produced a series of very powerful antiparasitic agents, combinations of a sulfonamide or sulfone together with a pyrimidine. The mixture is able sequentially to block an essential metabolic process within the parasite which leads to the formation of purines and eventually of DNA.

II. Historical

A. Sulfonamides

The foundation for a biochemical approach to chemotherapy was probably initiated in 1935 with the advent of Prontosil and the discovery by Tréfouel *et al.* (1935) and Colebrook *et al.* (1936) that its action was not due to the dye but to the *in vivo* formation of an active metabolite sulfanilamide. A description of the antimalarial activity of the sulfonamides soon followed; Díaz de León (1937, 1938, 1940) claimed to have produced a clinical cure of *Plasmodium vivax* using Rubiazol (6-carboxy-4-sulfamide-2′,4′-diaminoazobenzene). Hill and Goodwin (1937) treated 93 patients infected with *P. falciparum* with intramuscular doses of prontosil, producing a marked improvement in 48 hours. The following years saw a number of papers reporting the use and varying success of sulfonamides against both human and experimental malarias (Van der Weilen, 1937; Coggeshall, 1938a,b, 1940; Coggeshall *et al.*, 1941; Chopra *et al.*, 1939; Chopra, 1939; Chopra and Das

Gupta, 1938, 1939; Farinaud and Ragiot, 1938; Niven, 1938; Sorley and Currie, 1938; Farinaud and Eliche, 1939; Menk and Mohr, 1939; and Sinton *et al.* 1939).

Fairley (1945) found that 1 gm sulfadiazine or sulfamezathine daily for 23 days was able to suppress and in certain cases to eradicate *P. falciparum* in patients in New Guinea. Findlay *et al.* (1946) analyzing the results from 138 patients infected with *P. falciparum* in West Africa found some variation in the effect of certain sulfonamides; the drugs exerted an effect but their action was slow. Coatney *et al.* (1947) used large doses of the most effective sulfonamide of that time, sulfadiazine, against sporozoite-induced infections of *P. falciparum* and were able to prevent the development of a patent parasitaemia; but several complications were noted in patients receiving the highest doses.

The practical use of sulfonamides, as antimalarials with their short duration in the body, slow rate of action, and need for high dose levels coupled with the possibility of toxic manifestations, was reduced to one of academic interest with the advent of the more powerful synthetic antimalarials in the early 1950's.

B. Sulfones

The use of diaminodiphenyl sulfone, (dapsone, DDS), as an antimalarial has received comparatively little attention. Shortly after the antimalarial activity of the drug was discovered, the drug was discarded as too toxic for human use (Buttle *et al.*, 1937; Coggeshall *et al.*, 1941; Long, 1950). This was due in part to the assumption that the amount of sulfone required for treatment was comparable to that used with the sulfa drugs. During the first trials in humans (Patrono, 1943; Tarabini and Secreto, 1945), dapsone was shown to be effective against *P. falciparum*, but the introduction of the 4-aminoquinoline drugs together with the reports of the toxicity of dapsone led to the abandonment of the drug as an antimalarial.

Dapsone was used, however, by Ardias (1948) in the treatment of malaria. Two hundred and forty-three patients were treated with varying doses of drug. Ardias concluded that dapsone in doses of 9 gm had a marked action on stages of the development of the malarial parasite. Young trophozoites were especially vulnerable. Doses higher than 9 gm were no more effective and offered no advantage, while smaller doses were ineffective. The sulfone was no more effective than other antimalarial drugs in preventing relapses.

In 1949 Cochrane introduced dapsone for the treatment of leprosy (Cochrane *et al.*, 1949). It was Leiker (1956) who suggested that dapsone may have prophylactic properties against malaria which he found to be absent from leprosarium patients, treated with the drug, in contrast to the general population in a holoendemic area.

Archibald and Ross (1960) compared the antimalarial activity of dapsone relative to that of two chloroquine salts, the phosphate (Avochlor) and the diphosphate (Resoquin). Single doses of 200 mg of dapsone and 300 mg of chloroquine base were given orally, and the patients' blood was examined at intervals up to 96 hours. Dapsone appeared capable of clearing the blood of trophozoites of both *P. falciparum* and *P. malariae*, though at a slower rate than that achieved by chloroquine. It was also reported that the price of 100 mg tablets of dapsone was one-tenth of that of the standard 150-mg base chloroquine tablet, which is a very important aspect when considering eradication campaigns. Weekly doses of 100 mg to 200 mg of dapsone were found to produce a radical cure in semi-immune Africans with *P. falciparum* (Costa, 1960), and Basu *et al.* (1962) stated that a single dose of 200 mg dapsone was able to arrest a fever due to *P. falciparum* within 72 hours. Chin *et al.* (1966) reported that daily doses of 25 mg of dapsone were unable to protect volunteers against a sporozoite-induced Chesson strain of *P. vivax*.

Ramakrishnan and his colleagues (1962) after studies using *P. gallinaceum*, *P. knowlesi*, and *P. cynomolgi* concluded that dapsone did not possess any causal prophylactic, gametocytocidal, or sporonticidal properties.

Numerous workers beginning with Thurston (1950) have shown dapsone to be effective in treating *P. berghei* infections in mice. The studies against the rodent malarias, however, were mainly of academic interest and could only corroborate the results established against human infections.

C. Pyrimidines

Several pyrimidines had been prepared and tested for antimalarial activity in 1946 and 1947 (Curd *et al.*, 1946; Basford *et al.*, 1947) with relatively little success. It was found by Hitchings *et al.* (1948) that many 2,4-diaminopyrimidines are powerful antagonists of folic and folinic acids in the growth of *Lactobacillus casei* in culture. The formal structural analogy between the 2,4-diaminopyrimidines and the antimalarial proguanil, also a folic and folinic acid antagonist, suggested that the pyrimidines might also have a similar antiparasitic activity (Falco *et al.*, 1949). This proved to be the case, and Goodwin (1949) reported antimalarial activity within the group of pyrimidines. Then followed a period of intense activity when hundreds of related compounds were tested against *P. gallinaceum* infections in chicks and *P. berghei* in mice. The more active compounds were tested against *P. cynomolgi* infections in monkeys.

Many of the compounds were tested against laboratory infections of *Trypanosoma rhodesiense*, *T. congolense*, *T. cruzi*, *Leishmania donovani*, and *Entamoeba histolytica*. Apart from slight activity against *T. congolense*, the pyrimidines had no significant antiprotozoal activity. Diaveridine,

2,4-diamino-5-(3,4-dimethoxybenzyl)pyrimidine, was later shown by Hitchings and Bushby (1963) to have a coccidiostatic action. The main field of interest at that time was in the use of the drugs against malaria in man. Falco *et al.* (1951) found that pyrimethamine, 5-(*p*-chlorophenyl)-2,4-diamino-6-ethylpyrimidine, was active against the erythrocytic forms of *P. cynomolgi* in monkeys but had no effective action on the exoerythrocytic stages.

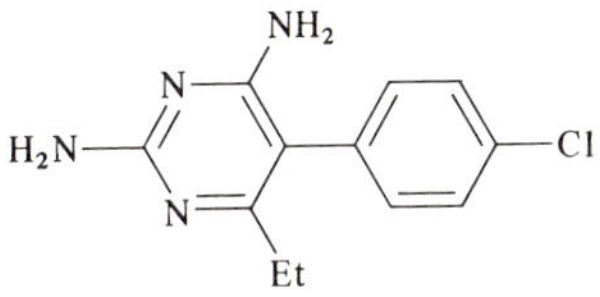

Pyrimethamine

Archibald (1951) was the first to try the drug against natural malarial infections. A single dose of 5 mg, the smallest dose he tried, was sufficient to cause the disappearance of asexual parasites of *P. falciparum* and *P. malariae* in African school children. Although the drug acted slowly, the action persisted for at least 1 month. McGregor and Smith (1952) in The Gambia used pyrimethamine in the treatment of overt malaria attacks. They found a single dose of 0.25 mg/kg to 0.5 mg/kg was sufficient to cause the disappearance of malaria parasites from the blood, although the speed of action in controlling the fever and parasitemia were slow. Mackerras and Ercole (1947) and Shute and Maryon (1948) demonstrated that proguanil affects the female gametocytes in such a way that they fail to develop to mature oocysts. Foy and Kondi (1952) demonstrated a similar action by pyrimethamine; gametocytes from a patient treated with the drug failed to develop to the sporozoite stage in mosquitoes fed on his blood up to a week after dosing.

So much has been written about pyrimethamine since these reported works, that it is too extensive to be included in this present review. It is now firmly established as an important prophylactic drug in the arsenal of antimalarials.

III. Mode of Action

A. Antagonism of *p*-Aminobenzoic Acid

It is evident that sulfonamides with their wide range of activity must interfere with some essential function which is common to widely diverse parasites. It is also clear that this same function is not essential to man. Woods (1940) was the first to mention that there was an antagonism between *p*-aminobenzoic acid (PABA) and a sulfonamide. Maier and Riley (1942) showed that the antimalarial action of many compounds also depends on a similar mechanism because the effect is reversed by the addition of *p*-aminobenzoic acid. This work although very interesting did not receive the attention it deserved. Thurston (1954) again demonstrated this antagonism in mice infected with *P. berghei*, and Rollo (1955) demonstrated it in chicks infected with *P. gallinaceum*.

It appears that the metabolic differences on which the selective toxicity of sulfonamides rests concern the method of folic acid utilization. In both parasites and man folic acid derivatives are essential for purine synthesis. Man is able to absorb his vitamin requirements directly via his diet; parasites on the other hand are unable to utilize the vitamins and they synthesize it from *p*-aminobenzoic acid. The parasites appear unable to differentiate between the structurally similar *p*-aminobenzoic acid and sulfonamides or sulfone. The drug is then accepted by and incorporated into the parasite and is able to arrest any future metabolism of folic acid.

B. Inhibition of Dihydrofolate Reductase

Details of the fine structure of dihydrofolate reductase vary from species to species, and a given inhibitor may show considerable selectivity as a result of looser or tighter binding to the corresponding enzyme of the parasite or host.

It was found by Hitchings *et al.* (1948) that essentially all derivatives of the 2,4-diaminopyrimidine series were antagonists of folic acid. Rollo (1955) suggested that the mode of action of pyrimethamine against experimental malarias was by interfering with the conversion of folic to folinic acid. This was firmly established by Hitchings (1960, 1962) and by Rollo (1964).

C. Potentiation

The recognition that combinations of sulfonamides and "antifolic" drugs were synergistic in action was first recorded by Greenberg (1949) and Greenberg and Richeson (1950, 1951) in the treatment of *P. gallinaceum* in chicks. The combination of pyrimethamine plus sulfonamide was shown by Eyles and Coleman (1953) to be effective against toxoplasmal infection in mice and by Ryan *et al.* (1954) in *Toxoplasma* infections in man. In the same year, Lux (1954) was able successfully to treat coccidiosis in chicks with mixtures of sulfaquinoxaline and either a pyrimidine or a dihydrotriazine; in 1955 Rollo studied the mode of action of sulfonamides and pyrimethamine on *P. gallinaceum* in chicks. He clearly showed that the actions of both sulfadiazine and pyrimethamine were competitively antagonized by folic acid. Sulfadiazine strongly potentiated the action of pyrimethamine against *P. gallinaceum*, but there was no such potentiation between pyrimethamine and proguanil. This dramatic potentiation, 1/8 of a dose of pyrimethamine plus 1/7 of a dose of sulfadiazine, produced the effect of a full dose of either drug given alone.

This work was followed by Hurley (1959) to discover if this potentiation could be reproduced in human malaria. The investigation was performed in The Gambia on African children who had a high degree of acquired immunity to malaria. The malaria infections in this area also reacted to much smaller doses of pyrimethamine than were used in other parts of West Africa. Seventy-two hours after treatment a group of children that had been treated either with pyrimethamine or sulfadiazine still had patent parasitaemias, whereas the two groups treated with a mixture of the two drugs were free from any obvious infection. It was found that 1/10 of the minimum effective dose of pyrimethamine plus 1/4 of the minimum effective dose of sulfadiazine was as effective against the asexual parasites of *P. falciparum*, *P. malariae*, and *P. ovale* as the minimum effective dose of either drug given alone.

Although this interesting work showed that combinations of pyrimethamine and sulfadiazine were very effective, there was no general acceptance of the mixture either as a prophylactic or as a means of therapy for malaria. At that time there was not the apparent need for such a drug, and the antimalarials available were able to deal with the problem.

Even so, a small number of workers continued to work in this field. One of the most difficult infections to cure, toxoplasmosis, was shown to respond to synergistic mixtures (Frenkel and Jacobs, 1958, and Hitchings, 1960). Basu *et al.* (1962) studied the effect of dapsone singly and in combination with pyrimethamine against *P. falciparum* and *P. vivax* in India. A single dose of dapsone at 250 mg or 200 mg was invariably effective in all the *P. falciparum* infections but was ineffective in clearing the asexual parasites in six out of 17 *P. vivax* infections. The trial lost some of its impact because the authors did not include a group that was treated with pyrimethamine alone, and therefore they had to refer to previous workers (Jaswant Singh *et al.*, 1952; Srivastava *et al.*, 1953), who showed that a single dose of 25 mg pyrimethamine was not only slow in its speed of action but not completely effective. When used in combination a dose of 50 mg dapsone plus 12.5 mg pyrimethamine was adequate for the treatment of both *P. vivax* and *P. falciparum* infections. The authors also stated that the speed of clearance of the asexual parasites as well as of the symptoms was comparable to that obtained with a single dose of 600 mg chloroquine base.

McGregor *et al.* (1963) treated an African child, who had not responded to three doses each of 50 mg of pyrimethamine, with 12.5 mg pyrimethamine combined with 1 gm of sulfadiazine; this treatment was repeated after 24 hours. After a further 48 hours the patient had no demonstrable parasites in the blood, and subsequent daily blood examinations failed to reveal any sign of infection. The conclusion drawn was that the potentiative effect of sulfadiazine effectively overcame the apparent resistance of the parasite to pyrimethamine.

Until 1960 there was no real need for another antimalarial. Pyrimethamine resistance had been established for a number of years, but chloroquine was still effective and it was used not only for therapy but also as a prophylactic. Potentiating mixtures were restricted in their use by the short half-life of the sulfonamides available at the time, which did not match that of pyrimethamine. This restricted treatment to a few patients at a time so that dosing schedules could be individually adjusted.

The first published report by Maberti (1960) of the failure of chloroquine to produce a radical cure of a *P. falciparum* infection went largely unnoticed, but that of Moore and Lanier (1961) demonstrated quite clearly that there was a pressing need for new antimalarial drugs. All the major antimalarial compounds had now shown some degree of failure in arresting malarial infections and quinine was again being used for therapy. Even so there was still no great interest in potentiating mixtures, due in part to the lack of balance in half-lives of the two component compounds. This was well demonstrated in the work of DeGowin and Powell (1964). Using sulfadiazine plus pyrimethamine they cured five out of six volunteers infected with the Malaya (Camp) strain of *P. falciparum* known to be resistant to chloroquine, chlorguanide, and pyrimethamine. The dosing schedule was 2 gm sulfadiazine daily for 5 days given concurrently with 50 mg pyrimethamine daily for 3 days. Previous trials with the same doses of sulfadiazine and pyrimethamine administered separately had been without success.

IV. The Long-Acting Sulfonamides

A. Sulfadoxine

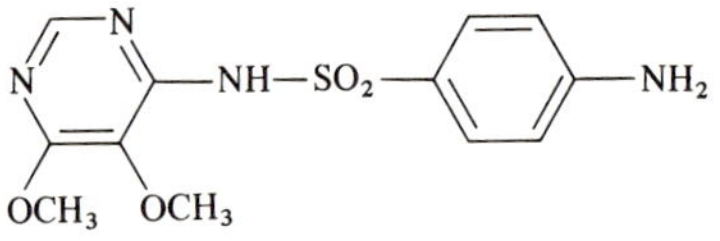

Sulfadoxine

In December 1964 Laing published the results of his first study of the antimalarial effects of sulfadoxine, 5,6-dimethoxy-4-sulfanilamidopyrimidine. This sulfonamide is markedly different from those previously available. It has a half-life of 100 to 200 hours as opposed to sulfadiazine which has only 17 hours. Oral absorption is as rapid as that of other antimalarials, and its slow elimination from the body allows therapeutically active blood levels to be maintained by weekly oral administration of the drug. Laing (1964) stated that sulfadoxine was chosen because of its sustained plasma concentration, which matched the plasma concentration of pyrimethamine better than any other sulfonamide. The trial was done in Tanzania where malaria was holoendemic and pyrimethamine resistance was established. Children were dosed with 25 mg pyrimethamine weekly for 2 months to eliminate all the sensitive parasites, and then treated weekly with 500-mg doses of sulfadoxine, either on its own or together with 25 mg pyrimethamine. After 6 weeks both these treated groups were free from infection; in a similar group treated with pyrimethamine along the asexual parasite rate was 26%, and the density of the infection was similar to that of a further group of untreated controls. Laing in his summary was surprised to find that sulfadoxine alone was as good as sulfadoxine plus pyrimethamine; it is possible, however, that there was still sufficient amount of pyrimethamine present in the plasma of the children to combine with the first dose of sulfadoxine with a resulting synergism. One thing was quite clear, there was now available a long acting sulfonamide which could be given together with pyrimethamine in a single oral dose.

B. Sulfadoxine and Pyrimethamine

1. *Experimental Malaria*

The effect of sulfadoxine on experimental malaria was not reported until 1966 by Richards. When used against a *P. berghei* infection, the drug was shown to have good antimalarial activity against normal and chloroquine-resistant strains (Richards, 1966). This activity was shown to be greatly enhanced when sulfadoxine was used in combination with pyrimethamine. The same effect was seen against a normal strain of *P. gallinaceum* in chicks (Figs. 1 and 2). When tested against triazine- and pyrimethamine-

Plasmodium berghei

$E.D._{50}$ mgm/kg × 7 orally

	Normal	Chloroquine resistant
Pyrimethamine	0.15	0.15
Fanasil	1.0	1.0
Pyrimethamine + Fanasil	0.0125 + 0.15	0.0125 + 0.15

FIG. 1. Antimalarial activity of pyrimethamine and sulfadoxine (Fanasil) against a normal and chloroquine-resistant isolate of *Plasmodium berghei* in mice. Results are expressed as the concentration of drug which reduces the parasitemia to 50% of that of the untreated controls.

	Plasmodium gallinaceum	
	E.D.$_{50}$ mgm/kg × 7 orally	
	Normal	Pyrimethamine resistant
Pyrimethamine	0.03	10
Fanasil	20	25
Pyrimethamine + Fanasil	0.004 + 2.6	0.02 + 5

FIG. 2. Antimalarial activity of pyrimethamine and sulfadoxine (Fanasil) against a normal and pyrimethamine-resistant isolate of *Plasmodium gallinaceum* in chicks. Results are expressed as the concentration of drug which reduces the parasitemia to 50% of that of the untreated controls.

resistant strains the mixture was still effective but needed increased amounts of drugs. The results suggested that the optimum potentiating ratio is ten parts of sulfadoxine plus one part of pyrimethamine. This same type of effect was elegantly demonstrated by Peters (1968), who also suggested that the potentiation, shown by the shorter acting compounds sulfadimethoxine and proguanil against *P. berghei* in mice, might form a logical combination for clinical trials against malaria in man.

Aviado *et al.* (1969) studied the antimalarial action of the sulfonamides, sulfadoxine, sulfadimethoxine, and sulfalene alone and in combination with the pyrimidine trimethoprim against *P. berghei* in rats. Although they were able to demonstrate antimalarial activity with the sulfonamides they were unsuccessful with trimethoprim. This was probably because the dose level used was too low. Richards (unpublished data) found that when trimethoprim at 100 mg/kg × 7 orally was given to mice infected with *P. berghei* it reduced the parasitemia to 50% of that of the untreated controls. Other findings by Aviado and his colleagues that are difficult to understand are, first, in rats they were unable to show antagonism of sulfonamide activity by folic acid or *p*-aminobenzoic acid although in mice this antagonism was seen, and, second, they were unable to demonstrate potentiation between the sulfonamides and trimethoprim; this is in direct contrast to the action of the combination of these compounds against *P. falciparum* in man (Martin and Arnold, 1968).

2. *Human Malaria*

Trials by Chin *et al.* (1966) used volunteers infected with multiresistant strains of *P. falciparum*. The infections were usually cured by treatment with combined pyrimethamine and a sulfonamide; the two drugs used in combination were more active than either alone, and single doses of pyrimethamine plus sulfadoxine appeared to hold the most promise. The infections induced in 40 volunteers was usually by blood inoculation. The drug regimens tested were (a) sulfadiazine, 0.5 gm every 6 hours for 5 days; (b) sulfadiazine, as in schedule (a) plus 50 mg of pyrimethamine on the first day; (c) sulfamethoxypyridazine, 2 gm on the first day, then 1 gm daily for 5 days; (d) sulfamethoxypyridazine, 1 gm plus pyrimethamine 50 mg on the first day, then the sulfonamide 0.5 gm daily for 4 days; (e) sulfadoxine, 1 gm as a single dose; and (f) sulfadoxine, 1 gm together with 50 mg pyrimethamine as a single dose. Treatment started before the parasite counts exceeded 10,000 cm^3 and the patients were observed for at least 60 days. The authors concluded that sulfadoxine was the most promising sulfonamide. One interesting point of this study was that the authors found the clinical and parasitological response to treatment was rather slow; this is different from that of later workers.

Laing continued his initial studies on the use of sulfadoxine in malaria and in 1965 treated 25 semi-immune Africans suffering from acute falciparum malaria each with a single dose of the sulfonamide (Laing, 1965a). The dose level used ranged from 250 mg in children to 1 gm in adults. Three of the 25 patients responded slowly to the drug, whereas the remaining cases responded as rapidly as they would have done had they been treated with chloroquine.

While still working in the same area of Tanzania, Laing (1966) once more assessed the activity of a single-dose treatment, comparing sulfadoxine 1 gm alone against sulfadoxine 500 mg combined with 12.5 mg pyrimethamine. There were 45 patients in each group, all suffering from *P. falciparum* infections. When the sulfonamide alone was used there were seven failures, whereas a single dose of the combined drugs was able to cure all 45 patients; the speed of action is also worth noting, as both the fever and the asexual parasitemia were reduced within 48 hours; this in an area where 25% of the asymptomatic malaria infections did not respond to weekly doses of pyrimethamine.

The effect of the combined drugs against strains of *P. falciparum* resistant to pyrimethamine was now clearly established. In 1968 Laing now working in southeast Asia was able to study the effect of sulfadoxine and pyrimethamine against chloroquine-resistant infections (Laing, 1968). Patients suffering with *P. falciparum* or *P. vivax* malaria were treated in hospital with various schedules including sulfadoxine, sulfadoxine and pyrimethamine, and chloroquine. When used against *P. falciparum* infections a single dose of sulfadoxine 1 gm cured eight out of nine cases although the response was slow (2 to 3 days). Various combinations of the sulfonamide with pyrimethamine were used to treat 49 patients: 200 mg to 1000 mg sulfadoxine combined with 12.5 mg to 50 mg of the pyrimidine. Five patients had not been cleared of parasites by the end of 7 days, although in the successful cases the duration of parasitemia after treatment was only 2.3 days and the fever 2 days.

Eleven out of 36 patients did not respond to treatment with chloroquine used in various dosages ranging from 600 mg in a single dose to a 4-day treatment when 2,580 mg was administered. In three of these cases sulfadoxine 1 gm combined with either 25 mg or 50 mg of pyrimethamine effected a cure within 48 hours. Another patient that had not responded to chloroquine was treated with a single dose of 25 mg of pyrimethamine; this, as was to be expected, had no effect and 3 days later 1 gm of sulfadoxine was given. Because of their long-lasting action in the body, the drugs were obviously able to combine effectively and within 2 days the young man was cured of his malaria.

In the treatment of patients with *P. vivax* infections chloroquine was able successfully to cure all 13 patients treated. Single-dose treatment of 1 gm sulfadoxine had five failures out of 13 cases, while combinations similar to these used for the treatment of *P. falciparum* malaria produced two failures out of 14 cases.

As a result of this trial Laing suggested that, until new antimalarials are available for the treatment of multiresistant *P. falciparum*, a single-dose treatment of sulfadoxine 1 gm plus pyrimethamine 50 mg is superior to any other form of treatment, with possibly the exception of quinine. He further suggested that such a combination should be restricted to radical cure of malaria.

Harinasuta *et al.* (1967) also studied the effects of sulfadoxine alone and in combination with pyrimethamine in patients who did not respond to treatment with chloroquine. The authors state that in Thailand chloroquine resistant *P. falciparum* has become widespread geographically and that resistance has extended to virtually all drugs commonly used to combat malaria. The report was a very good example of a hospital trial and demonstrated that using a combination of the long-acting sulfonamide, sulfadoxine and pyrimethamine for the treatment of chloroquine-resistant malaria the response was rapid, the cure rate high, and there were no obvious toxic side effects. The patients were first treated with chloroquine to demonstrate resistance to the drug; although the fever was controlled, the asexual parasites either persisted in the blood or returned after an initial clearance. Treatment with a single dose of sulfadoxine at 1 gm or 1.5 gm cleared the blood of parasites slowly, and only 11 out of 18 (61%) were cured. A lower dose of sulfadoxine 25 mg combined with 12.5 mg or 25 mg of pyrimethamine cured 11 patients out of 15, but when 1 gm of the sulfonamide was combined with 50 mg of pyrimethamine 17 out of 19 cases were cured. Apart from this much greater rate of cure with the higher dose of drugs, the response was quite rapid, the fever was cleared in just a little more than 24 hours, while the parasites had disappeared from the circulating blood in 2.9 days. Commenting on this work, Bruce-Chwatt (1967) thought it possible that "increasing the single dose of sulfadoxine to

1500/2000 mg and combining with 50 mg pyrimethamine may achieve a slightly higher proportion of radical cures"; Professor Harinasuta and her co-workers regarded this as far from certain.

Reviewing the treatment of chloroquine-resistant strains of *P. falciparum*, Clyde (1967a) favored the use of quinine, if chloroquine therapy fails, and suggests a combination of sulfadoxine 1 gm with pyrimethamine 50 mg as the third choice.

The investigations concerning the use of synergistic mixtures to cure malaria had involved semi-immunes only, but Bartelloni *et al.* (1967) were able to treat non-immune American soldiers. One group of 22 patients had had a clinical recurrence of *P. falciparum* after treatment with chloroquine. Ten received single doses of 50 mg pyrimethamine and 1 gm sulfadoxine; all became free from fever and parasites within 2 to 7 days and remained so for the 63-day observation period. The remaining 12 soldiers received 25 mg pyrimethamine every 8 hours for 3 days given concurrently with 0.5 gm sulfadiazine every 6 hours for 5 days. The fever was controlled in 2 to 8 days but two servicemen suffered a recrudescence after they had left Vietnam. Five nonimmune patients had a clinical cure of their primary infection with the sulfadoxine–pyrimethamine combination. In addition to the greater ease of administration, the overall cure rate of the long-acting sulfonamide when combined with pyrimethamine was far superior to that of sulfadiazine.

Kellett *et al.* (1968) had only one nonimmune serviceman to treat. This soldier had a *P. falciparum* infection acquired in Malaysia which was resistant to chloroquine and quinine. He was treated with 1 gm sulfadoxine plus 50 mg pyrimethamine, after which his fever rapidly subsided and his blood was free of parasites within 48 hours. Twenty-five days later he became ill with a *P. vivax* infection, which was cured with chloroquine and primaquine.

The treatment of drug-resistant malaria with sulfadoxine 1 gm and pyrimethamine 50 mg was recognized by Brooks *et al.* (1969), and used together with a 14-day course of quinine, 650 mg every 8 hours. The results were as previous workers results suggested: a prompt and complete disappearance of parasites. These workers, however, also studied the plasma concentrations and urinary excretion rates of the drugs tested. Sulfadoxine was shown to have a half-life of 200 hours with levels exceeding 8 mg per 100 ml for 4 days. Pyrimethamine plasma concentrations remained relatively stable for at least 14 days. The sustained plasma levels following a single dose was accounted for by a slow rate of urinary excretion. The results, the authors suggest, warrant further investigation.

All the workers using sulfadoxine combined with pyrimethamine have dealt mainly with the effects of a single dose or short courses of treatment. Little had been done about their performance when used for the suppression of malaria over a long period. Lucas *et al.* (1969) studied the prophylactic effect of sulfadoxine or dapsone in combination with pyrimethamine over a period of 1 year. The study was conducted at Ilora, a large Yoruba village, near Ibadan in Western Nigeria. The trial was very well controlled. All the clinical and laboratory investigations throughout the trial were made "blind", only one member of the team having knowledge of the code for the random allocation of drug. Various parameters were examined at intervals during the trial such as height and weight, hemoglobin genotype, packed cell volume, white cell count, spleen size, and urine examination.

The children were randomized into five groups having not less than 50 per group:

A. Control—placebo tablet
B. Pyrimethamine 25 mg
C. Pyrimethamine 12.5 mg + dapsone 100 mg
D. Pyrimethamine 12.5 mg + sulfadoxine 125 mg
E. Pyrimethamine 12.5 mg + sulfadoxine 250 mg

The drugs were administered weekly to all groups, and any child absent from school was visited at home to ensure that the treatment and investigations were not interrupted.

With pyrimethamine alone there was incomplete suppression of parasitemia with a parasite rate varying from 2% to 25%. The first dose of the drug combination sustained a virtually complete suppression parasitemia throughout the year. The drugs were very well tolerated, and no serious side effects were encountered among the treated children (Figs. 3–6, see pages 134–136).

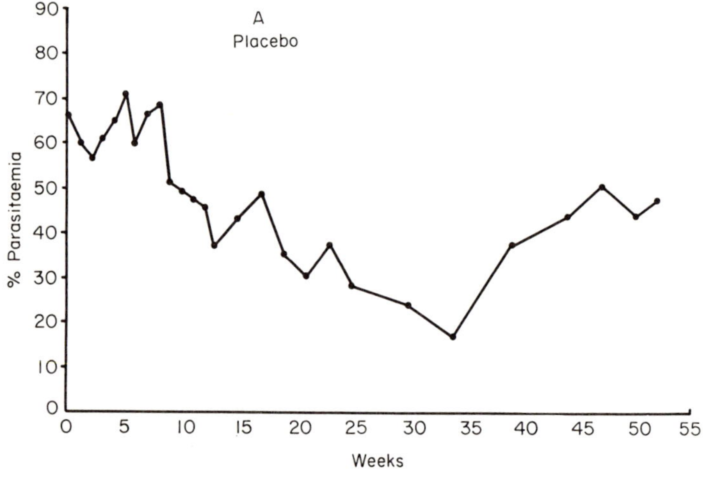

Fig. 3.

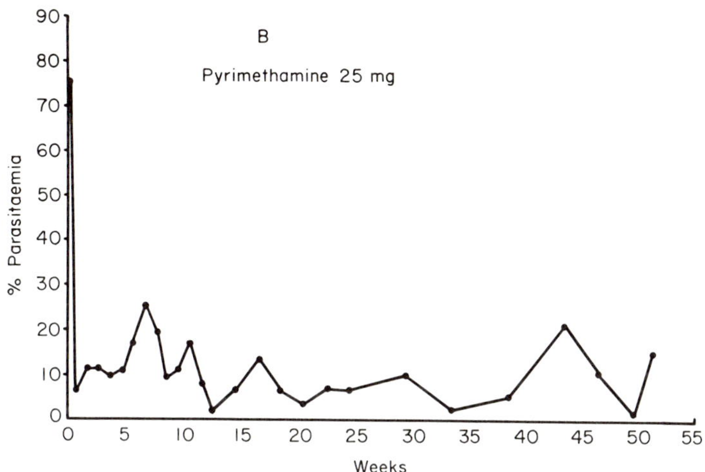

FIG. 4.

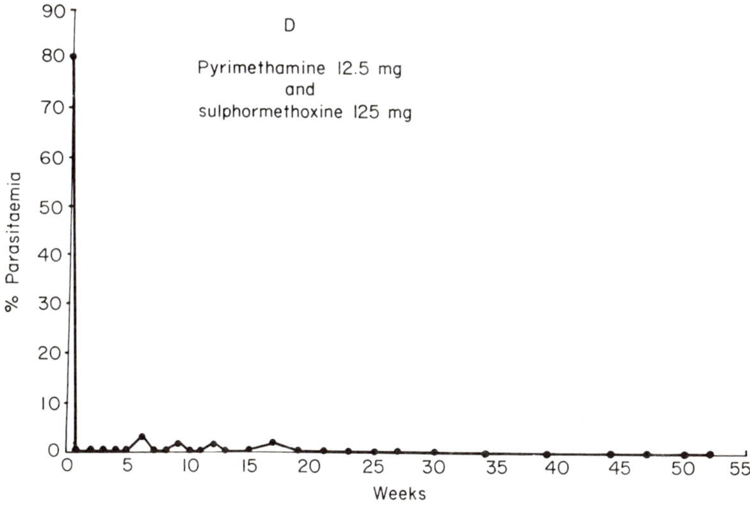

FIG. 5.

FIGS. 3–6 (pages 134–136). The suppressive effect of pyrimethamine and pyrimethamine plus sulformethoxine (sulfadoxine) on parasitemia in children. The frequency of asexual parasitemia in the treated groups is shown. All drugs were given as a single oral dose weekly to all groups. Figure 6 appears on page 136.

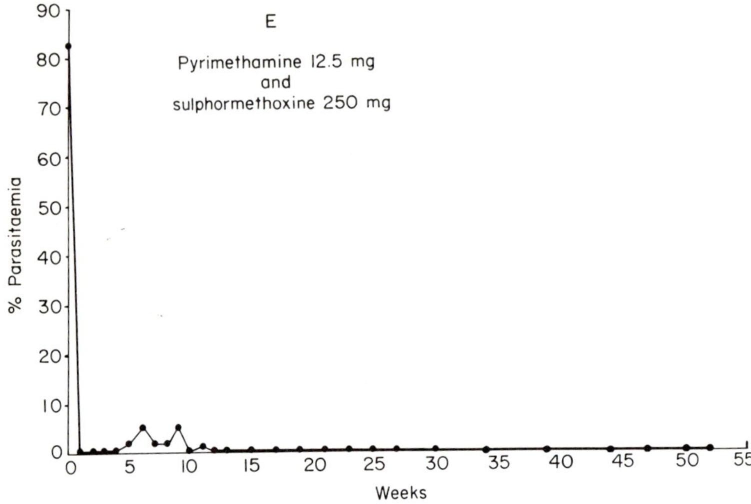

FIG. 6. See caption on page 135.

The persistent parasitemia in the pyrimethamine group in this trial causes some concern about the continued use of this drug alone for mass chemosuppression and at the same time raises the question of suitable alternatives. In the absence of an agreed policy about this matter there is the danger that the uncontrolled use of chloroquine for chemosuppression might result in the emergence of strains less susceptible to the drug. There is therefore an urgent need for further examination of pyrimethamine, in combination with sulfones or sulfadoxine, to determine their place relative to chloroquine in the mass chemosuppression and even in therapy of malaria.

C. SULFALENE

OCH

N

—NH · SO_2—

—NH_2

N

Sulfalene

Another new sulfonamide which has a relatively long plasma half-life is sulfalene, 2-sulfanilamido-3-methoxypyrazine. The therapeutic activity of this compound on *P. falciparum* infections in man has been reported by Baruffa (1966), Mazzoni (1967), and Catarinella (1967).

1. *Sulfalene and Pyrimethamine*

Marubini *et al.* (1968) found that the sulfonamide is active against *P. berghei* in mice and that this compound greatly enhanced the antimalarial action of pyrimethamine in mice. The same potentiation was observed by Aldighieri *et al.* (1968), although they judged the therapeutic result by the ability of the mice to survive for 34 days and not by blood examination. They also reported that a high environmental temperature improves the therapeutic efficiency of this drug treatment.

2. *Sulfalene and Trimethoprim*

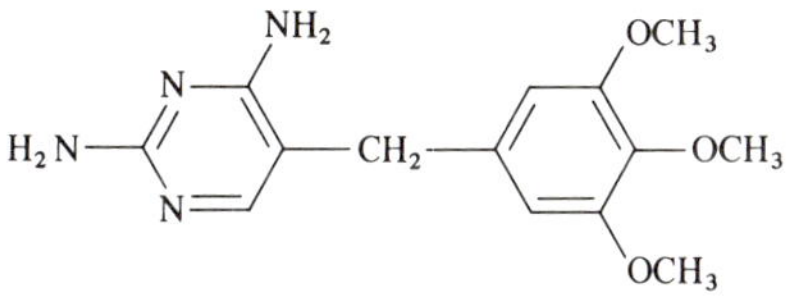

NH_2 OCH_3 N H_2N CH_2 OCH_3 N OCH_3

Trimethoprim

The combination of sulfalene with pyrimethamine received remarkably little attention; this may be due in part to the difference in half-lives of the two compounds, sulfalene being about 65 hours. Another pyrimidine, trimethoprim, has been used in combination with sulfalene, and it has a half-life of only 16 hours. Trimethoprim has been used with sulfonamides as an antibacterial agent; but recently Martin and Arnold (1967) studied its effect on malaria in man. The results suggested to them that, although not active enough on its own it might prove useful when combined with a sulfonamide. This they did, and in 1968 using sulfalene plus trimethoprim they were able successfully to treat infections of the Uganda I strain of *P. falciparum* induced by blood inoculation in human volunteers. They were also able, with a single-dose treatment, to cure 10 out of 11 patients infected with the multidrug-resistant Camp strain of *P. falciparum*, but a larger dose was required, viz., 750 mg sulfalene plus 500 mg trimethoprim. The same authors (Martin and Arnold, 1969) reported on the first trials of the combination of drugs against *P. vivax* in man. The volunteers were all infected by the intravenous injection of parasitized erythrocytes and were treated with dapsone, sulfadoxine, or sulfalene, all of which were ineffective. Trimethoprim, however, even in single doses of 500 mg caused a total and rapid suppression of the parasitemia, and, given daily for 5 days, it cured seven out of eight patients. Two or three doses of trimethoprim, 500 mg and sulfalene 1 gm, were able to produce radical cures in the nine patients studied, but when a single dose treatment was tried 7 out of 12 patients suffered a recrudescence of the infection. The authors state that such a mixture would produce a good clinical response in a mixed infection of *P. falciparum* and *P. vivax*, but the latter is likely to recrudesce unless two additional doses are given. These findings, however, were not corroborated by Clyde (1969a), who studied a recently isolated chloroquine-resistant strain (Poo) of *P. falciparum*. He even used twice the amount of drugs, sulfalene 1.5 gm and trimethoprim 1 gm, and yet two out of the three patients suffered a recrudescence. This is obviously a difficult strain of malaria to cure, and it would be interesting to study the effect of sulfadoxine and pyrimethamine against the infection.

Donno *et al.* (1969) compared the antimalarial activity of sulfalene plus either trimethoprim or pyrimethamine with that of chloroquine in field trials in Nigeria. The chloroquine-treated patients received 25 mg/kg of drug in 48 hours. The remaining groups all received a single dose of sulfalene at 20 mg/kg plus either pyrimethamine, at 0.2 mg/kg or 1 mg/kg, or trimethoprim at 10 mg/kg. All four groups showed a good initial response to treatment, although the parasitemia and fever appeared to be of shorter duration in the groups treated with the sulfonamide–pyrimidine mixture. Five days after treatment only the sulfalene–trimethoprim group were free of parasites. Certainly the combined drugs have an antimalarial effect equal to that of chloroquine. A longer period of observation would obviously have been more beneficial in assessing the results, and the results might have been a little closer if one of the pyrimethamine mixtures had been the accepted 10:1 ratio instead of the 100:1 that was used.

Although the activity of sulfalene and trimethoprim had been established in man against sensitive and drug-resistant strains of malaria, it was confirmed by Roth *et al.* (1969), who studied rhesus monkeys infected with *P. knowlesi*. Seven daily oral doses of 100 mg/kg of trimethoprim or 0.5 mg/kg sulfalene were effective in curing a normally lethal infection. Single doses of 25 mg/kg sulfalene or of 0.5 mg/kg trimethoprim were ineffective but when given as a combined treatment cured all animals. With the dose level used it was not possible to demonstrate strong potentiation but certainly the effect was at least additive.

D. Sulfadiazine

N N —NHSO$_2$— —NH$_2$

Sulfadiazine

A most valuable report by Walker and López-Antuñano (1967) underlines the extent to which chloroquine-resistant strains of *P. falciparum* are spreading in endemic areas of South America. A number of these strains were inoculated into volunteers and the response to drug treatment recorded. Pyrimethamine used on its own had a slow rate of clearance of parasites from the blood, and some patients suffered a recrudescence of the infection; when it was used in combination with sulfonamides all the strains tested were sensitive to treatment. A 4-day treatment with sulfadiazine 8 gm and pyrimethamine 200 mg eliminated the parasitemia in 48 hours, with no recurrence of infection.

Sulfadiazine was also used by Sheehy and Reba (1967) in the treatment of nonimmune American soldiers in Vietnam. The sulfonamide 1.5 gm given over 5 days was combined with 230 mg pyrimethamine in 3 days and 27.3 gm quinine in 14 days; this treatment was able to achieve a radical cure in 57/60 cases but a one- or two-dose treatment would have been more convenient. Sulfadoxine 1 g combined with 50 mg pyrimethamine and the 14-day course of quinine cured 54/55 cases; the one patient who had a recrudescence of his infection was cured after treatment with a further dose of sulfadoxine and 50 mg pyrimethamine. Quinine, the authors state, was used because at that time it was thought that the combination of sulfonamide and pyrimidine would act too slowly; this assumption proved incorrect; the clearance of asexual parasitemia was as rapid with the two drugs as it was with the three schizonticides. It was shown by Rieckmann *et al.* (1968) that, although the Malayan (Camp) strain of *P. falciparum* was cured by 500 mg sulfadiazine every 6 hours for 5 days together with 50 mg pyrimethamine daily for 3 days, this treatment did not exert a demonstrable gametocytocidal effect or a marked sporonticidal effect. Primaquine, however, although ineffective against the blood schizonts did exert a marked gametocytocidal and sporonticidal effect.

Sulfisoxazole (Gantrisin) was chosen by Berman (1969) "because of the ability of sulfonamides to potentiate pyrimethamine." It was difficult to assess the efficacy of the combination, as it was given together with chloroquine. Richards (unpublished results), showed that sulfisoxazole had little or no effect on *P. berghei* or *P. gallinaceum* infections.

E. Dapsone and Pyrimethamine

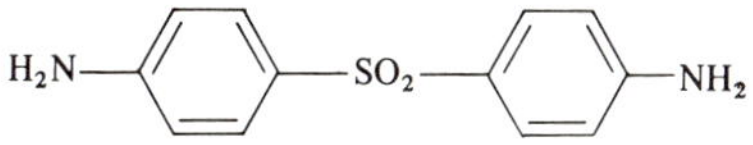

H_2N—⟨benzene ring⟩—SO_2—⟨benzene ring⟩—NH_2

Dapsone

A great deal of the early work using dapsone was done by Indian scientists. Ramakrishnan *et al.* (1963) showed that when the sulfone was given with pyrimethamine a synergistic effect was observed in the treatment of *P.*

gallinaceum. A combination 210 mg/kg of dapsone and 28 mg/kg pyrimethamine, both of which doses were ineffective by themselves, was able to potentiate the sporonticidal activity of pyrimethamine in addition to the schizonticidal activity. Basu *et al.* (1964) also demonstrated a potentiation between the two drugs against *P. gallinaceum* and *P. cynomolgi*. The lack of sporonticidal properties of dapsone used alone against *P. falciparum* infections was shown by Laing (1965b). He also considered that, although not a reliable drug for treating acute malaria, dapsone merits a place in malaria chemotherapy particularly as a potentiator of other drugs such as pyrimethamine. Similar findings were reported by DeGowin *et al.* (1966) and Clyde (1967b).

The real value of dapsone combined with pyrimethamine as a prophylactic was shown by Lucas *et al.* (1969), weekly doses of the combined drugs pyrimethamine 12.5 mg and dapsone 100 mg being sufficient to maintain suppression of infections for the whole period of study (one year). This was demonstrated in an area of Western Nigeria where *P. falciparum* was not completely controlled by pyrimethamine (see Figs. 4 and 7).

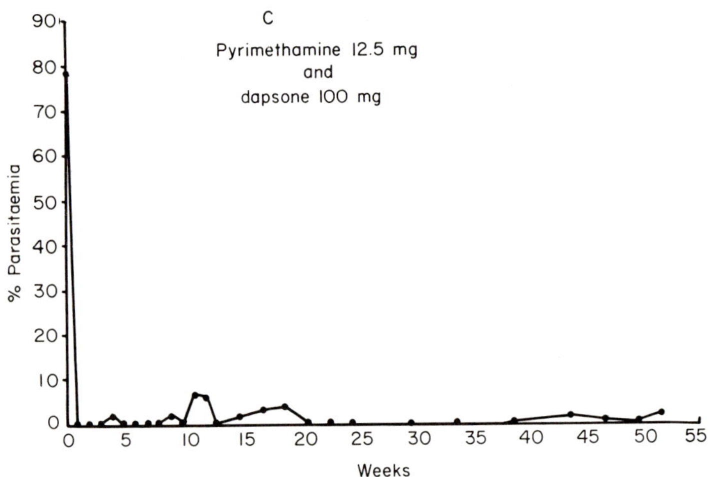

FIG. 7. The suppressive effect of pyrimethamine and pyrimethamine plus dapsone on parasitemia in children. The frequency of asexual parasitemia in the treated groups is shown. The drugs were given as a single oral dose weekly to all groups.

Verdrager *et al.* (1968) realizing that dapsone had antimalarial properties and that it was considerably cheaper than sulfadoxine tried the drug in combination with pyrimethamine in the treatment of Cambodian patients, most of whom were semi-immune. Two patients were given 100 mg or 200 mg dapsone and 50 mg pyrimethamine on one day: three were given one dose of

50 mg pyrimethamine and five daily doses of dapsone 100 mg and ten more were treated with one dose of pyrimethamine and five daily doses of 200 mg dapsone. In 13 out of 15 patients there was an immediate response, but two later relapsed. Further courses did not cure the relapsed patients, neither did they or the two originally resistant cases respond to sulfadoxine–pyrimethamine treatment, and quinine had to be used. The authors considered that for treatment dapsone–pyrimethamine is less effective than, and presents no advantage over, sulfadoxine–pyrimethamine.

F. Other Compounds

Thompson *et al.* (1965) studied the effects of dihydrotriazine and dapsone against experimental malaria infections. Clyde (1969b) notes that such a combination is able to protect against *P. falciparum* strains resistant to pyrimethamine or proguanil but not against similarly resistant *P. vivax*.

V. Toxoplasmosis

The treatment of toxoplasmosis has always proved difficult. Eyles and Coleman (1952, 1953), working with experimental infections in mice, found the organism was resistant to all chemotherapeutic substances except sulfonamides, sulfones, diaminopyrimidines, and aureomycin. The sulfones and aureomycin were of low activity, the sulfonamides little better, and the most effective of the pyrimidines was pyrimethamine. Ryan *et al.* (1954) treated 29 cases of congenital or acquired toxoplasmic choreoretinitis with 75 mg to 100 mg daily together with 0.5 gm to 1.5 sulfadiazine for 10 days. Such high doses caused nausea and had an effect upon hemopoiesis, but rapid recovery of the blood picture followed the cessation of treatment. Clinical evidence of improvement was seen in 25 cases; 17 of them showed obvious clearing of vitreous opacities.

Eyles and Coleman (1955) and later Eyles and Jones (1955), using experimental infections of *T. gondii* in rodents, showed a sixfold potentiation when using pyrimethamine and sulfadiazine in proportions of 22:78 in the diet.

Beverley and Fry (1957a) used sulfadimidine, pyrimethamine, and dapsone in the treatment of rabbits infected with *T. gondii* with doubtful results; but later (Beverley and Fry, 1957b) using mice they were able to show that both the sulfone and the sulfonamide when given together with pyrimethamine were synergistic in their action and able to protect the mice. It is difficult to know how much drug was given, as it was administered in the diet in quantities related to the amount that would arrest the growth of the animals!

A number of sulfones were tested by Eyles and Coleman (1957), and although the drugs were not very active when used alone against *Toxoplasma* infections in mice they were able to potentiate the effect of pyrimethamine.

Two human cases were successfully treated by Kayloe *et al.* (1957), using pyrimethamine 50 mg followed by 25 mg in 6 hours and 25 mg daily for 20 days together with triple sulfonamides, sulfadiazine, sulfamerazine and sulfamethazine, 1 gm every 4 hours, the blood level being maintained at 6.9 mg to 8.6 mg per 100 ml.

Following an accidental laboratory infection in a young woman, Frenkel *et al.* (1960) treated the patient with 25 mg pyrimethamine and 4 gm sulfadiazine daily. A rapid defervescence of fever followed the initiation of treatment, but 18 days later supplemental folic and folinic acid in the form of yeast had to be given to correct the blood picture. The cure was complete, as far as could be ascertained.

VI. Coccidiosis

The most important distinction between treating human infections and animal diseases is one of cost. A farmer has to relate the cost of treatment to that of his profit margin. Therefore, expensive compounds are not used for routine therapy. Several workers have found that synergistic mixtures of certain sulfonamides and pyrimethamine are effective against *Eimeria tenella* infections in chicks (Lux, 1954; Kendall, 1956; Kendall and Joyner, 1956a,b; Arundel, 1957; Ball, 1960). Ball (1964), using a diet mixture containing 0.01% each of sulfaquinoxaline and 2-amino-4-dimethylamino-5-(4-chlorophenyl)-6-ethyl pyrimidine, obtained good control of *E. tenella* infections in chicks. The mixture showed good potentiation between the two compounds.

Dapsone has also been studied for its effect against coccidiosis, and Ball and Warren (1965a) showed that inactive concentrations of dapsone 0.025% and pyrimethamine 0.005% in diet when mixed together could prevent mortality and morbidity from severe *E. tenella* infections in chicks.

A mixture containing 0.008% w/w sulfaquinoxaline and 0.001% w/w diaveridine, 2,4-diamino-5(3,4-dimethoxybenzyl) pyrimidine, in the food, was shown by Clarke (1962, 1964) to be effective in preventing infections caused by *E. tenella*, *E. necatrix*, *E. acervulina*, *E. brunetti*, or *E. maxima*, when medication was started before infection. Ball and Warren (1965b) used the same compounds in regimes likely to be suitable in practice. The medication was given in the drinking water as a solution containing sulfaquinoxaline 0.005% and diaveridine 0.0043%. Five days of treatment, beginning no later than 3 days after infection of chicks with *E. acervulina*, prevented the passage of oocysts until after the end of treatment. Good therapeutic control against. *E necatrix* was demonstrated only if treatment was not delayed for more than 2 days after infection and 3 days for *E. tenella*.

VII. Conclusions

The ability of sulfonamides to potentiate the antiprotozoal activity of pyrimidines has been recognized since 1949. The main interest at that period of time was concerned not so much with any practical application but with obtaining a greater knowledge of the mode of action of the compounds and why they proved synergistic when used in combination. The emergence of chloroquine-resistant strains of malaria demonstrated the lack of drugs available to combat the disease.

Strains of *P. falciparum* had now been shown to be resistant to all the major antimalarials, and new compounds are urgently needed.

The newer long-acting sulfonamides, produced in the early 1960's, with their extended plasma levels were able to match that of the pyrimidines and give a combination which was synergistic in its action. They were effective against normal and drug-resistant strains given in a single-dose treatment. Sulfones, especially dapsone, have been carefully reexamined and shown to possess the ability to potentiate pyrimethamine. Various workers have shown the efficacy of the combination of long-acting sulfonamides or sulfone and pyrimidines against experimental and human malarias.

A report of the W.H.O. Scientific Group on Chemotherapy of Malaria (World Health Organization, 1967) recognized the value of the therapeutic use of sulfadoxine and pyrimethamine for the treatment of *P. falciparum* infections resistant to 4-aminoquinolines, but the group could not yet recommend the combination of the two drugs either for prophylaxis or mass administration. There is no doubt that a combination of sulfadoxine or sulfalene in combination with pyrimethamine or trimethoprim is effective, and their use in the treatment of acute plasmodial infections would allow more time for research organizations to discover and develop more antimalarials.

The use of dapsone and pyrimethamine for prophylactic therapy in malarious areas must surely be the method of choice. It has been shown to be highly effective against not only normal but drug-resistant strains, it has no record of toxicity or adverse side effects, and it is reasonably cheap, a very important factor in mass administration of a drug.

There is obviously a risk of developing drug resistance to any drug or combination of drugs. Peters (1969) postulates that it is only a matter of time before chloroquine loses its effectiveness even in Africa and that "by the very nature of things" whatever new drug is developed it will be only a matter of time before the parasites are able to overcome that too. As experimental evidence, Richards (1968) suggests that resistance develops much more slowly when a sulfone or sulfonamide is used in combination with a pyrimidine than when either compound is used singly. If this proves to be the case when used against human infections, then this alone is a good reason for the use of such combinations. More work has still to be done, not only against malaria, but against all other infections where sulfonamides, sulfones, or pyrimidines are active and where combinations of the drugs should prove beneficial.

References

Aldighieri, J., Dupoux, R., Quilici, M., and Sautet, J. (1968). *Bull. Soc. Pathol. Exot.* **61** (5), 765–768.

Archibald, H. M. (1951). *Brit. Med. J.* **ii**, 821–823.

Archibald, H. M., and Ross, C. M. (1960). *J. Trop. Med. Hyg.* **63** (2), 25–27.

Ardias, A. (1948). *Arch. Ital. Sci. Med. Colon. Parassitol.* **29** (7/8), 115–133.

Arundel, J. H. (1957). *Aust. Vet. J.* **33**, 256–263.

Aviado, D. M., Singh, G., and Berkley, R. (1969). *Chemotherapy* **14**, 37–53.

Ball, S. J. (1960). *J. Comp. Pathol.* **70**, 249–256.

Ball, S. J. (1964). *J. Comp. Pathol.* **74** (4), 487–499.

Ball, S. J. and Warren, E. W. (1965a). *Vet. Rec.* **77**, 1028–1030.

Ball, S. J., and Warren, E. W. (1965b). *Vet. Rec.* **77**, 1252–1256.

Bartelloni, P. J., Sheehy, T. W., and Tiggert, W. D. (1967). *J. Amer. Med. Ass.* **199**, 173–177.

Baruffa, G. (1966). *Trans. Roy. Soc. Trop. Med. Hyg.* **60**, 222–224.

Basford, F. R., Curd, F. H. S., Hoggarth, E., and Rose, F. L. (1947). *J. Chem. Soc., London* pp. 1354–1364.

Basu, P. C., Mondal, M. M., and Chakrabarti, S. C. (1962). *Indian J. Malariol.* **16**, 157–175.

Basu, P. C., Singh, N. N., and Singh, N. (1964). *Bull. W. H. Org.* **31** (5), 699–705.

Berman, S. J. (1969). *J. Amer. Med. Ass.* **207**, 128–130.

Beverley, J. K. A., and Fry, B. A. (1957a). *Brit. J. Pharmacol. Chemother.* **12** (2), 185–188.

Beverley, J. K. A., and Fry, B. A. (1957b). *Brit. J. Pharmacol. Chemother.* **12** (2), 189–193.

Brooks, M. H., Malloy, J. P., Bartelloni, P. J., Sheehy, T. W., and Barry, K. G. (1969). *Clin. Pharmacol. Ther.* **10** (1), 85–91.

Bruce-Chwatt, L. J. (1967). *Lancet* **ii**, 216.

Buttle, G. A. H., Stephenson, D., Smith, S., Dewing, T., and Foster, G. E. (1937). *Lancet* **i**, 1331–1334.

Catarinella, G. (1967). *Gazz. Med. Ital.* **126**, 474–476.

Chin, W., Contacos, P. G., Coatney, G. R., and King, H. K. (1966). *Amer. J. Trop. Med. Hyg.* **15** (6), 823–829.

Chopra, R. N. (1939). *Indian Med. Gaz.* **74**, 658–660.

Chopra, R. N., and Das Gupta, B. M. (1938). *Indian Med. Gaz.* **73**, 395–396.

Chopra, R. N., and Das Gupta, B. M. (1939). *Indian Med. Gaz.* **74**, 201–202.

Chopra, R. N., Das Gupta, B. M., Sen, B., and Hayter, R. T. M. (1939). *Indian Med. Gaz.* **74**, 321–324.

Clarke, M. L. (1962). *Vet. Rec.* **74**, 845–849.

Clarke, M. L. (1964). *Vet. Rec.* **76**, 818–823.

Clyde, D. F. (1967a). *East Afr. Med. J.* **44** (6), 231–237.

Clyde, D. F. (1967b). *Amer. J. Trop. Med. Hyg.* **16** (1), 7–10.

Clyde, D. .F. (1969a). *J. Amer. Med. Ass.* **209**, 563.

Clyde, D. F. (1969b). *J. Trop. Med. Hyg.* **74** (4), 81–85.

Coatney, G. R., Clark Cooper, W., Young, M. D., and McLendon, S. B. (1947). *Amer. J. Hyg.* **46**, 84–104.

Cochrane, R. G., Ramanujam, K., Paul, H., and Russel, D. (1949). *Leprosy Rev.* **20** (4), 64–108.
Coggeshall, L. T. (1938a). *Proc. Soc. Exp. Biol. Med.* **38**, 768–773.
Coggeshall, L. T. (1938b). *Amer. J. Trop. Med.* **18**, 715–721.
Coggeshall, L. T. (1940). *J. Exp. Med.* **71**, 13–20.
Coggeshall, L. T., Maier, J., and Best, C. A. (1941). *J. Amer. Med. Ass.* **117**, 1077–1081.
Colebrook, L., Buttle, G. A. H., and O'Meara, R. A. Q. (1936). *Lancet* **ii**, 1323–1326.
Costa, F. C. (1960). *An. Inst. Med. Trop. Lisbon*, **17**, 737–752.
Curd, F. H. S., Richardson, D. N., and Rose, F. L. (1946). *J. Chem. Soc., London* pp. 378–384.
DeGowin, R. L., and Powell, R. D. (1964). *J. Lab. Clin. Med.* **64**, 851–852.
DeGowin, R. L., Eppes, R. B., Carson, P. E., and Powell, R. D. (1966). *Bull. W. H. Org.* **34**, 671–681.
Díaz de León, A. (1937). *Bol. Ofic. Sanit. Panamer.* **16**, 1039–1040.
Díaz de León, A. (1938). *Med. Mex.* **18**, 89–90.
Díaz de León, A. (1940). *Med. Mex.* **20**, 551–558.
Donno, L., Sanguineti, V., Ricciardi, M. L., and Soldati, M. (1969). *Amer. J. Trop. Med. Hyg.* **18**, 182–187.
Eyles, D. E., and Coleman, N. (1952). *Pub. Health Rep.* **67**, 249–252.
Eyles, D. E., and Coleman, N. (1953). *Antibiot. Chemother.* **3**, 483–490.
Eyles, D. E., and Coleman, N. (1955). *Antibiot. Chemother.* **5**, 529–539.
Eyles, D. E., and Coleman, N. (1957). *Antibiot. Chemother.* **7** (11), 577–585.
Eyles, D. E., and Jones, F. E. (1955). *Antibiot. Chemother.* **5**, 731–734.
Fairley, N. H. (1945). *Trans. Roy. Soc. Trop. Med. Hyg.* **38**, 311–365.
Falco, E. A., Hitchings, G. H., Russell, P. B., and Vanderwerff, H. (1949). *Nature (London)* **164**, 107–108.
Falco, E. A., Goodwin, L. G., Hitchings, G. H., Rollo, I. M., and Russell, P. B. (1951). *Brit. J. Pharmacol. Chemother.* **6** (2), 185–200.
Farinaud, M. E., and Eliche, J. (1939). *Bull. Soc. Pathol. Exot.* **32**, 674–681.
Farinaud, M. E., and Ragiot, C. H. (1938). *Bull. Soc. Pathol. Exot.* **31**, 907–910.
Findlay, G. M., Maegraith, B. G., Markson, J. L., and Holden, J. R. (1946). *Ann. Trop. Med. Parasitol.* **40**, 358–367.
Foy, H., and Kondi, A. (1952). *Trans. Roy. Soc. Trop. Med. Hyg.* **46**, 370.
Frenkel, J. K., and Jacobs, L. (1958). *AMA Arch. Ophthalmol.* **59**, 260–279.
Frenkel, J. K., Weber, R. W., and Lund, M. N. (1960). *J. Amer. Med. Ass.* **173**, 1471–1476.
Goodwin, L. G. (1949). *Nature (London)* **164**, 1133.
Greenberg, J. (1949). *J. Pharmacol. Exp. Ther.* **97**, 238–242.
Greenberg, J., and Richeson, E. M. (1950). *J. Pharmacol. Exp. Ther.* **99**, 444–449.
Greenberg, J., and Richeson, E. M. (1951). *Proc. Soc. Exp. Biol. Med.* **77** (1), 174–176.
Hackett, L. W. (1937). "Malaria in Europe: An Ecological Study." Oxford Univ. Press, London.
Harinasuta, T., Viravan, C., and Reid, H. A. (1967). *Lancet* **i**, 1117–1119.
Hill, R. A., and Goodwin, H. M., Jr. (1937). *5th Med. J. Nashville* **30**, 1170–1172.
Hitchings, G. H. (1960). *Clin. Pharmacol. Ther.* **1**, 570–589.
Hitchings, G. H. (1962). *In* "Drugs, Parasites and Hosts" (L. G. Goodwin, and R. H. Nimmo-Smith, eds.), pp. 196–210. Churchill, London.
Hitchings, G. H., and Bushby, S. R. M. (1963). *Proc. 5th Int. Congr. Biochem., Moscow, 1961*, p. 165.
Hitchings, G. H., Elion, G. B., Vanderwerff, H., and Falco, E. A. (1948). *J. Biol. Chem.* **174**, 765–766.

Hurley, M. G. D. (1959). *Trans. Roy. Soc. Trop. Med. Hyg.* **53**, 412–413.

Jaswant Singh, Ray, A. P., Misra, B. G., and Basu, P. C. (1952). *Indian J. Malariol.* **6**, 441.

Kayloe, D. E., Jacobs, L., Beye, H. K., and McCullough, N. B. (1957). *New Engl. J. Med.* **257** (26), 1247–1254.

Kellett, R. J., Cowan, G. O., and Parry, E. S. (1968). *Lancet* **ii**, 946–948.

Kendall, S. B. (1956). *Proc. Roy. Soc. Med.* **49**, 874–877.

Kendall, S. B., and Joyner, L. P. (1956a). *Vet. Rec.* **68**, 119–121.

Kendall, S. B., and Joyner, L. P. (1956b). *J. Comp. Pathol.* **66**, 145–150.

Laing, A. B. G. (1964). *Brit. Med. J.* **ii**, 1439–1440.

Laing, A. B. G. (1965a). *Brit. Med. J.* **i**, 905–907.

Laing, A. B. G. (1965b). *J. Trop. Med. Hyg.* **68**, 251–253.

Laing, A. B. G. (1966). *Bull. W. Org.* **34** (2), 308–311.

Laing, A. B. G. (1968). *Med. J. Malaya* **23** (1), 5–19.

Leiker, D. L. (1956). *Leprosy Rev.* **27**, 66–69.

Long, P. H. (1950). *Int. J. Lepr.* **18**, 247.

Lucas, A. O., Hendrickse, R. G., Okubadejo, O. A., Richards, W. H. G., Neal, R. A., and Kofie, B. A. K. (1969). *Trans. Roy. Soc. Trop. Med. Hyg.* **63** (2), 216–229.

Lux, R. E. (1954). *Antibiot. Chemother.* **4**, 971–977.

Maberti, S. (1960). *Archos Venez. Med. Trop. Parasitol. Med.* **3**, 239–259.

McGregor, I. A., and Smith, D. A. (1952). *Brit. Med. J.* **i**, 730–732.

McGregor, I. A., Williams, K., and Goodwin, L. G. (1963). *Brit. Med. J.* **ii**, 728–729.

Mackerras, M. J., and Ercole, Q. N. (1947). *Trans. Roy. Soc. Trop. Med. Hyg.* **41**, 365–376.

Maier, J., and Riley, E. (1942). *Proc. Soc. Exp. Biol. Med.* **50**, 152–154.

Martin, D. C., and Arnold, J. D. (1967). *J. Clin. Pharmacol. J. New Drugs* **7**, 336–341.

Martin, D. C., and Arnold, J. D. (1968). *J. Amer. Med. Ass.* **203**, 476–480.

Martin, D. C., and Arnold, J. D. (1969). *J. Clin. Pharmacol. J. New Drugs* **9**, 155–159.

Marubini, E., Soldati, M., and Ghione, M. (1968). *Chemotherapy* **13**, 232–241.

Mazzoni, P. (1967). *Panminerva Med.* **9**, 139–141.

Menk, W., and Mohr, W. (1939). *Arch. Schiffs- Tropen-Hyg.* **43**, 117–125.

Moore, D. V., and Lanier, J. E. (1961). *Amer. J. Trop. Med. Hyg.* **10**, 5–9.

Niven, J. C. (1938). *Trans. Roy. Soc. Trop. Med. Hyg.* **32**, 413–418.

Patrono, V. (1943). *G. Med. Mil.* **417**, 427–437.

Peters, W. (1968). *Ann. Trop. Med. Parasitol.* **62** (4), 488–493.

Peters, W. (1969). *Trans. Roy. Soc. Trop. Med. Hyg.* **63** (1), 25–40.

Ramakrishnan, S. P., Basu, P. C., Singh, H., and Singh, N. (1962). *Bull. W. H. Org.* **27** (2), 213–221.

Ramakrishnan, S. P., Basu, P. C., Harwant, S., and Wattal, B. L. (1963). *Indian J. Malariol.* **17**, 141–148.

Richards, W. H. G. (1966). *Nature* (*London*) **212**, 1494.

Richards, W. H. G. (1968). *MRC* (*Med. Res. Counc.* (*Gt. Brit.*)), *Malaria Semin., London.*

Rieckmann, K. H., McNamara, J. V., Frischer, H., Stockert, T. A., Carson, P. E., and Powell, R. D. (1968). *Bull. W. H. Org.* **38**, 625–632.

Rollo, I. M. (1955). *Brit. J. Pharmacol. Chemother.* **10** (2), 208–214.

Rollo, I. M. (1964). *In* "Biochemistry and Physiology of Protozoa" (S. H. Hutner, ed.), Vol. 3, pp. 525–561. Academic Press, New York.

Roth, W. E., Jacobus, D. P., and Walter, W. G. (1969). *Amer. J. Trop. Med. Hyg.* **18** (4), 491–494.

Ryan, R. W., Hart, W. M., Culligan, J. J., Gunkel, R. D., Jacobs, L., and Cook, M. K. (1954). *Trans. Amer. Acad. Ophthalmol. Otolaryngol.* **58**, 867.

Sadun, E. H. (1964). *Amer. J. Trop. Med.* **13**, Suppl., 145–146.

Sheehy, T. W., and Reba, R. A. (1967). *Ann. Intern. Med.* **66** (3), 616–622.

Shute, P. G., and Maryon, M. (1948). *Parasitology* **38**, 264–270.

Sinton, J. A., Hutton, E. L., and Shute, P. G. (1939). *Ann. Trop. Med. Parasitol.* **33**, 37–44.

Sorley, E. R., and Currie, J. G. (1938). *J. Roy Nav. Med. Serv.* **24**, 322–325.

Srivastava, R. S., Chakrabarti, A. K., and Mukherjee, S. K. (1953). *Indian J. Malariol.* **7**, 5–12.

Tarabini, G., and Secreto, E. (1945). *Boll. Soc. Med.- Chir Modena* **1**, 19–31.

Thompson, P. E., Oiszewski, B., and Waitz, J. A. (1965). *Amer. J. Trop. Med. Hyg.* **14**, 343–353.

Thurston, J. P. (1950). *Brit. J. Pharmacol. Chemother.* **5**, 409–416.

Thurston, J. P. (1954). *Parasitology* **44**, 99–110.

Tréfouël, J., Tréfouël, J., Nitti, F., and Bovet, D. (1935). *C. R. Soc. Biol.* **120**, 756–758.

Van der Weilen, Y. (1937). *Ned. Tijdschr. Geneesk*, **81**, 2905–2906.

Verdrager, J., Riche, A., and Chhoeum Mun Chheang (1968). *Med. Trop.* (*Marseilles*) **28** (5), 663–671.

Walker, A. J., and López-Antuñano, F. J. (1967). Pan American Health Organization Malaria Eradication Branch Report.

Woods, D. D. (1940). *Brit. J. Exp. Pathol.* **21**, 74–90.

World Health Organization (1967). *World Health Organ. Tech. Rep. Ser.* No. 375.

Chemotherapeutic Compounds Affecting DNA Structure and Function

B. A. NEWTON

Medical Research Council Biochemical Parasitology Unit
The Molteno Institute, University of Cambridge
Cambridge, England

I. Introduction

Our understanding of drug action can never be in advance of our knowledge of the biochemistry of cells and organisms.

During the last 15 years we have seen a more rapid advance in knowledge of cell structure and metabolism than in any previous period and many gaps in our understanding of the processes of growth and cell division have been filled. In parallel with this advance there has been an increase in our knowledge of the mechanisms of action of chemotherapeutic agents so that, in some cases, it is now possible to identify a specific enzyme or cell component as the primary site of a drug's action. Perhaps one of the most striking, and unexpected, findings to come from studies on the mechanism of drug action is that a number of antibiotics and synthetic drugs do not act by inhibiting a reaction, or combining with a cell component which is unique to a particular microorganism, but block such universal processes as the synthesis of proteins or nucleic acids. In the case of some drugs, which inhibit the replication of DNA or interfere with its function, there is now good evidence that they achieve their effect by combining with DNA itself, rather than with sites on DNA-dependent polymerases or by blocking the synthesis of nucleic acid precursors. It is with some of these compounds that the present review is concerned.

In the last 5 years there have been many reports of the interaction of drugs and antibiotics, often of unknown structure, with nucleic acids. It must be emphasized at the outset that the author has made no attempt to produce a comprehensive review of such studies. The discussion which follows has been limited to compounds whose structure has been unequivocally established and whose interaction with DNA has been critically studied. The compounds discussed have also been selected to illustrate different types of binding to DNA.

Identification of DNA as the primary binding site of a chemotherapeutic agent and the discovery that the drug selectively interferes with the synthesis or function of this nucleic acid *in vivo* does not, of course, mean that the investigator of drug action has achieved his goal. These findings immediately pose new questions, the most important of which are: Why are drugs which bind to DNA effective chemotherapeutic agents? What is the basis of their selective toxicity? How do organisms become resistant to such drugs? In no case can we provide complete answers to these questions. Some antibiotics and drugs which are known to interact with DNA *in vivo* are so generally cytotoxic that they have little practical value as chemotherapeutic agents. Others, such as the phenanthridinium compounds and certain aminoquinoline derivatives, are vital drugs in the present day control and treatment of diseases such as trypanosomiasis and malaria. As yet we know little about the basis of the selective activity of these compounds but recent work, which will be discussed, is beginning to throw some light on this question.

II. Combination with DNA by Intercalation

A. Acridines and Phenanthridines

The historical association between acridine and phenanthridine drugs in present-day use and Paul Ehrlich's pioneer work on chemotherapy is too well known to be discussed at length here. Investigations of the chemotherapeutic properties of dyestuffs which led to the development of today's trypanocidal and antimalarial drugs and studies on the relationships between the structure and biological activity of these compounds have been the subject of many comprehensive reviews (e.g., see Williamson, 1962; Browning, 1964; Hawking, 1963; Albert, 1968).

The first of these compounds to attract attention on biological grounds was Ehrlich's "trypaflavin" (I) (Ehrlich and Benda, 1913). Half a century later the same compound, in the form of its base (proflavine II) was studied

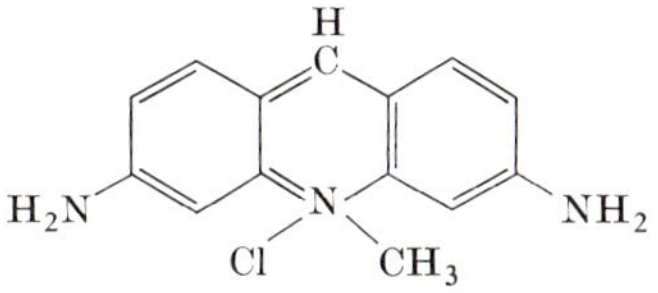

H C H₂N N NH₂ Cl CH₃

(I)

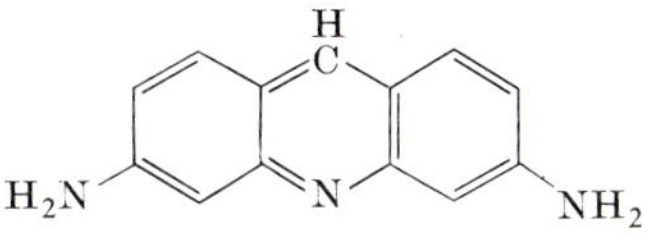

H C H₂N N NH₂

(II)

by Lerman (1963). His work provided the kind of information that is sought by all investigators of drug action, namely, how the geometry and stereochemistry of a drug molecule combine to give a structure which precisely fits into and disorganizes the function of a "biological molecule" (in this case DNA).

The phenanthridine nucleus (III) is isomeric and analogous to acridine, and Morgan and Walls (1931) directed attention to the possibility that derivatives of this substance might be useful trypanocides. Their work

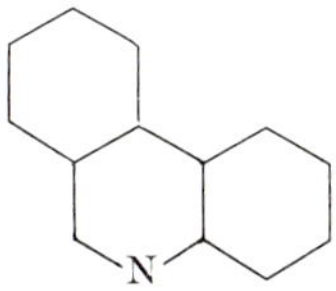

N

(III)

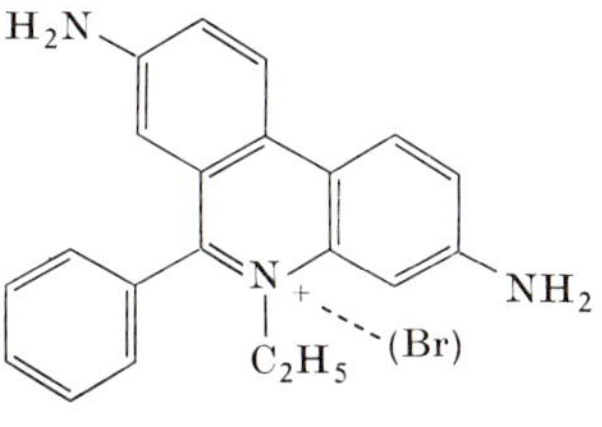

H_2N N+ NH_2 C_2H_5 (Br)

(IV)

triggered off a program of research which is still being pursued and which has yielded a number of valuable drugs such as ethidium (homidium) bromide (IV). We know now that ethidium interacts with DNA in a very similar way to proflavine (Waring, 1964).

The ability of acridines and phenanthridines to interact with nucleic acids has long been known. McIlwain (1941) found that the antibacterial action of amino acridines is annulled by nucleic acid and Seaman and Woodbine (1953) have reported a similar effect for phenanthridine drugs. Albert and co-workers (1945, 1949) showed that the antimicrobial activity of both types of compound is dependent upon their existence as cations and can be correlated with the "area of flatness" of the molecules. This requirement for planarity can now be explained in terms of the interaction of these compounds with DNA.

The Intercalation Hypothesis

As a result of studies on the complex formed between proflavine and purified DNA, Lerman (1961) proposed that planar heterocyclic molecules such as acridines can intercalate between adjacent base pairs in the DNA double helix. He observed that the combination of proflavine with DNA resulted in an increased viscosity of DNA solutions, a decreased sedimentation coefficient, and a change in the X-ray diffraction patterns of the DNA. To explain these changes Lerman suggested that interaction between such a drug molecule and DNA resulted in a local unwinding of the double helix so that a space, large enough to accommodate a single drug molecule, was produced between the stacked base pairs (Fig. 1). Such unwinding of the

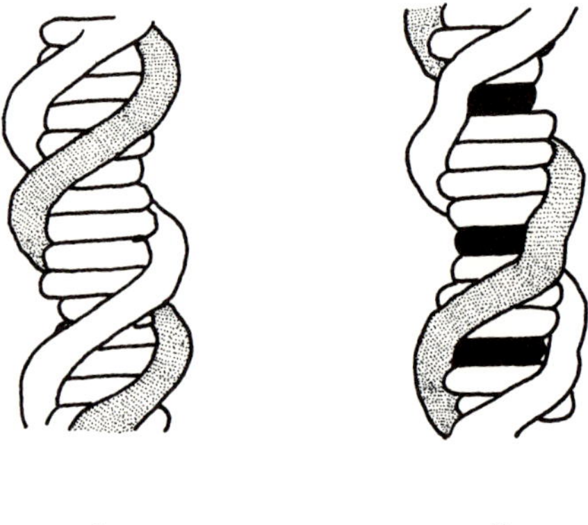

FIG. 1. Intercalation of drug molecules into DNA. (A) A diagram to illustrate the secondary structure of normal DNA. (B) A distorted DNA structure resulting from intercalation of drug molecules. (Based on original drawings by Lerman, 1964).

helix can be achieved without affecting the hydrogen bonding between bases, and the orientation of the base pairs perpendicular to the axis of the helix is maintained. A proflavine molecule intercalated in this way also lies in a plane perpendicular to the helix axis, and it has been calculated that the space it occupies, about 3.4 Å, is equivalent to the normal distance between successive base pairs. Thus, an unwinding of the helix and insertion of a drug molecule results in the base pairs above and below this drug molecule becoming separated by twice their normal distance. According to Lerman (1964) the helix has to be uncoiled by a turn of 36 degrees to permit the insertion of a proflavine molecule. Similar calculations by Fuller and Waring (1964) for the insertion of a phenanthridine molecule indicated that in this case an unwinding of only 12 degrees is necessary.

Intercalated drug molecules are thought to be held firmly in position by strong electronic interactions with base pairs above and below the drug. It is also possible that, in the case of drug molecules containing amino groups, hydrogen bonding may occur between these groups and the charged oxygen atoms in the adjacent phosphate groups of the polynucleotide (Fuller and Waring, 1964). Certainly the combination of both acridines and phenanthridines with double-stranded DNA results in a stabilization of the helix as judged by the temperature required to denature the molecule. Lerman (1964) found that the increase in T_m (the midpoint in the thermal transition of helical to coiled DNA) is directly proportional to the logarithm of the acridine concentration. Presumably this increase in melting temperature of drug-treated DNA corresponds to the extra energy needed to dissociate the bound drug molecules from the helix in addition to separating the polynucleotide strands of the DNA molecule.

Clearly, an unwinding of the DNA helix, as suggested in Lerman's hypothesis, must result in an extension of the molecule. Direct evidence of this was obtained by Cairns (1962) soon after the publication of Lerman's results. In Cairn's experiment bacteriophage T_2 DNA was labeled with thymine-^{3}H and then treated with proflavine. Autoradiographs were prepared and measurement of control and proflavine-treated DNA molecules revealed that the drug-treated molecules were longer than molecules in control preparations. Cairns also observed that the density of silver grains per unit length of the DNA was lower in autoradiographs of molecules containing proflavine. An increase in length, as observed in these experiments could explain the changes in viscosity, sedimentation coefficient, and X-ray diffraction produced by the combination of proflavine with DNA.

Further evidence in support of the intercalation hypothesis has come from a number of different approaches. Luzzati *et al.* (1961) used a low-angle X-ray scattering technique to detect a decrease in mass per unit length of DNA when combined with proflavine. The measured decrease was found to agree with estimates based on the intercalation model. Lerman (1963), from measurements of flow dichroism, obtained evidence that the planes of purine and pyrimidine bases in DNA remain perpendicular to the helix axis after combination with acridine and that the bound acridine molecules are parallel to the bases. Measurements of the fluorescence of DNA–drug complexes (Lerman, 1963; Le Pecq *et al.*, 1964) also indicate that drug molecules are orientated in positions perpendicular to the helix axis.

Intercalation of the type proposed in Lerman's model would be expected to shield the drug molecule from the surrounding medium and, in the case of proflavine, protect the amino groups from attack by reagents such as nitrous acid. Such protection was observed by Lerman (1964) when he measured the diazotization rates of proflavine free in solution or bound to DNA. He found that combination with a number of polyanions reduced the reactivity of proflavine amino groups but the reduction in the presence of DNA was greater than with any other polymer studied.

Direct evidence of uncoiling of the DNA helix in the presence of ethidium bromide has been obtained by Crawford and Waring (1967). These workers used DNA from polyoma virus, which is a circular supercoiled molecule (Vinograd *et al.*, 1965), and measured its sedimentation coefficient in the presence of increasing amounts of ethidium bromide. They found that the sedimentation coefficient of the DNA–drug complex fell, reached a minimum and then increased again as increasing amounts of drug became bound. Supercoiling is thought to occur in circular molecules in which the two complimentary strands of DNA are twisted round each other to either a greater or lesser extent than is required to form a stable Watson-Crick helix (Vinograd *et al.*, 1965). This results in the molecule developing supercoils which are superimposed upon the circular double helical structure in an attempt to attain a stable form. Supercoiled molecules are more compact than molecules lacking supercoils and consequently sediment faster. In the case of polyoma DNA, Crawford and Waring (1967) conclude that supercoiling results from a strain imposed by a deficiency of turns: they believe that as drug molecules are bound this strain is lessened and the number of supercoils diminishes until, at a certain ratio of drug to DNA, the untwisting caused by the bound drug just balances the initial shortage of turns in the circular DNA double helix. At this point the sedimentation coefficient will be at a minimum, and then as further drug is bound the circular molecule will become strained in the opposite sense causing supercoils to reappear and the sedimentation coefficient to increase again.

The results which have been outlined provide considerable evidence in favor of the intercalation hypothesis; nevertheless, acridines and phenanthridines can bind to DNA in another way. Intercalation is a first order reaction which reaches equilibrium when one molecule of proflavine per

4 or 5 nucleotides has been bound. Further drug can be bound by a weaker, higher order process that leads to the fixation of one molecule of proflavine per nucleotide (Peacocke and Skerrett, 1956). This secondary binding, which is thought to consist of an adsorption of acridine molecules onto those already bound by intercalation, is a relatively weak binding in which the drug molecules are probably "stacked" on the surface of the nucleic acid (Stone and Bradley, 1961). The secondary binding results eventually in an electrically neutral complex being formed which precipitates from solution. It seems possible that secondary binding may have contributed to the results described by Mason and McCaffery (1964), which are at variance with the intercalation hypothesis. These workers studied a DNA–acridine orange complex and measured circular dichroism bands in molecules partially aligned by flow. Their results indicated that the dye molecules were organized into a left-handed super helix and were not oriented perpendicular to the helix axis as suggested by Lerman (1961). On the other hand, these findings are difficult to interpret because the complexes used contained one dye molecule per base pair, and thus only about half of the total dye bound would be expected to be intercalated, the remainder presumably being "stacked" on the surface of the nucleic acid.

Although the general concept of intercalation now seems to be well supported by experimental findings it is perhaps premature to assume that the model proposed by Lerman is correct in all its details. Pritchard *et al.* (1966), assessing the evidence, pointed out that in Lerman's model proflavine was located over a base pair (Fig. 2). If this is so they suggest that denaturation

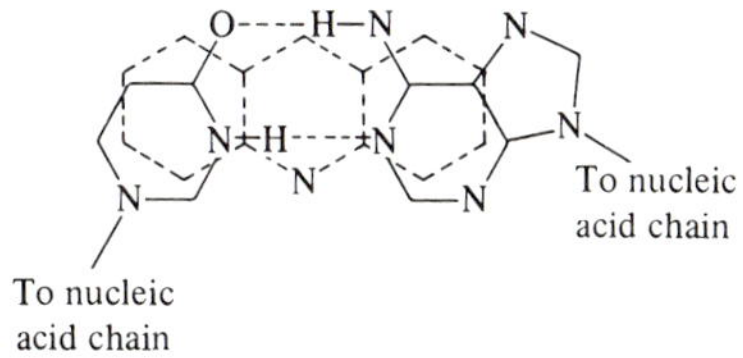

To nucleic acid chain

To nucleic acid chain

FIG. 2. The interrelationship between an intercalated acridine molecule (dotted) and a hydrogen-bonded base pair of DNA as proposed by Lerman (1961).

of DNA, which disrupts the ordered arrays of base pairs in the double helix (apart from limited local renaturation), would be expected to remove, or at least greatly reduce, the strong primary binding. The results of Drummond *et al.* (1965) and Liersch and Hartmann (1965) suggest that this is not so. Pritchard *et al.* (1966) have therefore proposed a modified intercalation model, which they consider satisfies the criteria of intercalation already discussed and also explains how binding can occur to the same extent on native or denatured DNA. The basis of their model is that acridine does not interact with a hydrogen-bonded base pair but reacts with two adjacent bases in the same polynucleotide chain. They suggest that increasing the spacing between the two base pairs to approximately 6.8 Å would allow room for an acridine molecule without greatly reducing the angle of rotation between the two base pairs. An important difference between their model and Lerman's is that a negatively charged atom on the phosphate group between the two bases can move to the inside of the chain where it would be adjacent to the positively charged ring nitrogen of the aminoacridine. This, the authors suggest, would explain the marked effect which ionic strength has on intercalation. Also, because it is proposed that binding takes place between a drug molecule and adjacent bases on the same polynucleotide chain strand, separation by thermal denaturation would not be expected to reduce greatly the overall binding.

Neville and Davies (1966) have reported quantitative discrepancies between optical transformations based on Lerman's model and X-ray diffraction patterns of the acridine–DNA complex. They point out that these discrepancies could be resolved if the untwisting of the helix during complex formation was considerably less than that proposed by Lerman and if the bound dye were not situated wholly over a base pair. Pritchard and co-workers (1966) believe that these structural requirements are met by their modified intercalation model. They also point out that a number of experimental observations are incompatible with Lerman's model. For example, substitution of a side chain in position 9 on the acridine molecule, as in the antimalarial compound mepacrine (V), does not reduce binding to DNA as might be expected from Lerman's model. Also, hydrogenation of acridine, to form a tetrahydro derivative, reduces the flat area of the molecule and causes the planar acridine ring to buckle in a way which might be expected to prevent intercalation of the type proposed by Lerman. Nevertheless, some binding of the reduced compound still occurs (Drummond *et al.*, 1965). Pritchard and co-workers (1966) consider that these findings are more easily explained in terms of their modified intercalation model.

Further evidence against the complete intercalation model of Lerman (1961) has come from the recent work of Roth and Manjon (1969) who have studied the specific association between acriflavine and DNA in intact cells from buccal mucosa. These workers found that denaturation, ultraviolet irradiation, and base analog substitution significantly reduce the ability of DNA to bind acriflavine. Predictable modifications of DNA structure were correlated with quantitative alterations in dye absorption by the cells. They conclude that their results support the views of Pritchard *et al.* (1966) and a number of other workers (Tubbs *et al.*, 1964; Gersch and Jordan, 1965; Neville and Davies, 1966) and point away from the original intercalation model. They favor a model in which diaminoacridines associate preferentially with adjacent thymine-containing base pairs in a strong bond which is disposed toward one of the DNA strands. They also suggest that the preferred binding site is situated between two adjacent thymine molecules whose 5-methyl groups endow the interaction with its specificity. Acriflavine was found to have a low affinity for nucleohistone and nucleoprotamine, a finding which is in general agreement with the view that phosphate groups of the sugar moieties play an important role in nucleic acid–acridine interactions.

B. Chloroquine and Related Antimalarial Drugs

Parker and Irvin (1952) first reported that the absorption spectrum of chloroquine (VI) is altered in the presence of DNA. In the same year Clarke (1952) and later Schellenberg and Coatney (1961) showed that three important antimalarials, chloroquine, mepacrine (V), and quinine (VII) inhibit the incorporation of phosphate-^{32}P into the DNA and RNA of *Plasmodium gallinaceum* and *Plasmodium berghei*. These observations have since been

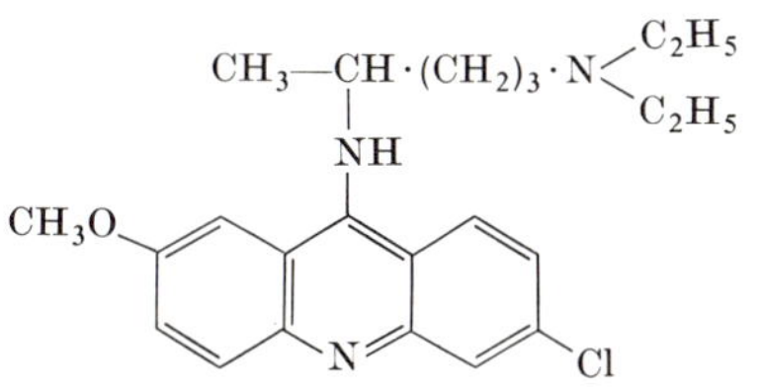

(V)

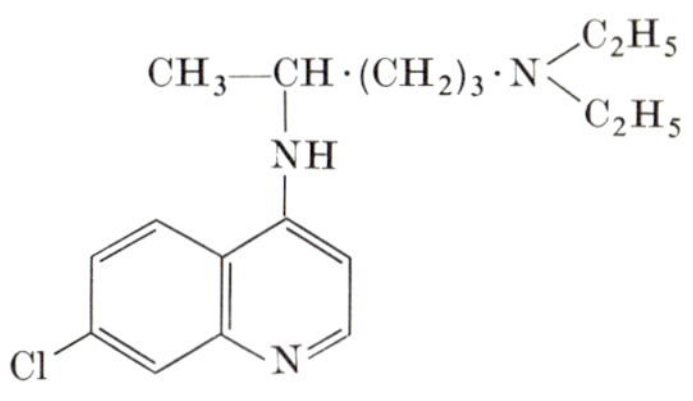

(VI)

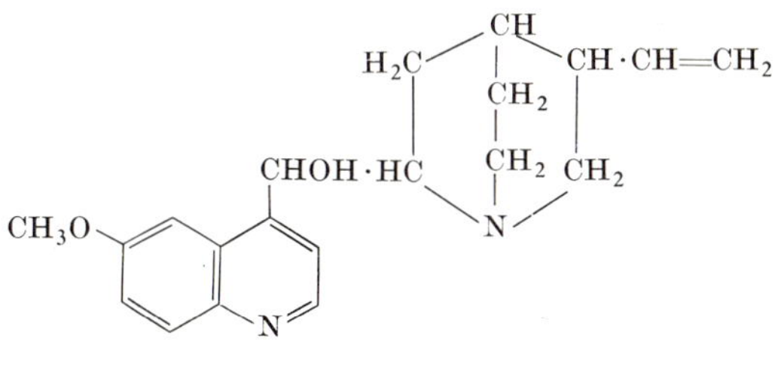

(VII)

followed up by a number of other workers (Kurnick and Radcliffe, 1962; Cohen and Yielding, 1965; Allison *et al.*, 1965, 1966), and it has now been established that chloroquine and related 4-aminoquinolines are potent inhibitors of DNA polymerase in cell-free systems and form complexes with double-stranded DNA. More recently (Whichard *et al.*, 1968) a number of

8-aminoquinoline drugs, including primaquine (VIII) and pamaquine (IX), have also been reported to form complexes with DNA, but the mechanism of binding remains unknown.

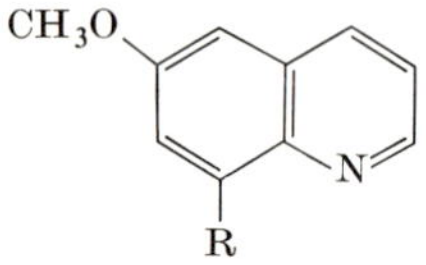

CH_3O (quinoline ring, N; substituent R at position 8)

(VIII) $R = —NH \cdot CH(CH_3) \cdot (CH_2)_3 \cdot NH_2$

(IX) $R = \cdot NH \cdot CH(CH_3) \cdot (CH_2)_3 \cdot N \langle {}^{C_2H_5}_{C_2H_5}$

Hahn and associates (1966) have made a detailed study of the chloroquine–DNA complex and consider that their hydrodynamic and optical measurements provide evidence for an intercalation of the quinoline ring between bases of DNA. They also report, from a study of the interaction of chloroquine with a number of synthetic polymers, that guanine is essential for binding of this drug, and they suggest that this may reflect a specific attraction between the 7-chloro substituent of the intercalated quinoline ring and the 2-amino group of guanine. These studies do not give any indication of the way the 1,4-diaminopentane side chain of chloroquine is bound to DNA, but Hahn *et al.* (1966) suggest that aliphatic diamines and spermine might be considered as models for the side chain of chloroquine.

Aliphatic diamines stabilize DNA, and the effect is related to the distance between the two primary amino groups (Mahler and Mehrotra, 1963). Spermine, which contains two secondary amino groups separated by four carbon atoms is, on a molar basis, as effective as chloroquine in elevating the melting temperature of DNA (Tabor, 1962), and like chloroquine it inhibits DNA and RNA polymerase. It has been suggested that aliphatic amines bind ionically to DNA phosphate groups (Suwalsky *et al.*, 1969), and O'Brien and Hahn (1966) speculate that side chain of chloroquine falls outside the contour of the DNA base pairs when the quinoline ring intercalates and, like spermine, interacts with phosphate groups of the complementary strands of DNA across the minor groove of the double helix. The presence of the side chain in chloroquine is necessary for strong binding (Cohen and Yielding, 1965), and a study of chloroquine analogs has shown that both antimalarial activity and affinity for DNA vary with the length of the side chain on the drug molecule. Hahn *et al.* (1966) point out that the distance across the minor groove of DNA between two phosphoric acid groups in complementary strands is 10.5 Å. They calculate that the distance between the centers of the two nitrogen atoms in the 1,4-diaminopentane side chain of chloroquine is 7.5 Å, which, taking the ionic radii of the amino groups into account, is optimal for electrostatic bonding between two phosphate groups.

A comparison of the interactions of chloroquine mepacrine and quinine with DNA has revealed significant differences in the types of DNA–drug complexes formed. There is some evidence (Parker and Irvin, 1952; Cohen and Yielding, 1965; Hahn *et al.*, 1966) that the acridine ring structure of mepacrine intercalates in much the same way as proflavine producing the characteristic changes in viscosity and sedimentation coefficient of DNA solutions. In contrast to chloroquine, mepacrine does not exhibit any base specificity. The formation of both chloroquine and mepacrine–DNA complexes is markedly affected by the ionic strength of the environment but little affected by the presence of urea (6 *M*). In contrast, the interaction of quinine with DNA is greatly reduced in the presence of urea suggesting that hydrogen bonding plays a more important part in complex formation between this drug and DNA than in the case of chloroquine and mepacrine (Hahn *et al.*, 1966). The way in which the side chains of mepacrine and quinine interact with DNA is still a matter for speculation.

C. Miracil D

Miracil D (X) is a 10-theaxanthenone which is bacteriostatic (Weinstein *et al.*, 1967), carcinostatic (Hirschberg *et al.*, 1959), and an effective agent in the treatment of Schistosomiasis in man (Newsome, 1951). The drug is a potent inhibitor of RNA synthesis in *Bacillus subtilis* (Weinstein *et al.*, 1965) and DNA-directed RNA synthesis in a cell-free system (Weinstein *et al.*, 1967). As will be seen from its structural formula miracil shares certain similarities with the acridines and actinomycin D (XI), and, in keeping with this, it has

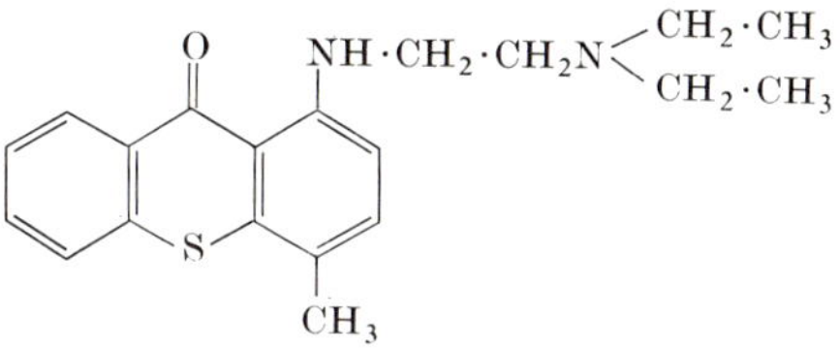

O $NH \cdot CH_2 \cdot CH_2N<^{CH_2 \cdot CH_3}_{CH_2 \cdot CH_3}$

S

CH_3

(X)

been found to stabilize DNA against heat denaturation and to increase the viscosity of DNA solutions. A study of derivatives of miracil has shown that an intact three-ring system and an unsubstituted proximal nitrogen in the side chain are important for the interaction with DNA and for the drug's growth inhibitory activity (Weinstein *et al.*, 1965; Carchman *et al.*, 1969). The effects of miracil on intact cells and isolated DNA can be reversed by spermine, and there is evidence that this amine can affect both cellular uptake of drug and its interaction with DNA. Discussing these results Carchman *et al.* (1969) suggest two possible types of interaction between this drug and DNA. First, the terminal nitrogen of the side chain may anchor the drug by electrostatic bonding to the DNA backbone while the three ring system inserts between adjacent base pairs, the quinoidal group of the ring and the proximal nitrogen of the side chain becoming hydrogen bonded to purine or pyrimidine bases. Second, the proximal nitrogen may bind electrostatically to negatively charged phosphate groups on the DNA backbone while the ring system intercalates and reacts with adjacent base pairs in a dipole-dipole manner. The experimental data are consistent with either of these explanations.

Miracil is less active, on a molar basis, than actinomycin D, but it is a more potent inhibitor of purified RNA polymerase than proflavine. As a tool for the investigation of macromolecular biosynthesis miracil has the disadvantage of being less specific in its action than actinomycin; concentrations which inhibit RNA synthesis in intact *E. coli* also partially inhibit DNA and protein synthesis, the effect on protein synthesis probably being due to combination of miracil with RNA.

D. Some Effects of Intercalating Agents on Cell Growth and Metabolism

The initial effect of intercalating agents on the growth of microorganisms can generally be reversed by transferring organisms to a drug-free medium (Newton, 1957; Albert, 1968; Tomchick and Mandel, 1964), but long exposure or treatment with high concentrations of drug is lethal (Seaman and Woodbine, 1953). In the case of ethidium bromide acting on the flagellate *Crithidia oncopelti*, the drug causes a progressive reduction in growth rate over a period of at least one generation time before multiplication is irreversibly blocked. The irreversible action of ethidium (Newton, 1957) and acriflavine (Steinert and Van Assel, 1967) is observed only with growing organisms. A study of the kinetics of ethidium-^{14}C uptake by resting and growing organisms (Newton, 1957) has indicated that two types of binding occur: a rapid combination with "primary binding sites" which is readily reversible and a slower "secondary binding" with sites which only become available during growth. Examination of drug-treated organisms by fluorescence microscopy, and fractionation of ethidium-^{14}C-treated organisms, suggests that, in the case of trypanosomatid flagellates, the primary binding of this drug occurs mainly in the nucleus and kinetoplast whereas the secondary binding sites are located in the cytoplasm, particularly on ribosomes (Newton, unpublished observations). These findings are in keeping with the observed effects of phenanthridines on biosynthesis in flagellates. DNA synthesis is rapidly inhibited, while RNA and protein synthesis are blocked only after longer periods in contact with the drug. This differential effect of phenanthridines on DNA and RNA synthesis has not been observed in bacteria. Ethidium, like proflavine, rapidly suppresses the uptake of radioactive precursors into RNA by bacteria (Gale and Folkes, 1958; Woese *et al.*, 1963; Chantrenne, 1964). Proflavine also inhibits inducible β-galactosidase synthesis by *E. coli* (Kepes, 1963) and ethidium blocks the formation of a lytic enzyme by *Bacillus subtilis* at concentrations well below those required to cause a significant inhibition of total protein synthesis (Richmond, 1959). These and other known effects of intercalating drugs *in vivo* have led to the conclusion that they act primarily on DNA replication and transcription. All the same, other possibilities cannot at present be ruled out. For example, Allison and Young (1964) have studied the uptake of acridines and related compounds by living cells in culture and have shown that they are rapidly concentrated in lysosomes. Following this observation Williamson and Macadam (1965) found that ethidium and a number of other cationic trypanocidal drugs cause damage to all intracellular membranes except lysosome membranes. It has been suggested by these workers that these compounds bind to and stabilize lysosome membranes. Allison and Mallucci (1964) have proposed that lysosome dissolution may be responsible for the initiation of mitosis; if so, stabilization of lysosomal membranes could result in the inhibition of cell division. These ideas are purely speculative at the present time, but they serve to emphasize that the *in vivo* action of cationic heterocyclic drugs, such as phenanthridines and acridines is not limited to intercalation into the DNA double helix.

III. Interaction of Actinomycin with DNA

The actinomycins are bright red compounds containing a phenoxazone ring system coupled to two cyclic peptide side chains (Brockmann, 1960; Johnson, 1960). The first observations on the mode of action of these antibiotics were made by Kirk (1960) who showed that in *Staphylococcus aureus*, actinomycin D (XI) rapidly inhibited RNA synthesis but allowed DNA synthesis to continue for a limited time. Kirk also observed that when DNA, but not RNA, is added to solutions of actinomycin the absorption spectrum of the antibiotic is changed; the peak in the visible region is reduced and shifted to longer wavelengths. Subsequent work (Hurwitz *et al.*, 1962) showed

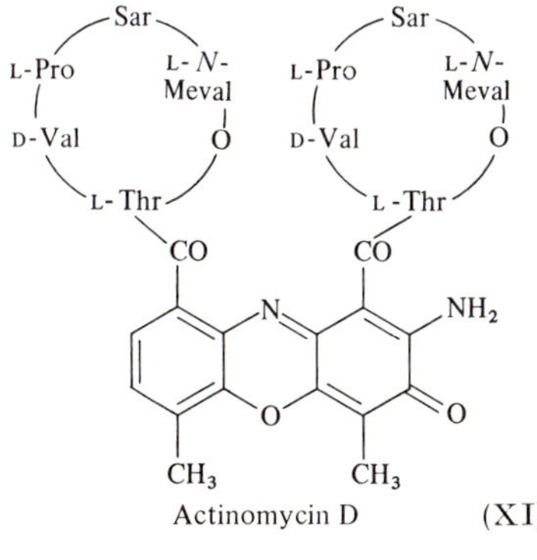

Sar, L-Pro, L-*N*-Meval, D-Val, O, L-Thr, CO; Sar, L-Pro, L-*N*-Meval, D-Val, O, L-Thr, CO; N, NH_2, O, O, CH_3, CH_3

Actinomycin D (XI)

that actinomycin is a powerful inhibitor of purified DNA synthesis. Inhibition of these systems was shown to be unaffected by variations in the concentration of enzyme, substrate, or cofactors in the reaction mixture, but was markedly affected by the concentration of DNA primer. The synthesis of RNA by RNA polymerase in the presence of templates which do not bind actinomycin (e.g., oligopolythymidylate) was found to be completely insensitive to the antibiotic.

Since these early observations cytochemical studies by many workers have shown that actinomycin has a profound effect on the nuclear structure of a wide variety of cells. Autoradiographic techniques have clearly demonstrated that actinomycin-^{3}H becomes localized in the DNA of chromosomes and in extranuclear DNA (Camargo and Plaut, 1967; Ebstein, 1967). All these findings lead to the conclusion that many of the biological activities of actinomycin are related to its ability to form complexes with DNA.

A. Factors Affecting Complex Formation

Actinomycin has been reported to interact specifically with helical deoxypolynucleotides which contain guanine. Synthetic deoxypolynucleotide polymers which lack this base do not bind the antibiotic (Goldberg *et al.*, 1962; Kahan *et al.*, 1963; Reich, 1964) except in the case of a deoxyadenine/thymine (dAT) copolymer containing diaminopurine residues in place of some of the adenine residues. This copolymer was synthesized by Cerami *et al.* (1967) and shown to have the chemical and biochemical properties of poly-dAT with the exception that the 2-amino group of the diaminopurine residues (which are in the same position as the 2-amino group of guanine) permits actinomycin binding. Goldberg *et al.* (1962) showed that the maximal amount of actinomycin bound by a particular species of DNA parallels the guanine content of that DNA. Even the very small amount of guanine (less than 2%) in "crab dAT" is sufficient to permit some actinomycin binding.

Studies of the interaction of actinomycin with polymers such as apyrimidinic DNA or single-stranded DNA from the bacteriophage ΦX174 have shown that they have a lower affinity for the antibiotic than native DNA (Goldberg *et al.*, 1962), suggesting that a helical configuration is important in the binding. The complexes formed with DNA can be isolated in a number of ways, for example, by electrophoresis (Kawamata and Imanishi, 1961), by centrifugation (Rauen *et al.*, 1960), or by chromatography on Sephadex (Hartmann *et al.* 1962). They are more stable than native DNA to increased temperature and decreased pH, but they are dissociated by treatments which destroy the helic structure of the DNA and also by low concentrations of urea which do not denature DNA (Hartmann *et al.*, 1962).

The groups on the actinomycin molecule which are essential for its biological activity and for DNA binding have been identified as the amino group and the quinoidal oxygen on the phenoxazone chromophore and the cyclic pentapeptide lactones. Mauger and Wade (1966) replaced the two pentapeptide lactones with a single neutral decapeptide (Gramicidin S) and Reich *et al.* (1967) found that this derivative had lost the characteristic properties of actinomycin. These workers have also reported that replacement of the pentapeptide by a hexapeptide sequence or substitution of the C-terminal L-*N*-methylvaline by L-valine results in a loss of biological activity. Thus it is clear that the actinomycin–DNA complex is formed as the result of highly specific molecular interaction which is dependent upon the stereochemical properties of the antibiotic and DNA.

B. The Nature of the Actinomycin–DNA Complex

In 1963 Hamilton *et al.* proposed a molecular model for the actinomycin–DNA complex which was based on X-ray and model-building studies. They suggested that the antibiotic was located in the minor groove of helical DNA and was held in place by up to seven hydrogen bonds. These included bonds between the 2-NH_2, N-3 and deoxyribose ring oxygen of deoxyguanosine and the quinoidal oxygen and amino group of the antibiotics chromophore. The geometry of these bonds has been studied and found to be stereochemically satisfactory. In this model the peptide chains pack into the small groove of the helix and so would be in a position to form further hydrogen bonds with the oxygen atoms of phosphate groups in the DNA strand opposite the guanine which is binding the chromophore. This model is represented diagrammatically in Fig. 3. Hamilton *et al.* (1963) believed that this model accounts for most of the known facts concerning the reaction of actinomycin with DNA and the resulting inhibition of DNA dependent RNA synthesis. They point out that the model depends entirely on the relative position of DNA constituents as they occur in the B-configuration of helical DNA and so would explain the fact that actinomycin binds very poorly to single-stranded DNA and does not bind to tRNA or reovirus RNA which are believed to exist in the A-configuration (Shatkin, 1965). Measurements of the dissociation constant of the actinomycin–DNA complex (Gellert *et al.*, 1965) suggest that interaction of the peptides with DNA makes a major contribution to the stability of the complex, but we still know little about the nature of this part of the interaction.

The mandatory requirement for the 2-amino group of guanine in the formation of an actinomycin–DNA complex has been used by Reich and co-workers as an argument in favor of their model, and against intercalation of the phenoxazone ring system into the DNA helix. Also against intercalation is the finding that binding of actinomycin causes a decrease, rather than an increase, in the viscosity of DNA solutions. Nevertheless, Müller and Crothers (1968) have recently reinvestigated the system and reported that the formation of an actinomycin–DNA complex does result in an increase in viscosity, and a decrease in sedimentation coefficient, if the molecular weight of the DNA is reduced by sonication before adding the antibiotic. With DNA of high molecular weight a decrease in viscosity and an increase in sedimentation was

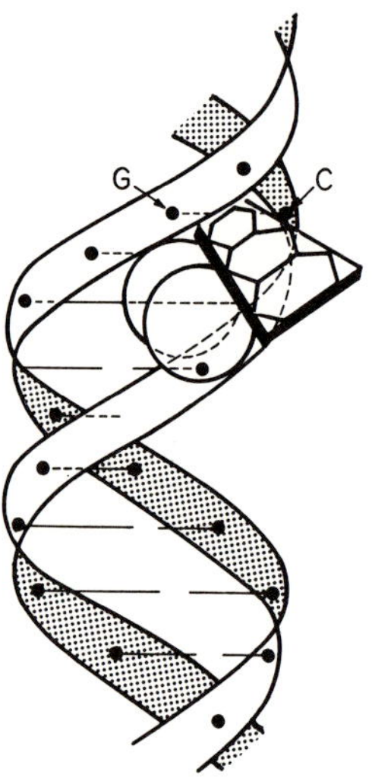

FIG. 3. Diagrammatic representation of the actinomycin–DNA complex based on the molecular model proposed by Hamilton *et al.* (1963). The cyclic peptide chains of the antibiotic are represented as circles filling the minor groove of the DNA helix for a distance of about three base pairs. The chromophore in this model is hydrogen bonded to a guanine residue.

observed. Their interpretation of these results is that the length of DNA molecules is increased by complex formation (as proposed in the intercalation theory) and that this is the only effect seen with DNA of low molecular weight. They also suggest that actinomycin increases the tendency of parts of the DNA molecule to interact with each other leading to a kind of cross-linking of the randomly coiled chain and a resultant decrease in viscosity of solutions. This cross-linking would not, they believe, occur with low molecular weight DNA because the shorter, more rigid, molecules could not double back on themselves. These and other findings lead Müller and Crothers to conclude that the chromophore of actinomycin does intercalate between adjacent base pairs. They propose the following points: (1) Binding can occur adjacent to any GC pair, but, binding at a given site distorts the helix so much that binding of another actinomycin molecule is unlikely to occur nearer than six base pairs away. This could explain why the apparent number of binding sites is much less than the number of GC pairs. (2) Hydrogen bonding occurs between the deoxyribose ring oxygens and the —CO, NH— groups attached to the chromophore. (3) The specificity for guanine results from electronic interactions in the π-complex formed in the intercalated structure. (4) Several forms of the complex can exist at equilibrium due to changes in conformation of the pentapeptide rings. From a comparison of the binding properties of actinomycin derivatives lacking peptide rings, and other modified structures, Müller and Crothers (1968) have speculated that the difference between actinomycin and simpler derivatives, which lack biological activity, is due to the very slow dissociation of the actinomycin–DNA complex, which may be a result of a slow reversal of conformational changes in the peptide rings.

A recent report (Wells, 1969) has raised further doubts about the validity of existing models of the actinomycin–DNA complex. Wells has shown that little or no actinomycin is bound by the double-stranded DNA polymer polydeoxy(adenylyl-thymidylyl-cytidylyl)·polydeoxy(guanidylyl-adenylyl-thymidylyl) or poly-d(ATC)·poly-d(GAT). This high molecular weight (0.3 million daltons) polymer, which contains 33% G + C, was synthesized by a combination of chemical and enzymatic techniques (Wells *et al.*, 1967). Ability of this DNA to bind actinomycin was very carefully studied by spectroscopy, equilibrium dialysis, buoyant density measurements, absorbance-temperature transitions, and inhibition of *in vitro* DNA-dependent synthesis of RNA. No significant binding of actinomycin was detected by any of these methods. This is the first example of a double-stranded DNA which contains guanine failing to bind actinomycin and is contrary to the predictions of Cerami *et al.* (1967). The reason for the inability of poly-d-(ATC)·poly-d(GAT) to bind the drug is at present unknown. Wells (1969) points out that physical and enzymatic studies have shown that this DNA has slightly different characteristics from its sequence isomer poly-d-(TAC)·poly-d(GAT), and this latter polymer does bind the antibiotic (Wells *et al.*, 1967; Wells and Blair, 1967). He suggests that the difference in ability of these two polymers to bind actinomycin may be due to changes in configuration resulting from the differences in base sequence, or to a requirement for a specific base sequence not present in poly-d(ATC)·poly-d(GAT). It seems that poly-d(ATC)·poly-d(GAT) may not have a DNA B-configuration (Wells, 1969), but this is thought to be unimportant because polymers with configurations other than B have now been found to bind actinomycin. Wells (1969) suggests that the observed mandatory guanine requirement for actinomycin binding may be due to this base, inducing a suitable configuration in most DNA's but not poly-d(ATC)·poly-d(GAT). This remains to be established, but whatever the explanation proves to be it is clear that, at the present time, the precise nature of the actinomycin–DNA complex is still a controversial question.[1]

Even more controversial is the nature of actinomycin binding *in vivo*: Intracellular DNA molecules are present in the form of complexes with the protein and metal ions, and we know little of the factors which influence the binding of actinomycin in the cell nucleus. Ringertz and Bolund (1969) have recently reported that preparations of deoxyribonucleoprotein bind only one molecule of actinomycin per 35–140 nucleotides whereas, under their conditions, DNA preparations bind one molecule of antibiotic per 14–20 nucleotides. Proteins therefore appear to block potential binding sites. These workers also found that divalent cations had a marked inhibitory effect on the *in vitro* binding of actinomycin to DNA, and they suggest that in the chromatin of the intact cell nucleus, actinomycin binding may be greatly modified by the presence of divalent metal ions.

C. Selective Inhibition of Gene Expression

Actinomycin inhibits gene expression to a much greater extent than gene replication, and any theory which attempts to explain the mechanism of action of this antibiotic must explain the observed differences in sensitivity of the two nucleotide polymerizations.

Reich (1964) has proposed that enzymes which catalyze reactions involving DNA may combine with sites at different parts of the surface of the DNA helix. He has suggested, as a speculative hypothesis, that actinomycin inhibits RNA polymerase directly by blocking sites (possibly in the minor groove) at which this enzyme acts. In contrast, DNA polymerase, he suggests, is only affected indirectly at much higher actinomycin concentrations and when enough molecules of the antibiotic have been bound to cause physical changes in the template and inhibit strand separation. Richardson (1966) considers that actinomycin may block RNA synthesis by preventing the progression of RNA polymerase along the DNA template, rather than by prevention of binding to the template. More recent discussion of the question (Müller and Crothers, 1968) has led to the suggestion that DNA synthesis is less sensitive than RNA synthesis because the replicative mechanism involved is somehow able to cause actinomycin to dissociate from the template, perhaps by a localized denaturation during the formation of daughter helices. These workers suggest that RNA polymerase may be unable to catalyze the removal of actinomycin from DNA, perhaps because the mechanism of action of this enzyme does not involve strand separation in the template.

It seems unlikely that the mechanism of actinomycin action will be defined more precisely until we know the exact nature of the interaction of the

[1] See Note Added in Proof, page 184.

pentapeptide portions of the antibiotic with DNA and until we have a complete understanding of the mechanisms of action of the two polymerases.

D. Actinomycin as a Biochemical Tool

Drugs cannot be used as effective tools in biochemical investigations until their mechanism of action is thoroughly understood. Actinomycin has been used more widely as a selective inhibitor of DNA-primed RNA synthesis than any other antibiotic. It has been used in the study of the kinetics of decay of unstable RNA in many cell types (Reich and Goldberg, 1964) and has proved to be a particularly valuable tool in the demonstration of DNA-independent RNA synthesis in RNA viruses (Montagnier, 1968). All the same, in the author's opinion the need for caution in interpreting the results obtained with actinomycin-inhibited systems cannot be overstressed. This antibiotic is a highly toxic compound, and at concentrations which inhibit transcription many cell processes, which are only remotely connected with transcription of DNA, may cease. It seems particularly dangerous to make deductions about the life of messenger-RNA from measurements of rates of protein synthesis in the presence of actinomycin. Inhibition of protein synthesis may occur for reasons other than template decay (Honig and Rabinowitz, 1965), and there is evidence that actinomycin may induce degradation of all types of cellular RNA (Wiesner *et al.*, 1965; Schwartz and Garofalo, 1967; Stewart and Farber, 1968). If, however, a synthetic process continues in the presence of high concentrations of actinomycin, which inhibits RNA synthesis, it suggests that the synthesis is not immediately dependent on the transcription of DNA. Even so, there is need for caution in the interpretation of results, and it must be borne in mind that it is very difficult to obtain 100% inhibition of transcription.

This view has also been strongly stated by Harris (1968): ". . . with actinomycin, only the positive result, the persistence of function in the absence of RNA synthesis, has probative value; the negative result, the impairment of function, is, without other evidence, uninterpretable."

IV. Chromomycins and Anthracyclines

In addition to the actinomycins a number of other antibiotics are now known selectively to inhibit DNA-dependent RNA synthesis by binding to the DNA template. These include members of the chromomycin and anthracycline groups of antibiotics. The properties and actions of these compounds have been reviewed in detail (Di Marco, 1967; Gause, 1967; Bhuyan, 1967; Hartmann, *et al.*, 1968). Space does not permit a full recapitulation of these data, and only a summary of the general conclusions will be presented here.

A. Chromomycin A_3, Mithramycin, and Olivomycin

These three closely related antibiotics have been found to inhibit DNA-primed RNA polymerase almost as strongly as actinomycin (Berlin *et al.*, 1966; Kaziro and Kamiyama, 1965) and are without effect on the RNA-primed reaction (Ward *et al.*, 1965). Like actinomycin the interaction of chromomycin (XII) with DNA depends on the guanine content and the double-stranded state of the DNA (Kaziro and Kamiyama, 1965). A 2-aminopurine group in DNA is required in the chromophore of these antibiotics

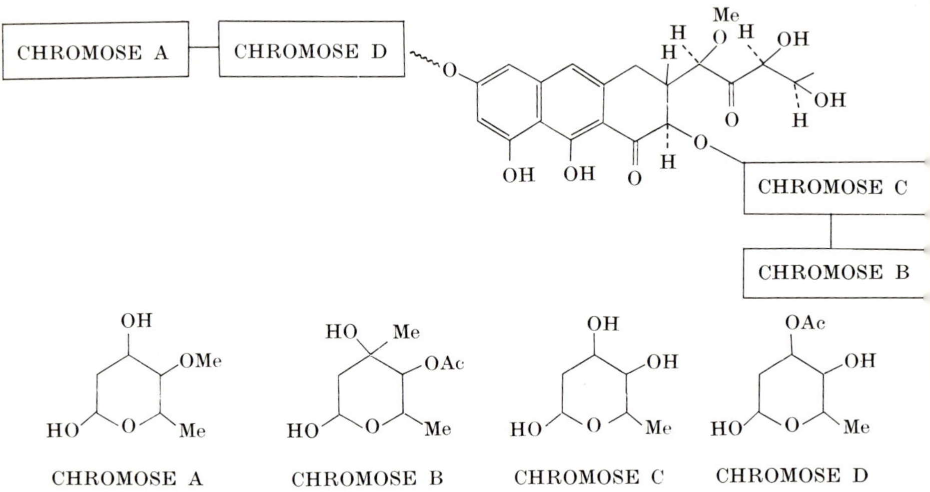

CHROMOSE A CHROMOSE D CHROMOSE C CHROMOSE B

CHROMOSE A CHROMOSE B CHROMOSE C CHROMOSE D

(XII)

(Müller and Crothers, 1968). Kersten *et al.* (1966) have studied the interaction of this group of antibiotics with DNA in some detail and have reported that they differ in a number of ways from actinomycin. In particular, they do not cause the changes which characterize intercalating drugs, and only increase the melting temperature of DNA when present in very high concentrations (>100 μg/ml) and in the presence of $MgCl_2$ (10^{-4} M). Kersten *et al.* suggest that under these conditions the antibiotics are able to form thermostable bridges between complementary strands of DNA.

B. Daunomycin, Nogalamycin, and Cinerubin

These representatives of the anthracycline group inhibit DNA-primed RNA polymerase (Brockmann, 1963; Tulinsky, 1964; Arcamone *et al.*, 1968) but are considerably less active than the actinomycins and chromomycins. Their action appears to be relatively independent of the base composition of DNA (Ward *et al.*, 1965), and they will inhibit RNA-primed polymerase reactions. The anthracyclines contain the chromophore shown in (XIII), but some details of their structures remain to be established. Studies of the

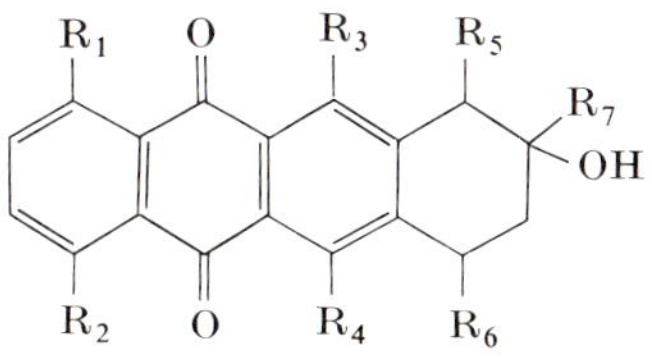

Sugar components may be:
Rhodosamine
Rhodinose
Daunosamine
2·Desoxy-L-fucose

R_1 = H or OH or OCH_3
R_2 = H or OH or OCH_3
R_3 = H or OH
R_4 = H or OH

R_5 = H or OH or $COOCH_3$
R_6 = H or OH
R_7 = C_2H_5 or $COCH_3$

(XIII)

interaction of these compounds with DNA (Hartmann *et al.*, 1964; Kersten and Kersten, 1965; Calendi *et al.*, 1965; *Kersten et al.*, 1966; Di Marco, 1967) have shown that, like the acridines, they increase the viscosity and decrease the sedimentation coefficient of DNA. They also cause a considerable increase in the melting temperature of DNA. Unlike acridines the binding of these compounds persists at high ionic strengths. It appears that amino sugar residues are responsible for the stabilization of the antibiotic–DNA complex inasmuch as acetylation of these causes a profound decrease in affinity for DNA (Calendi *et al.*, 1965). This group of antibiotics also has been found to decrease the buoyant density of DNA (Kersten *et al.*, 1966), nogalamycin producing the greatest effect of the compounds tested. It has been suggested that the magnitude of this effect may be related to the number of sugar residues in the antibiotic (Kersten *et al.*, 1966), but this remains to be established.

A detailed knowledge of the structure of these antibiotics and the nature of the complex which they form with DNA is necessary before they can become important as tools for the investigation biosynthetic mechanisms.

V. Cross-Linking by Mitomycins

Mitomycin C was first isolated from *Streptomyces caespitosus* by Wakiki and co-workers in 1956 (Wakiki *et al.*, 1958); it attracted interest because of its antitumor activity. Since that time a number of related antibiotics have been obtained from several *Streptomyces* species and are now known to be similar in structure (Fig. 4) and biological activity (Szybalski and Iyer, 1964). For simplicity these compounds will be referred to in this section by the general name "mitomycin."

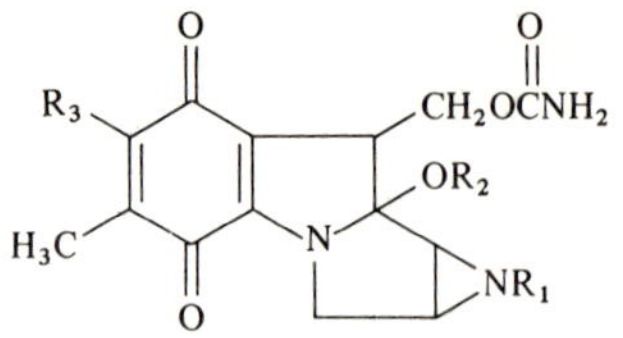

		R_1	R_2	R_3
Mitomycin	A	H	CH_3	H_3CO
	B	CH_3	H	H_3CO
	C	H	CH_3	H_2N
Porfiromycin		CH_3	CH_3	H_2N

FIG. 4. Structure of mitomycins and porfiromycin.

In addition to antitumor activity, mitomycins have antibacterial activity and are characterized by a rapid and irreversible action. Early investigations by Shiba and co-workers (1958, 1959) led to the suggestion that mitomycin is a specific inhibitor of DNA synthesis and, consequently, during the last 10 years the actions of this group of antibiotics have been extensively studied. This work has been comprehensively reviewed by Szybalski and Iyer (1967).

The ability of mitomycin to inhibit DNA synthesis selectively, without concomitant inhibition of RNA or protein synthesis, has been observed by many workers using a variety of cell systems. In some, but not all organisms, inhibition of DNA synthesis is accompanied by a massive breakdown of the preexisting DNA with an accumulation of mononucleotides and free bases in the pool of the cells or in the medium (Reich *et al.*, 1961) but Terawaki and Greenberg (1966) have provided convincing evidence that the breakdown is not directly related to the lethal effects of mitomycin. They found no evidence of DNA depolymerization in radiation sensitive *Escherichia coli* mutants which were hyposensitive to mitomycin, whereas radiation and mitomycin-resistant mutants showed considerable breakdown of DNA in the presence of bactericidal concentrations of the antibiotic. These and other experiments have led to the view that the breakdown of DNA may be associated with either the appearance of new nucleases resulting from mitomycin induction of lysogenic bacteriophages or with the excision and repair of alkylated DNA.

A. Evidence for Cross-Linking

The investigations of Iyer and Szybalski (1963) and Matsumoto and Lark (1963) showed that the lethal effects of mitomycin on bacterial and mammalian cells are associated with dramatic changes in the structure of the cells' DNA. Exposure of organisms to the antibiotic for periods as short as 1 minute, followed by extraction of DNA, revealed that mitomycin had become covalently linked to the DNA. This combination occurs in such a way as to form cross-links between complementary strands of the DNA helix.

The existence of cross-links was elegantly demonstrated by Iyer and Szybalski (1963) by heating DNA from normal and from mitomycin-treated cells to 100°C and then rapidly cooling to 0°C. This procedure normally yields single-stranded DNA, but it was found that the DNA which had been isolated from mitomycin-treated cells retained its double-stranded form, indicating the presence of abnormal heat-stable cross-links. The breakdown in the helical structure of DNA and the separation of the two strands which occurs at the "melting temperature" is accompanied by a substantial increase in absorption at 260 nm. The complementary strands of DNA, once they have separated, lose their proper alignment so that "renaturation" is a trial-and-error process which is almost completely prevented if denatured DNA is rapidly cooled (Marmur *et al.*, 1963). Iyer and Szybalski (1963) studied the thermal denaturation and renaturation profiles of DNA from *E. coli* grown in the presence or absence of mitomycin C (10 μg/ml). DNA from control organisms, after denaturation, showed little fall in absorbancy when cooled, whereas the absorbance of DNA from mitomycin-treated cells fell rapidly, indicating the presence of a spontaneously renaturing fraction. Iyer and Szybalski's interpretation of these findings is shown schematically in Fig. 5.

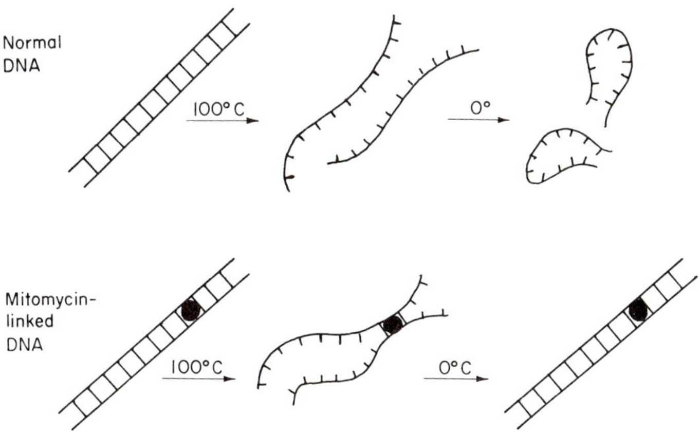

FIG. 5. Schematic presentation of the effects of heat denaturation followed by rapid cooling on normal and mitomycin-linked DNA. (Based on Iyer and Szybalski, 1963.)

The renatured, cross-linked, DNA has many properties in common with native helical DNA and can be distinguished from the denatured, single-stranded material by its behavior in cesium chloride density gradients and by a number of other techniques (reviewed by Szybalski, 1967).

The degree of cross-linking by mitomycin depends on temperature, the concentration of the antibiotic, and the duration of its contact with organisms. It seems that the physiological state of the bacteria has little effect on the susceptibility of the DNA to cross-linking. Szybalski and Iyer, (1964) have shown that the rate of cell death correlated well with the degree of DNA cross-linking and have calculated that one cross-link per genome is sufficient to cause cell death.

B. Activation of Mitomycin

The changes in DNA produced by the treatment of intact cells with mitomycin do not occur when purified DNA is treated with the antibiotic. All the same, *in vitro* cross-linking can be obtained if a DNA-mitomycin mixture is supplemented with a cell lysate of mitomycin-sensitive bacteria (Iyer and Szybalski, 1963, 1964). This suggests that mitomycin must be activated in some way before cross-linking can occur. More detailed study of the role of the cell lysate has indicated that the activation process is the result of a reduction of mitomycin to its hydroquinone derivative by a TPNH-dependent diaphorase (Fig. 6). Activation can also be achieved by chemical-reducing agents such as potassium borohydride, sodium hydrogen sulfite, or molecular hydrogen in the presence of paladium as a catalyst. The activated form of mitomycin is very unstable and rapidly loses its capacity to cross-link purified DNA. The cross-linking reaction clearly requires at least two reactive sites on the mitomycin molecule. Iyer and Szybalski (1964) have discussed the probable location of these and suggest that reactive sites 1 and 2 (Fig. 6) are sufficient

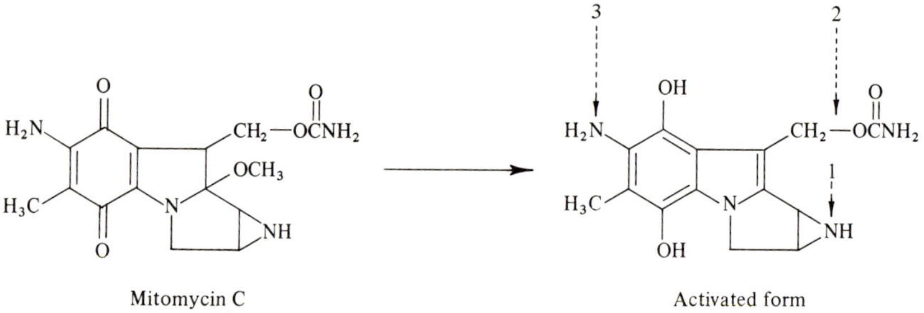

Mitomycin C → Activated form

Fig. 6. Reduction of mitomycin to its hydroquinone derivative. The location of three possible reactive sites suggested by Iyer and Szybalski (1964) are indicated by arrows 1, 2, and 3.

to explain the necessary bifunctional alkylating properties of the activated molecule. They point out that they cannot yet exclude the possibility of a third active site (3) at the C-7 position in the molecule. Murakami (1966) has outlined, in a theoretical paper, possible electronic mechanisms for mitomycin activation which involve the formation of an intermediate semiquinoid form of the antibiotic. However, Szybalski and Iyer (1967) point out that this is not confirmed by the results of Patrick *et al.* (1964) who did not observe any secondary rearrangements upon reduction of mitomycin to a semiquinone.

C. Binding Sites on DNA

Direct evidence of covalent binding of mitomycins to DNA has been obtained by Szybalski and Iyer (1964) and by Weissbach and Lisio (1965) who used labeled porfiromycin (prepared by methylation of mitomycin C with methyl iodide-^{14}C) and mitomycin C-^{3}H. They found that DNA, isolated after incubation with labeled antibiotic under reducing conditions *in vitro*, had bound as much as one antibiotic molecule per 500 nucleotides. The amount bound *in vitro* was dependent upon the antibiotic/DNA ratio in the incubation and was much greater than the amount bound when intact organisms were treated with antibiotic (Iyer and Szybalski, 1963). These investigations indicate that only about one in five to ten antibiotic molecules bound forms a cross-link, while, the others attach to a single base of one DNA strand by a monofunctional alkylation.

This work was carried a stage further by Lipsett and Weissbach (1965) who investigated the alkylation of a number of synthetic polyribonucleotides by labeled antibiotic. They found that guanine residues were alkylated four times as fast as other bases and suggested that the N-7 position of guanine was the site of attack, inasmuch as guanine residues in poly-GU are alkylated to a greater extent than those in poly-G where the N-7 position is protected by hydrogen bonding. These findings are consistent with Iyer and Szybalski's (1964) finding that cross-linking increases with the guanine plus cytosine content of DNA. Nevertheless, the exact nature of the cross-linking sites on DNA is not yet established and other possibilities exist. Murakami (1966) has suggested that cross-linking occurs among O-6 of guanine, N-4 and O-5 of mitomycin, and N-4 of cytosine, but no evidence for the formation of dicytidyl or cytidylguanyl porfiromycin was found by Lipsett and Weissbach (1965) during the treatment of s-RNA with reduced porfiromycin.

As Iyer and Szybalski (1963) have pointed out, it may prove difficult to establish the precise nature of the cross-linking since the number of links occurring *in vivo* appears not to exceed 1 per 10^3 nucleotide pairs.

D. Mitomycin Action *in Vivo*

The results described in the above sections have led to the postulate that the lethal action of the mitomycin group of antibiotics can be accounted for by the cross-link between complementary strands of DNA preventing strand separation during the semiconservative replication process. Certainly there is good evidence for the formation of such cross-links *in vitro* and *in vivo*. On the other hand, it should perhaps be stressed that, although the inhibition of synthesis of RNA and certain proteins becomes evident only a long time after the suppression of DNA synthesis, alkylation by mitomycin is not restricted to DNA. Weissbach and Lisio (1965) fractionated *E. coli* which had been treated with porfiromycin-^{14}C and found that 60–80% of the antibiotic was bound to protein and 25% was located in the ribosome fraction of cells. Also, ribosomes and t-RNA are known to be alkylated *in vitro* by mitomycin. It has been suggested (Kersten *et al.*, 1964) that damage to sRNA and ribosomes may lead to unmasking of latent nucleases. Clearly, all these findings must be borne in mind when considering the mode of action of this group of antibiotics.

VI. Diamidines, Polyamines, and Related Compounds

A. Aromatic Diamidines

Aromatic diamidines such as stilbamidine (XIV) and pentamidine (XV) inhibit the growth of protozoa, bacteria, fungi, and neoplastic cells, generally at concentrations well below those found to be toxic in host tissues. The pharmacology and action of these compounds has been reviewed in detail by Schoenbach and Greenspan (1948), Williamson (1962), Newton (1963), and Hawking (1963). The biological activity of these compounds is known to be markedly affected by alterations in chain length and by modification of the guanyl group. Early work (Bichowsky-Slomnitzki, 1948) showed that nucleic acid can reverse the bacteriostatic action of pentamidine. This finding, together with the observations that stilbamidine gives rise to basophilic granules in myeloma cells (Snapper *et al.*, 1947) and is concentrated in the kinetoplast

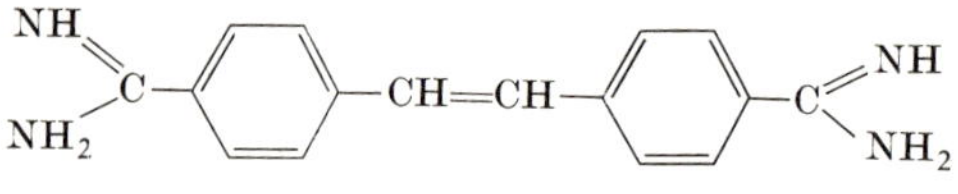

(XIV)

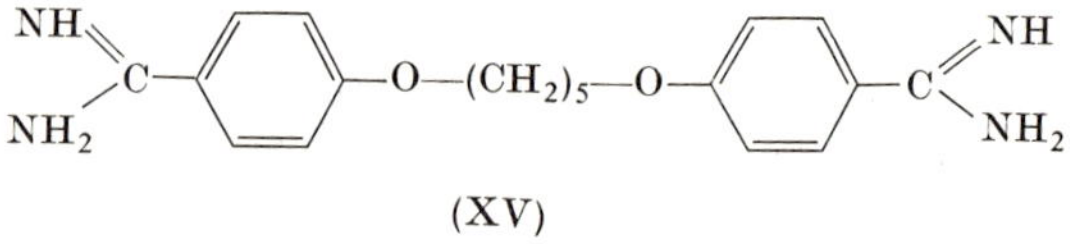

(XV)

and cytoplasmic granules of trypanosomes (Hawking and Smiles, 1941; Ormerod, 1951, 1952), led to the suggestion that the growth inhibitory actions of aromatic diamidines may be due to a direct interaction with nucleic acid. More recent work tends to support this view: Pentamidine inhibits DNA-primed RNA polymerase *in vitro* by combining with the DNA primer (Waring, 1965) and also blocks the incorporation of amino acids in a cell-free system by combining with ribosomes (Chesters, 1966).

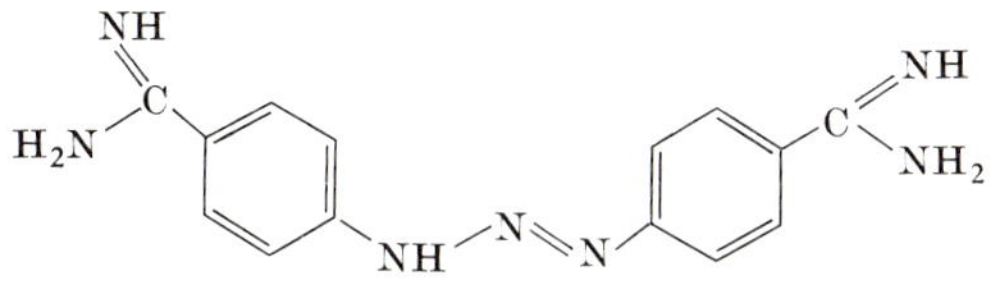

(XVI)

The trypanocidal drug berenil (XVI) has also been shown to form complexes with DNA both *in vivo* and *in vitro* (Newton and Le Page, 1967). Addition of DNA to solutions of drug causes a shift in the absorption spectrum to longer wavelengths and quantitative studies based on this spectral shift have shown that one molecule of drug is bound by native DNA for every four to five nucleotides; heat denaturation of the DNA results in a doubling of the amount of drug bound. Berenil also raises the helix-coil transition point of DNA and decreases the buoyant density, but there is no evidence that the drug can intercalate or form "mitomycin-like" cross-links. Comparison of the effects of berenil on DNA of various base compositions has established a positive correlation between the adenine plus thymine content of DNA and the decrease in buoyant density produced by the drug, (Newton, 1967). In neutral solution the berenil molecule undergoes a rearrangement (Fig. 7) which results in the

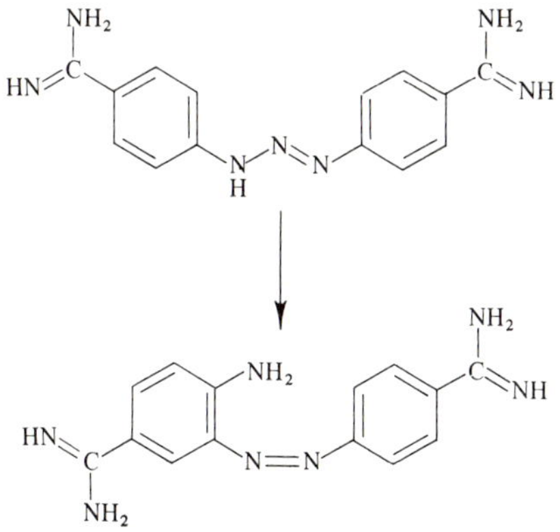

FIG. 7. Breakdown of berenil in neutral solution to form an *O*-aminoazo derivative. (Based on a personal communication from Dr. H. Loewe.)

formation of an *O*-aminoazo derivative from the original triazine structure (Dr. H. Loewe, personal communication). The breakdown product is without trypanocidal activity and has no effect on the buoyant density of DNA. This suggests that the spacing of the amidino groups of berenil may be critical in the formation of a complex with DNA, but the exact nature of the complex remains to be defined.

B. Polyamines and Derivatives

Polyamines, such as spermine and spermidine, and diamines, such as putrescine, have long been recognized as widely distributed constituents of biological materials (for a comprehensive review see Tabor *et al.*, 1961; Tabor and Tabor, 1964). Polyamines are associated with nucleic acids in cells and combine with isolated nucleic acid. In particular, diamines have been found to protect infective nucleic acid prepared from T_2 bacteriophage against heat denaturation (Fraser and Mahler, 1958). A detailed study of nucleic acid–diamine interactions by Mahler and Mehrotra (1963) has shown that with primary aliphatic diamines of the type $H_2N—(CH_2)_n—NH_2$ optimal binding to DNA occurs when $n = 5$. They suggest that binding involves bridging between the phosphate residues of one DNA strand and the adenine and/or thymine of the other. These findings are relevant to the subject of this review because the biological activity of diamidine drugs is also closely related to the chain length of the molecules and because the work of Bachrach and collaborators has drawn attention to oxidized spermine (XVII) and related iminodialdehydes as growth inhibitors for bacteria (Tabor *et al.*, 1964),

$$\mathrm{OHC(CH_2)_2NH(CH_2)_4NH(CH_2)_2CHO}$$

(XVII)

bacteriophages (Bachrach and Persky, 1964; Bachrach *et al.*, 1963), viruses (Bachrach *et al.*, 1965), and tumor cells (Katz *et al.*, 1967).

Oxidized spermine is a potent inhibitor of nucleic acid synthesis in both intact cells and cell-free systems (Bachrach and Persky, 1969). DNA synthesis is somewhat more sensitive to the drug than RNA synthesis and its action is the result of binding to the DNA primer and not to its interaction with either enzymes or substrates. *In vitro* oxidized spermine had a greater effect on DNA replication when primers with a high guanine plus cytosine content are used.

There is now evidence (Bachrach and Eilon, 1967) that oxidized spermine is bound to DNA by electrostatic and covalent bonds and induces the formation of cross-links between paired strands of DNA. Thus, the drug resembles other bifunctional alkylating agents such as mitomycin and it is suggested that it inhibits DNA synthesis by preventing separation (Goldacre *et al.*, 1949; Kohn *et al.*, 1966; Bachrach and Persky, 1966). Oxidized spermine, however, is not a selective inhibitor for RNA synthesis, and its use as a biochemical tool is open to some criticism.

VII. Speculations on the Basis of Selective Toxicity

It was pointed out in the introduction to this review that many of the synthetic drugs and antibiotics which are known to interact with DNA are too generally toxic to be of any practical importance as chemotherapeutic agents. Some, however, hold promise as antiviral or carcinostatic agents and others are valuable drugs, widely used for the control of trypanosomiasis and malaria. At the present time we do not know the basis of the selective toxicity of any of these compounds, but recent work is beginning to throw some light on this question.

A. Differential Binding to DNA

It has been seen that the formation of drug–DNA complexes may be markedly influenced by the composition and the tertiary structure of the nucleic acid. Since the base composition of DNA from different cell types is known to vary widely, and the conformation of nuclear and extranuclear DNA is known to differ, it is possible that these factors may influence the amount of a drug that is bound by a particular organism or organelle.

There is evidence that acridines (Steinert and Van Assel, 1967; Hill and Anderson, 1969), phenanthridines (Steinert *et al.*, 1969), and berenil (Newton and Le Page, 1967) selectively inhibit the synthesis of extranuclear DNA in the kinetoplast of trypanosomatid flagellates. Ethidium produces "petite" mutants in yeasts with almost 100% efficiency (Slonimski *et al.*, 1968). Radloff and co-workers (1967) and Hudson *et al.* (1969), have studied the binding of ethidium to nuclear DNA and to closed circular duplexes of the type found in mitochondria. The maximum amount of drug that can be bound by closed circular DNA was found to be smaller than with linear DNA or "nicked" circular DNA, but circular DNA appeared to have a higher affinity for ethidium than did linear DNA. These workers suggest that this difference in affinity may explain the selective inhibition of mitochondrial DNA synthesis that has been observed with both acridines and phenanthridines. On the other hand, other factors which may contribute to the selective action of these drugs must be considered. These include the following factors: (1) The lack of histone in the kinetoplast (Steinert, 1965), and possibly in mitochondria, may mean that the DNA of these organelles is more readily available for combination with drug molecules than is nuclear DNA. (2) Differences may exist in the permeability of mitochondrial, kinetoplast, and nuclear membranes to drugs. Some evidence that ethidium may not penetrate to all parts of Ehrlich ascites carcinoma cells has been obtained by Kandaswamy and Henderson (1963). (3) The concentration of divalent cations in nuclei and mitochondria may differ. Mg^{++} concentration is known to affect the binding of a number of drugs to DNA and a high concentration of such ions in the nucleus might be sufficient to account for the higher resistance of this organelle to such drugs (Steinert and Van Assel, 1967). (4) There may be differences in the drug sensitivity of enzymes involved in DNA replication in different organelles. Acridines are known to cause the irreversible loss of episomes in bacteria (Hirota, 1960; Marmur *et al.*, 1961; Rogolsky and Slepecky, 1964), and Jacob *et al.* (1963), discussing the loss of the F episome from *E. coli*, suggested that it may be explained by a differential sensitivity of replication enzymes. Some support for this hypothesis has come from the recent work of Meyer and Simpson (1969), who found that DNA polymerase from rat liver mitochondria is more sensitive to ethidium and acriflavine than the polymerase from rat liver nuclei.

While one or other of these various possibilities may explain the selective inhibition of DNA synthesis in an organelle of a particular cell, there is no evidence that any of them are of importance in explaining the selective killing of a parasite within a host. DNA's from parasitic protozoa and from mammalian cells appear to have the same affinity for trypanocidal drugs such as ethidium or antimalarial compounds such as chloroquine (Newton, unpublished observations). These findings direct our attention to the membranes and osmotic barriers of host cells and parasites and suggest that the selective activity of drugs which affect the structure and function of DNA may depend upon differential permeability of cells.

B. Differences in Cell Permeability

Although a great deal is known about relationships between the chemical structure and biological activity of compounds such as acridines, phenanthridines, and diamidines (reviewed by Sexton, 1963; Albert, 1968), we have little detailed knowledge of cell structures which control the permeability of organisms to these drugs. We can offer no satisfactory explanation for the fact that acriflavine readily penetrates the flagellate *Bodo candatus* but is unable to enter *Crithidia oncopelti* (Robertson, 1963) or for the fact that *E. coli* is impermeable to actinomycin. Our understanding of selective toxicity can not advance far until such phenomena have been adequately explained.

Recent studies (Hollingshead *et al.*, 1963; Vickerman, 1969) are beginning to yield some information about the surface structures of trypanosomes which may be of importance to our understanding of drug action. The bloodstream forms of trypanosomes have been found to differ from other freely circulating cells in the bloodstream, in that they have either no net charge or are slightly positively charged at a physiological pH; lymphocytes and red blood cells carry a net negative charge. The lack of a net negative charge on trypanosomes will undoubtedly affect the nature of the primary interaction of the organisms with cationic drugs such as ethidium. Watkins (1952) has suggested that this drug may enter the cell in the neutral pseudo-base form (Fig. 8) which has a much greater liposolubility than the cation from which it

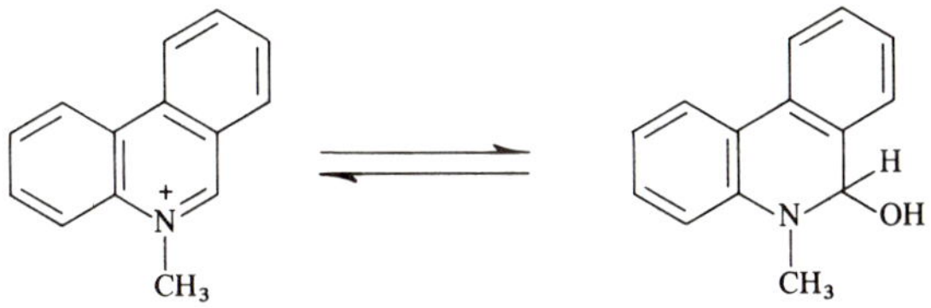

CH_3 CH_3 H OH

FIG. 8. The structure of cationic and pseudo-base forms of a heterocyclic quaternary compound.

is derived. With this possibility in mind it is interesting to note that ethidium is a much more effective trypanocidal drug than the methyl quaternary homolog dimidium (XVIII). Ethidium and dimidium show the same affinity

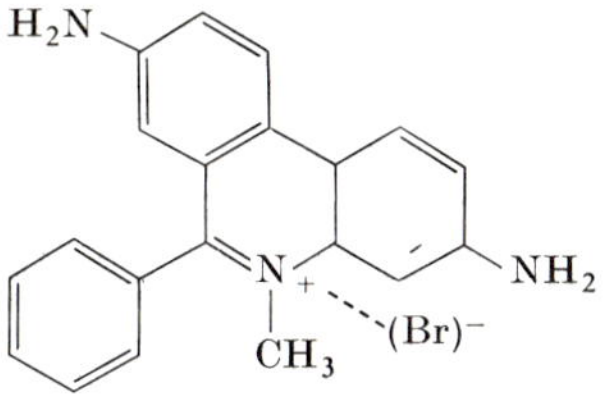

H_2N NH_2 CH_3 $(Br)^-$

(XVIII)

for DNA *in vitro* (Newton, unpublished observations) but, at a physiological pH, ethidium forms twice as much pseudo-base as dimidium (Watkins, 1952). This fact may explain the superior trypanocidal activity of the ethyl homolog.

These findings emphasize the need for more information about the interaction of drugs with cell surfaces, and about factors which influence the penetration of drug molecules through lipoprotein membranes, if we are to understand the basis of the selective toxicity of chemotherapeutic agents which combine with DNA.

References

Albert, A. (1968). "Selective Toxicity," 4th Ed. Methuen, London.

Albert, A., Rubbo, S., Goldacre, R., Davey, M., and Stone, J. (1945). *Brit. J. Exp. Pathol.* **26,** 160.

Albert, A., Rubbo, S., and Burvill, M. (1949). *Brit. J. Exp. Pathol.* **30,** 159.

Allison, A. C., and Mallucci, L. (1964). *Lancet* **ii,** 1371.

Allison, A. C., and Young, M. R. (1964). *Life Sci.* **3,** 1407.

Allison, J. L., O'Brien, R. L., and Hahn, F. E. (1965). *Science* **149,** 1111.

Allison, J. L., O'Brien, R. L., and Hahn, F. E. (1966). *Antimicrob. Ag. Chemother.* 1965, p. 310.

Arcamone, F., Cassinelli, G., Franceschi, G., Orezzi, P., and Mandelli, R. (1968). *Tetrahedron Lett.* p. 3353.

Bachrach, U., and Eilon, G. (1967). *Biochim. Biophys. Acta* **145,** 418.

Bachrach, U., and Persky, S. (1964). *J. Gen. Microbiol.* **37,** 195.

Bachrach, U., and Persky, S. (1966). *Biochem. Biophys. Res. Commun.* **24,** 135.

Bachrach, U., and Persky, S. (1969). *Biochim. Biophys. Acta* **179,** 484.

Bachrach, U., Tabor, C. W., and Tabor, C. W. (1963). *Biochim. Biophys. Acta* **78,** 768.

Bachrach, U., Rabina, S., Loebenstein, G., and Eilon, G. (1965). *Nature (London)* **208,** 1095.

Berlin, Y. A., Esipov, S. E., and Kolosov, M. N. (1966). *Tetrahedron Lett.* p. 1431.

Bhuyan, B. K. (1967). *In* "Antibiotics. I: Mechanisms of Action" (D. Gottlieb and P. D. Shaw, eds.), pp. 173–180. Springer, Berlin.

Bichowsky-Slomnitzki, L. (1948). *J. Bacteriol.* **55,** 27.

Brockmann, H. (1960). *Ann. N.Y. Acad. Sci.* **89,** 323.

Brockmann, H. (1963). *Fortschr. Chem. Org. Naturst.* **21,** 121.

Browning, C. H. (1964). *In* "Experimental Chemotherapy" (R. J. Schnitzer and F. Hawking, eds.), Vol. 2, Pt. I, pp. 1–36. Academic Press, New York.

Cairns, J. (1962). *Cold Spring Harbor Symp. Quant. Biol.* **27,** 311.

Calendi, E., Di Marco, A., Reggiani, M., Scarpinato, B., and Valentini, L. (1965). *Biochim. Biophys. Acta* **103,** 25.

Camargo, E. P., and Plaut, W. (1967). *J. Cell Biol.* **35,** 713.

Carchman, R. A., Hirschberg, E., and Weinstein, I. B. (1969). *Biochim. Biophys. Acta* **179,** 158.

Cerami, A., Reich, E., Ward, D. C., and Goldberg, I. H. (1967). *Proc. Nat. Acad. Sci. USA* **57,** 1036.

Chantrenne, H. (1964). *J. Cell. Comp. Physiol.* **64,** Suppl. 1, 149.

Chesters, J. K. (1966). *Biochim. Biophys. Acta* **114,** 385.

Clarke, D. H. (1952). *J. Exp. Med.* **96,** 451.

Cohen, S. M., and Yielding, K. L. (1965). *J. Biol. Chem.* **240,** 3123.

Crawford, L. V., and Waring, M. (1967). *J. Mol. Biol.* **25,** 23.

Di Marco, A. (1967). *In* "Antibiotics. I: Mechanisms of Action" (D. Gottlieb and P. D. Shaw, eds.), pp. 190–210. Springer, Berlin.

Drummond, D. S., Simpson-Gildemeister, V. F. W., and Peacocke, A. R. (1965). *Biopolymers* **3,** 135.

Ebstein, B. S. (1967). *J. Cell Biol.* **35,** 709.

Ehrlich, P., and Benda, L. (1913). *Ber. Deut. Chem. Ges.* **46,** 1931.

Fraser, D., and Mahler, H. R. (1958). *J. Amer. Chem. Soc.* **80,** 6456.

Fuller, W., and Waring, M. (1964). *Ber. Bunsenges. Phys. Chem.* **68,** 805.

Gale, E. F., and Folkes, J. P. (1958). *Biochem. J.* **69,** 620.

Gause, G. F. (1967). *In* "Antibiotics. I: Mechanisms of Action" (D. Gottlieb and P. D. Shaw, eds.), pp. 246–258. Springer, Berlin.

Gellert, M., Smith, C. E., Neville, D., and Felsenfeld, G. (1965). *J. Mol. Biol.* **11**, 445.

Gersch, N. F., and Jordan, D. O. (1965). *J. Mol. Biol.* **13**, 138.

Goldacre, R. J., Loveless, A., and Ross, W. C. J. (1949). *Nature* (*London*) **163**, 667.

Goldberg, I. H., Rabinowitz, M., and Reich, E. (1962). *Proc. Nat. Acad. Sci. U.S.A.* **48**, 2094.

Hahn, F. E., O'Brien, R. L., Ciak, J., Allison, J. L., and Olenick, J. G. (1966). *Mil. Med.* **131**, Suppl., 1071–1089.

Hamilton, L., Fuller, W., and Reich, E. (1963). *Nature* (*London*) **198**, 538.

Harris, H. (1968). "Nucleus and Cytoplasm." Oxford Univ. Press (Clarendon) London and New York.

Hartmann, G., Coy, U., and Kniese, G. (1962). *Hoppe-Seyler's Z. Physiol. Chem.* **330**, 227.

Hartmann, G., Goller, H., Koschel, K., Kersten, W., and Kersten, H. (1964). *Biochem. Z.* 341, 126.

Hartmann, G., Behr, W., Beissner, K. A., Honikel, K., and Sippel, A. (1968). *Angew. Chem. Int. Ed. Engl.* **7**, 693.

Hawking, F. (1963). *In* "Experimental Chemotherapy" (R. J. Schnitzer and F. Hawking, eds.), Vol. 1, pp. 131–208. Academic Press, New York.

Hawking, F., and Smiles, J. (1941). *Ann. Trop. Med. Parasitol.* **35**, 45.

Hill, G. C., and Anderson, W. A. (1969). *J. Cell Biol.* **41**, 547.

Hirota, Y. (1960). *Proc. Nat. Acad. Sci. U.S.A.* **46**, 57.

Hirschberg, E., Gellhorn, A., Murray, M. R., and Elslager, E. F. (1959). *J. Nat. Cancer Inst.* **22**, 567.

Hollingshead, S., Pethica, B. A., and Ryley, J. F. (1963). *Biochem. J.* **89**, 123.

Honig, G. R., and Rabinowitz, M. (1965). *Science* **149**, 1504.

Hudson, B., Upholt, W. B., Devinny, J., and Vinograd, J. (1969). *Proc. Nat. Acad. Sci. U.S.A.* **62**, 813.

Hurwitz, J., Furth, J. J., Malamy, M., and Alexander, M. (1962). *Proc. Nat. Acad. Sci. U.S.A.* **48**, 1222.

Iyer, V. N., and Szybalski, W. (1963). *Proc. Nat. Acad. Sci. U.S.A.* **50**, 355.

Iyer, V. N., and Szybalski, W. (1964). *Science* **145**, 55.

Jacob, F., Brenner, S., and Cuzin, F. (1963). *Cold Spring Harbor Symp. Quant. Biol.* **28**, 329.

Johnson, A. W. (1960). *Ann. N.Y. Acad. Sci.* **89**, 336.

Kahan, E., Kahn, F., and Hurwitz, J. (1963). *J. Biol. Chem.* **238**, 2491.

Kandaswamy, T. S., and Henderson, J. F. (1963). *Cancer Res.* **23**, 250.

Katz, E., Goldblum, T., Bachrach, U., and Goldblum, N. (1967). *Isr. J. Med. Sci.* **3**, 575.

Kawamata, J., and Imanishi, M. (1961). *Biken J.* **4**, 13.

Kaziro, Y., and Kamiyama, M. (1965). *Biochem. Biophys. Res. Commun.* **19**, 433.

Kepes, A. (1963). *Biochim. Biophys. Acta* **55**, 558.

Kersten, H., Kersten, W., Leopold, G., and Schnieders, B. (1964). *Biochim. Biophys. Acta* **80**, 521.

Kersten, W., and Kersten, H. (1965). *Biochem. Z.* **341**, 174.

Kersten, W., Kersten, H., and Szybalski, W. (1966). *Biochemistry* **5**, 236.

Kirk, J. M. (1960). *Biochim. Biophys. Acta* **42**, 167.

Kohn, K. W., Spears, C. L., and Doty, P. (1966). *J. Mol. Biol.* **19**, 266.

Kurnick, N. B., and Radcliffe, I. E. (1962). *J. Lab. Clin. Med.* **60**, 669.

Le Pecq, J. B., Yot, P., and Paoletti, C. (1964). *C. R. Acad. Sci.* **259**, 1786.

Lerman, L. S. (1961). *J. Mol. Biol.* **3**, 18.

Lerman, L. S. (1963). *Proc. Nat. Acad. Sci. U.S.A.* **49**, 94.

Lerman, L. S. (1964). *J. Mol. Biol.* **10**, 367.

Liersch, M., and Hartmann, G. (1965). *Biochem. Z.* **343**, 16.
Lipsett, M. N., and Weissbach, A. (1965). *Biochemistry* **4**, 206.
Luzzati, V., Masson, F., and Lerman, L. S. (1961). *J. Mol. Biol.* **3**, 634.
McIlwain, H. (1941). *Biochem. J.* **35**, 1311.
Mahler, H. R., and Mehrotra, B. D. (1963). *Biochim. Biophys. Acta* **68**, 211.
Marmur, J., Rownd, R., Falkow, S., Baron, L. S., Schildkraut, C., and Doty, P. (1961). *Proc. Nat. Acad. Sci. U.S.A.* **47**, 972.
Marmur, J., Rownd, R., and Schildkraut, C. L. (1963). *Progr. Nucl. Acid Res.* **1**, 231.
Mason, S. F., and McCaffery, A. J. (1964). *Nature (London)* **204**, 468.
Matsumoto, I., and Lark, K. G. (1963). *Exp. Cell Res.* **32**, 192.
Mauger, A. B., and Wade, R. (1966). *J. Chem. Soc.* p. 1406.
Mehrotra, B. D., and Mahler, H. R. (1964). *Biochim. Biophys. Acta* **91**, 78.
Meyer, R. R., and Simpson, M. V. (1969). *Biochem. Biophys. Res. Commun.* **34**, 238.
Montagnier, L. (1968). *Symp. Soc. Gen. Microbiol.* **18**, 125.
Morgan, G. T., and Walls, L. P. (1931). *J. Chem. Soc., London* p. 2447.
Müller, W., and Crothers, D. M. (1968). *J. Mol. Biol.* **35**, 251.
Murakami, H. (1966). *J. Theor. Biol.* **10**, 236.
Neville, D. M., and Davies, D. R. (1966). *J. Mol. Biol.* **17**, 57.
Newsome, J. (1951). *Trans. Roy. Soc. Trop. Med. Hyg.* **44**, 611.
Newton, B. A. (1957). *J. Gen. Microbiol.* **17**, 718.
Newton, B. A. (1963). *In* "Metabolic Inhibitors" (R. M. Hochster and J. H. Quastel, eds.), Vol. 2, pp. 285–310. Academic Press, New York.
Newton, B. A. (1967). *Biochem. J.* **105**, 50P.
Newton, B. A., and Le Page, R. W. F. (1967). *Biochem. J.* **105**, 50P.
O'Brien, R. L., and Hahn, F. E. (1966). *Antimicrob. Ag. Chemother.* 1965, p. 315.
Ormerod, W. E. (1951). *Brit. J. Pharmacol.* **6**, 334.
Ormerod, W. E. (1952). *Brit. J. Pharmacol.* **7**, 674.
Parker, F. S., and Irvin, J. L. (1952). *J. Biol. Chem.* **199**, 897.
Patrick, J. B., Williams, R. P., Meyer, W. E., Fulmor, W., Cosulich, D. B., Broschard, R. W., and Webb, J. S. (1964). *J. Amer. Chem. Soc.* **86**, 1889.
Peacocke, A. R., and Skerrett, J. N. H. (1956). *Trans. Faraday Soc.* **52**, 261.
Pritchard, N. J., Blake, A., and Peacocke, A. R. (1966). *Nature (London)* **212**, 1360.
Radloff, R., Bauer, W., and Vinograd, J. (1967). *Proc. Nat. Acad. Sci. U.S.A.* **57**, 1514.
Rauen, H. M., Kersten, H., and Kersten, W. (1960). *Hoppe-Seyler's Z. Physiol. Chem.* **321**, 139.
Reich, E., (1964). *Science* **143**, 684.
Reich, E., and Goldberg, I. H. (1964). *Prog. Nucl. Acid Res. Mol. Biol.* **3**, 184.
Reich, E., Shatkin, A. J., and Tatum, E. L. (1961). *Biochim. Biophys Acta* **53**, 132.
Reich, E., Cerami, A., and Ward, D. C. (1967). *In* "Antibiotics. I: Mechanisms of Action" (D. Gottlieb and P. D. Shaw, eds.), pp. 714–725. Springer, Berlin.
Richardson, J. P. (1966). *J. Mol. Biol.* **21**, 83.
Richmond, M. H. (1959). *Biochim. Biophys. Acta* **34**, 325.
Ringertz, N. R., and Bolund, L. (1969). *Biochim. Biophys. Acta* **174**, 147.
Robertson, M. (1963). *J. Gen. Microbiol.* **33**, 177.
Rogolsky, M., and Slepecky, R. A. (1964). *Biochem. Biophys. Res. Commun.* **16**, 204.
Roth, D., and Manjon, M. L. (1969). *Biopolymers* **7**, 695.
Schellenberg, K. A., and Coatney, G. R. (1961). *Biochem. Pharmacol.* **6**, 143.
Schoenbach, E. B., and Greenspan, E. M. (1948). *Medicine (Baltimore)* **27**, 327.
Schwartz, H. S., and Garofalo, M. (1967). *Mol. Pharmacol.* **3**, 1.
Seaman, A., and Woodbine, M. (1953). *Atti 6th Congr. Int. Microbiol., Rome* **1**, 636.
Sexton, W. A. (1963). "Chemical Constitution and Biological Activity." Spon, London.

Shatkin, A. J. (1965). *Biochem. Biophys. Res. Commun.* **19**, 506.
Shiba, S., Terawaki, A., Taguchi, T., and Kawamata, J. (1958). *Biken J.* **1**, 179.
Shiba, S., Terawaki, A., Taguchi, T., and Kawamata, J. (1959). *Nature (London)* **183**, 1056.
Slonimski, P., Perrodin, G., and Craft, G. H. (1968). *Biochem. Biophys. Res. Commun.* **30**, 232.
Snapper, I., Mirsky, A. E., Ris, H., Schneid, B., and Rosenthal, M. (1947). *Blood* **2**, 311.
Steinert, M. (1965). *Exp. Cell Res.* **39**, 69.
Steinert, M., and Van Assel, S. (1967). *J. Cell Biol.* **34**, 489.
Steinert, M., Van Assel, S., and Steinert, G. (1969). *Exp. Cell Res.* **56**, 69.
Stewart, G. A., and Farber, E. (1968). *J. Biol. Chem.* **243**, 4479.
Stone, A. L., and Bradley, D. F. (1961). *J. Amer. Chem. Soc.* **83**, 3627.
Suwalsky, M., Traub, W., Shmueli, U., and Subirana, J. A. (1969). *J. Mol. Biol.* **42**, 363.
Szybalski, W. (1967). *In* "Thermobiology" (A. H. Rose, ed.), Ch. 4. Academic Press, New York.
Szybalski, W., and Iyer, V. N. (1964). *Fed. Proc. Fed. Amer. Soc. Exp. Biol.* **23**, 946.
Szybalski, W., and Iyer, V. N. (1967). *In* "Antibiotics. I: Mechanisms of Action" (D. Gottlieb and P. D. Shaw, eds.), pp. 211–245. Springer, Berlin.
Tabor, C. W., Tabor, H., and Bachrach, U. (1964). *J. Biol. Chem.* **239**, 21904.
Tabor, H. (1962). *Biochemistry* **1**, 496.
Tabor, H., and Tabor, C. W. (1964). *Pharmacol. Rev.* **16**, 245.
Tabor, H., Tabor, C. W., and Rosenthal, S. M. (1961). *Annu. Rev. Biochem.* **30**, 579.
Terawaki, A., and Greenberg, J. (1966). *Biochim. Biophys. Acta* **119**, 540.
Tomchick, R., and Mandel, H. G. (1964). *J. Gen. Microbiol.* **36**, 225.
Tubbs, R. K., Ditmars, W. E., and Van Winkle, Q. (1964). *J. Mol. Biol.* **9**, 545.
Tulinsky, A. (1964). *J. Amer. Chem. Soc.* **86**, 5368.
Vickerman, K. (1969). *J. Cell Sci.* **5**, 163.
Vinograd, J., Lebowitz, J., Radloff, R., Watson, R., and Laipis, P. (1965). *Proc. Nat. Acad. Sci. U.S.A.* **53**, 1104.
Wakiki, S., Marumo, H., Tomioka, K., Shimizu, G., Kato, E., Kamada, S., and Fujimoto, Y. (1958). *Antibiot. Chemother. (Washington, D.C.)* **8**, 228.
Ward, D., Reich, E., and Goldberg, I. H. (1965). *Science* **149**, 1259.
Waring, M. J. (1964). *Biochim. Biophys. Acta* **87**, 358.
Waring, M. J. (1965). *Mol. Pharmacol.* **1**, 1.
Watkins, T. I. (1952). *J. Chem. Soc., London* p. 3059.
Weinstein, I. B., Chernoff, R., Finkelstein, I., and Hirschberg, E. (1965). *Mol. Pharmacol.* **1**, 297.
Weinstein, I. B., Carchman, R., Marner, E., and Hirschberg, E. (1967). *Biochim. Biophys. Acta* **142**, 440.
Weissbach, A., and Lisio, A. (1965). *Biochemistry* **4**, 196.
Wells, R. D. (1969). *Science* **165**, 75.
Wells, R. D., and Blair, J. E. (1967). *J. Mol. Biol.* **27**, 273.
Wells, R. D., Jacob, T. M., Narang, S. A., and Khorana, H. G. (1967). *J. Mol. Biol.* **27**, 237.
Whichard, L. P., Morris, C. R., Smith, J. M., and Holbrook, D. J. (1968). *Mol. Pharmacol.* **4**, 630.
Wiesner, R., Acs, G., Reich, E., and Shafiq, A. (1965). *J. Cell Biol.* **27**, 47.
Williamson, J. (1962). *Exp. Parasitol.* **12**, 274.
Williamson, J., and Macadam, R. F. (1965). *Trans. Roy. Soc. Trop. Med. Hyg.* **59**, 367.
Woese, C., Naona, S., Soffer, R., and Gros, F. (1963). *Biochem. Biophys. Res. Commun.* **11**, 435.

Note Added in Proof: Since this article was completed there have been numerous papers dealing with drug–DNA interactions. Time and space do not permit a complete survey of these, but recent work on actinomycin D, summarized below, is important in relation to Section III of this review. Anthramycin can now be added to the list of drugs which form complexes with DNA and is of interest since it does not resemble any previously described DNA-binding compound in structure.

A. Actinomycin D

Wells and Larson (1970) studying the binding of actinomycin D to DNA and DNA model polymers have confirmed that the presence of deoxyguanylic acid in a DNA is not necessary for complex formation. A marked nucleotide sequence preference exists for the binding reaction. These results are contrary to the predictions of Reich and Goldberg (1964). Wells and Larson discuss their results in relation to two models for the actinomycin–DNA complex, the hydrogen bonded "outside-binding" model and the intercalation model, and conclude that the data are not consistent with the former. Further support for the intercalation model has been obtained by Waring (1970) who has found that actinomycin decreases and then increases the sedimentation coefficient of closed circular ϕX 174 (R.F.) DNA in a manner similar to ethidium bromide. Hycanthone, daunomycin, nogalamycin, and chloroquine gave similar results whereas drugs which are believed not to intercalate (spermine, berenil, streptomycin, chromomycin, and mithramycin) did not uncoil supercoiled molecules.

Further investigation of the effect of actinomycin D on DNA-directed transcription by RNA polymerase (Hyman and Davidson, 1970), suggests that the main effect of the antibiotic is to inhibit the rate of chain growth by preferentially inhibiting the incorporation of guanine and cytosine, rather than by inhibiting initiation or termination steps.

B. Anthramycin

Anthramycin has antibacterial and antitumor activity and inhibits DNA and RNA synthesis in mammalian cells (Kohn *et al.*, 1968). Its structure (XIX) has been confirmed by total synthesis (Leimgruber *et al.*, 1968).

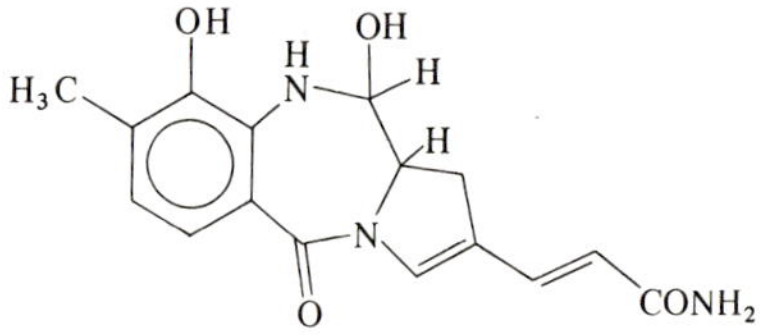

(XIX)

Kohn and Spears (1970) report that this antibiotic complexes with DNA by the formation of a labile covalent bond. The reaction is highly selective for native DNA and it appears to be influenced by base sequence. The high degree of specificity and near irreversibility of the anthramycin–DNA interaction suggests that this compound may prove to be a useful tool for the study of DNA-containing structures.

References

Hyman, R. W., and Davidson, N. (1970). *J. Mol. Biol.* **50**, 421.

Kohn, K. W., Bono, V. H., and Kann, H. E. (1968). *Biochim. Biophys. Acta* **155**, 121.

Kohn, K. W., and Spears, C. L. (1970). *J. Mol. Biol.* **51**, 551.

Leimgruber, W., Batcho, A. D., and Czajkowski, R. C. (1968). *J. Amer. Chem. Soc.* **90**, 5641.

Waring, M. J. (1970). *J. Mol. Biol.* (in press).

Wells, R. D., and Larson, J. E. (1970). *J. Mol. Biol.* **49**, 319.

Interactions of Monoamine Oxidase Inhibitors, Amines, and Foodstuffs

E. Marley and B. Blackwell*

Institute of Psychiatry
De Crespigny Park
London, England

I. Introduction

Interest in intolerance to foodstuffs in man is as old as medicine; Hippocrates remarked that "I certainly hold it necessary for every physician to know this much at least about nature; namely what are a man's

*Present Address: Department of Psychiatry and Pharmacology, University of Cincinnati, Ohio.

relations to food and drink . . . and how each person is affected by each" (Brock, 1929).

The medieval practice of purgation to cleanse the body of evil humors gained scientific credance when Metchnikoff (1903) declared the large intestine "a reservoir of waste which stagnates long enough to putrefy" and suggested that "ptomaines" produced within it by bacterial fermentation were "the cause of serious misfortune and the greatest disharmony in the constitution of man." The symptoms which were often vague or ill-defined included headaches or fluctuations in blood pressure. Arbuthnot Lane, a surgeon, established a reputation by removing the colon for such complaints in patients with chronic constipation (Tanner, 1946).

Controversy over this drastic implementation of what Bernard Shaw (in the *Doctor's Dilemma*) described as "Metchnikoff's fanciful biological romances" led to a series of meetings at the Royal Society of Medicine in London during 1913 (*Proc. Roy. Soc. Med.*, 1913). Here it was speculated that "the end products of protein digestion may reach the general circulation if the quantity absorbed is larger than the liver can deal with" (Harley, 1913). This possibility was discounted unless there was "some inability on the part of the oxidising machinery to keep pace with the formation of putrefactive products" (Somerville, 1913).

Such a protective oxidative mechanism was not elucidated until 15 years later when "tyramine oxidase" was isolated from liver (Hare, 1928) and later renamed "monoamine oxidase." Presence of this enzyme in the gut was considered to be "an enigma" (Davison, 1958), but in 1952 Blaschko speculated that it might serve as a "detoxicating agent, particularly if the food has been exposed to putrefaction and amines are already in it when eaten" (Blaschko, 1952).

That such foods existed was well known, and cheese was among the first to be singled out. Hippocrates had observed that "cheese is a bad article of food, in that it gives pain to anyone eating it in excess." In the search for new chemical substances during the early nineteenth century many naturally occurring foodstuffs were analyzed and Liebig (1846) isolated a white crystalline substance from cheese. He named this new amino acid "tyrosine" after the Greek word meaning cheese. By the turn of the century its amine derivative, tyramine, had been isolated from the same source (Van Slyke and Hart, 1903) so that when the "intestinal toxemia" controversy broke out soon afterward cheese became suspect. Thus Dixon (1913) noted how "the simplest way in which harmless amino acids are made toxic is by decarboxylation. Tyramine has been shown to occur in ripened cheese, being in this case produced by bacterial action."

The potent effects of such naturally occurring amines had been demonstrated by Dale and Dixon (1909). They found that tyramine obtained from putrid meat produced hypertension in man and animals; two years later Findlay (1911) showed that tyramine injected intramuscularly produced large rises in pressure accompanied by "excruciating headaches."

By the time monoamine oxidase inhibitors were first used in medicine in 1952 the potential toxicity of cheese had been recognized. Its major constituent amine and its physiological actions were known, the protective oxidative gut mechanisms were identified, and the likely consequences of their destruction had been predicted.

II. Amines in Foodstuffs

Amines are formed in animal and plant tissues when amino acids are decarboxylated either by endogenous enzymes during life or by bacterial contaminants after death. Such decarboxylating enzymes are widely distributed in animal tissues (Blaschko, 1945). Analysis of foodstuffs for amines may be by chemical or biological methods.

A. Chemical Analysis

Most of the amines in foodstuffs have been detected and estimated by chromatographic or spectrofluorimetric methods. Some of the findings are shown in Tables I and II. Clearly a large number of edible plants or plant products

TABLE I

Concentration of Amines in Foods (in μg/gm unless otherwise stated)

Foodstuff	5-HT	Tryptamine	Tyramine	Dopamine	Dopa	Nad	Histamine	Ref.[a]
Banana (peel)	50–150	0	65	700	—	122	—	1
Banana (pulp)	28	0	7	8	—	2	—	1
Plaintain(pulp)	45	—	—	—	—	—	—	1
Tomato	12	4	4	0	—	0	—	1
Red plum	10	0–2	6	0	—	+	—	1
Blue-red plum	8	2	—	—	—	—	—	1
Blue plum	0	5	—	—	—	—	—	1
Avocado pear	10	0	23	4–5	—	0	—	1
Potato	0	0	1	0	—	0.1–2		1
Spinach	0	0	1	0	—	0	—	1
Grape	0	0	0	0	—	0	—	1
Orange (pulp)	0	0.1	10	0	—	+	—	1
Eggplant	2	0.5–3.0	3	0	—	0	—	1
Broadbeans	—	—		—	+	—	—	2
Passion fruit	1–4	—	—	—	—	—	—	3

(*Cont.*)

TABLE I (*Cont.*)

Foodstuff	5-HT	Tryptamine	Tyramine	Dopamine	Dopa	Nad	Histamine	Ref.[a]
Pawpaw	1–2	—	—	—	—	—	—	3
Pineapple (green)	50–60	—	—	—	—	—	—	4
Pineapple (ripe)	19	—	—	—	—	—	—	4
Pineapple, canned juice	23–25 μg/ml	—	—	—	—	—	—	5
Pineapple, fresh juice	12 μg/ml	—	—	—	—	—	—	5
Sauerkraut juice	—	—	—	—	—	—	40 μg/ml	6
Camembert cheese	—	—	2000	—	—	—	—	7
Stilton cheese	—	—	466	—	—	—	—	8
Brie cheese	—	—	180	—	—	—	—	8
Emmenthal cheese	—	—	225	—	—	—	—	8
N.Y. State Cheddar	—	—	1416	—	—	—	—	8
Gruyere	—	—	516	—	—	—	—	8
Processed American	—	—	50	—	—	—		8
Cream	—	—	0	—	—	—	—	8
Cottage	—	—	0	—	—	—	—	8
Beer	—	—	1.8 μg/ml	—	—	—	—	8
Sherry wine	—	—	3.6 μg/ml	—	—	—	—	8
Sauterne wine	—	—	0.4 μg/ml	—	—	—	—	8
Riesling wine	—	—	0.6 μg/ml	—	—	—	—	8
Chianti wine	—	—	24.5 μg/ml	—	—	—	—	8
English Cheddar	—	—	0–953	—	—	—	—	9
Canadian Cheddar	—	—	251–535	—	—	—	—	9
New Zealand Cheddar	—	—	417–580	—	—	—	—	9
Australian Cheddar	—	—	226	—	—	—	—	9
Kraft (Cracker Barrel)	—	—	214	—	—	—	—	9
Marmite[b]	—	—	1087–1639	—	—	—	976–2832	10
Yex[b]	—	—	506	—	—	—	1344	10
Befit[b]	—	—	419	—	—	—	272	10
Barmene[b]	—	—	152	—	—	—	208	10
Yeastrel[b]	—	—	101	—	—	—	256	10
Pickled herring	—	—	3030	—	—	—	—	11
Chicken livers	—	—	94–113	—	—	—	—	12

[a] References: 1, Udenfriend *et al.*, 1959; 2, Hodge *et al.*, 1964; 3, Foy and Parratt, 1960; 4, Foy and Parratt, 1961; 5, Bruce, 1960; 6, Keil and Kritter, 1934; 7, Asatoor *et al.*, 1963; 8, Horwitz *et al.*, 1964; 9, Blackwell and Mabbitt, 1965; 10, Blackwell *et al.*, 1968; 11, Nuessle *et al.*, 1965; 12, Hedberg *et al.*, 1966.

[b] Yeast extracts.

TABLE II

HISTAMINE CONTENT OF FISH PRODUCTS ON THE JAPANESE MARKET[a]

Kind of product	Amount of histamine: μg/gm product	Amount of histamine: μg/gm dry matter
Canned fish		
Oil sardine	57.9	113.1
Seasoned sardine	13.1	48.0
	81.6	203.1
Seasoned mackerel	1.8	6.3
	49.3	148.6
Seasoned tuna	63.8	162.1
	99.8	275.0
Seasoned bonito	59.9	156.3
	156.9	489.5
Seasoned whale	11.3	34.9
Pink salmon	2.3	6.6
Dried fish		
Sardine	124.3	150.9
Herring	300.9	366.2
Sand eel	39.5	48.5
Squid	26.0	34.5
Shark fin	1.8	2.0
Salted fish		
Herring	98.3	200.7
Trout	22.5	48.8
Herring roe	5.1	11.7
Salted dried fish		
Mackerel pike	297.8	522.8
Gutted cod	0.7	1.0
Sardine	15.0	23.3
Seasoned dried fish		
Pressed squid	10.2	11.7
Globefish	2.4	3.6
Broiled sardine	398.9	471.8
Fish boiled in soy sauce		
Sand eel	1.8	2.5
Goby	5.3	7.2
Smoked fish		
Herring	345.2	520.2
Salmon	16.6	24.9
Salted fish gut		
Bonito	24.7	59.8
Sea cucumber	107.2	292.2
Fish cake		
Kamaboko	0.4	1.6
Kamaboko	0.7	2.3

[a] From Kimata, 1961.

contain significant quantities of amines which are metabolized by amine oxidase, although there is disagreement in some instances about the amount present. For example, Bruce (1960) found the 5-HT (5-hydroxytryptamine) in canned pineapple juice to be 23 to 25 μg/ml, whereas Foy and Parratt (1961) recorded it as 2.8 to 8 μg/ml. The point at issue was not the potentiation of 5-HT by amine oxidase inhibition but an erroneous diagnosis of carcinoid tumor following pineapple ingestion. Apart from plants, certain molluscs, e.g., octypus contain 5-HT (Kimata, 1961).

If the amine-containing food is a staple part of the diet, large quantities of amine may be ingested. The plantain, a banana-like fruit, contributes largely to the West African's diet. Plantains are fried and eaten as a vegetable, an average of 6 to 15 being eaten each week. A plantain fruit can weigh over 300 gm, containing an estimated 12 mg 5-HT (Foy and Parratt, 1960), so that the oral ingestion of 5-HT may be from 70 to 180 mg a week. There appears to have been no instances of adverse reactions attributable to 5-HT in foods eaten by patients on monoamine oxidase inhibitors.

In contrast, there have been many hypertensive incidents in patients on monoamine oxidase inhibitors attributable to tyramine in cheese. Asatoor *et al.* (1963) chromatographed several types of fermented cheese and found tyramine to be the only pressor amine consistently present in significant amounts. On feeding Camembert or Stilton cheese, which are rich in this amine, to healthy adults, they were able to demonstrate an increase in the urinary excretion of *p*-hydroxyphenylacetic acid, a metabolic end product of tyramine. If an average portion of a matured cheese eaten at a meal is 50 gm (about 2 oz), the portion could contain between 2.5 and 100 mg tyramine apart from other pressor amines, a quantity sufficient to provoke a hypertensive crisis in a subject treated with a monoamine oxidase inhibitor. Portions of cheese that came to analysis and which had provoked a hypertensive crisis in man contained substantial quantities of tyramine (Blackwell and Mabbitt, 1965). There is no evidence, as was once thought, that cheeses with visible and olfactory evidence of putrefaction necessarily contain most tyramine, although unmatured "cottage" style cheeses contain least (Table I). This sort of cheese is more commonly eaten in the U.S.A. and may account for the fewer adverse reactions reported there. Other dairy products that have been incriminated include cream and chocolate. Cheeses contain pressor amines in addition to those listed in Table I—phenethylamine in Gouda cheese and typtamine as well as phenethylamine in Stilton (Asatoor *et al.*, 1963). The diamines cadaverine, putrescine, and histamine have been found in cheeses, but these amines lower blood pressure.

Yeast extracts are ingredients of foods such as canned soups, sauces, relishes, or moulded meat products (Lyall, 1963), and at least five extracts are sold in Britain as sandwich spreads or beverages. Their tyramine content is at least as high as that in cheese (Table I). Hypertensive attacks have been provoked in patients treated with a monoamine oxidase inhibitor and who ingested 4 gm of the extract Marmite estimated to contain about 6 mg tyramine (Blackwell *et al.*, 1965). As with cheeses, the tyramine content differed substantially from one yeast extract to another.

Substantial quantities of histamine are present in some yeast extracts (Blackwell and Marley, 1966a; Blackwell *et al.*, 1968) and in some animal tissues (Tabor, 1954), particularly fishes (Kimata, 1961). The histamine content of fish products on the Japanese market are given in Table II and apply to preserved fish, e.g. dried, smoked, and tinned. The higher values for histamine (0.3 mg/gm) in fish approximate those for yeast extracts such as Befit, Barmene, and Yeastrel which had the lowest histamine values of a series of yeast extracts examined by Blackwell *et al.* (1968) and are about one tenth those found for Marmite. Canned tuna and sardine as well as smoked cod and herring on sale in Britain were assayed biologically; the highest value for histamine was 0.01 mg/gm in the case of sardine, the concentration in the other fishes being substantially lower (Blackwell and Marley, unpublished). Histamine may appear in spoiled fish meat (Kimata, 1961), but this aspect was not tested.

L-Dopa (dihydroxyphenylalanine) has been incriminated in interactions between foodstuffs and monoamine inhibitors, although its natural occurrence in significant quantities seems to be confined to the pods and seeds of certain leguminous plants (Sealock, 1949). Chromatographic examination of ethanol-soluble extracts of bean pods revealed dopa to be the predominant amino acid and the only one with pressor activity; sympathomimetic amines were not present (Hodge *et al.*, 1964). Amino acid precursors of biologically active amines occur in some foodstuffs; tyrosine is present in cheese (Liebig, 1846), histidine in many fishes (Kimata, 1961), and histidine as well as tyrosine in yeast extracts. Conversion of the amino acid to the corresponding amine can occur during ripening or storage. The 5-HT content of bananas was measured during ripening and found to be considerably increased (Udenfriend *et al.*, 1959), although that in pineapples was diminished (Foy and Parratt, 1961). Cheeses, with the exception of the unmatured varieties, are ripened for at least 3 months and the concentration of tyrosine rises steadily as protein break-down proceeds during maturation. Because some bacteria (coliforms and streptococci group D) in cheeses have tyrosine decarboxylase activity the tyramine concentration also increases. Little is known about decarboxylation enzymes in fungi and yeasts which might produce amines during their autolysis, as in preparation of yeast extracts. A possible source of amines after ingestion of the foodstuffs is decarboxylation of its amino acid components by gut commensals. There are many microorganisms capable of amino acid decarboxylation in the human gut (Wilson and Miles, 1955), where the pH of the lower ileum and colon with anaerobic conditions and constant temperature provide an ideal environment for bacterial growth coupled with a ready supply of amino acids produced by enzymatic proteolysis. Much of the earlier evidence for the bacterial production of amines from amino acids in the gut is discussed by Gale (1940), and additional evidence derived from the use of antibiotics which suppress bacterial activity and limit amine formation in the bowel is described by Melnykowycz and Johannson (1955). Only 41% of ^{14}C-labeled protein fed orally to rats and cats is transported across the intestine in the form of amino acids, and the appearance of $^{14}CO_2$ in the expired air suggests that some of the amino acids are catabolized in the gut or intestinal wall (Dawson and Porter, 1962). In rats treated with mebanazine such a possibility was unlikely to account for the effects of cheese because large amounts (250 to 1000 μmole/kg intraduodenally) of tyrosine, phenylalanine, and tryptophan, amino acid precursors of the three amines in cheese with greatest pressor activity, were ineffective on the blood pressure (Blackwell and Marley, 1966b).

B. Pharmacological Analysis

Pharmacological methods were well suited for estimating histamine in yeast extracts. The presence of histamine was strongly indicated by contraction of isolated guinea pig ilea evoked by the yeast extracts in the presence of hyoscine (Fig. 1A, B) and of abolition of the contractions due to histamine and to the yeast extract by mepyramine (Fig. 1D) when the effect of another contractor substance, 5-HT, was scarcely altered (compare Fig. 1C, D). Antagonism was surmounted by a 100-fold increase in the doses of histamine and of the extract (Fig. 1E, F).

Assay of 5-HT in pineapple and plantain extracts has been done using isolated rat uterus and rat colon preparations. Contractions were evoked by these extracts in the presence of atropine (10^{-7}) and were antagonized by bromolysergic acid diethylamide, a selective 5-HT antagonist (Foy and Parratt, 1960, 1961). Tyramine in pickled herring was identified by chemical methods, and its pharmacological properties tested on isolated rat atria before and after pretreatment of rats with reserpine (Nuessle *et al.*, 1965). If the substance was tyramine or allied congener then its chronotrophic properties would be abolished by reserpine pretreatment, which proved to be the case.

Inasmuch as phenethylamine and tryptamine as well as tyramine occur in some cheese and as other foods contain other pressor substances like 5-HT, dopamine, or its precursor L-dopa, pressor effects caused by intravenous injection of saline extracts of the food are less meaningful than the specific biological test for histamine. Nevertheless, an estimate of the pressor content of saline extracts of cheese or yeast products in terms of "tyramine equivalents" on the blood pressure of pithed rats was helpful (see Fig. 6A). The presence of tryptamine was excluded by the abolition of pressor activity by phenoxybenzamine, an antagonist which prevents the action of noradren-

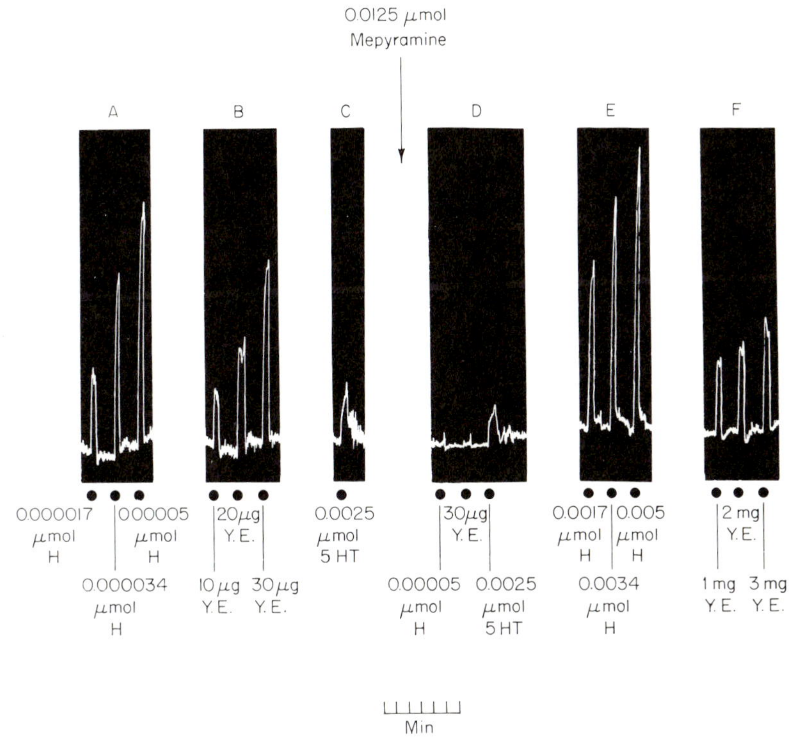

FIG. 1. Contractions of the isolated guinea pig ileum produced (A) by histamine (H), (B) by the yeast extract salt-free Marmite (Y.E.), and (C) by 5-hydroxytryptamine (5-HT) in the presence of hyoscine (10^{-7}). (D) Antagonism to histamine and to the yeast extract by mepyramine (0.0125 μmole) placed in the bath for 5 minutes and then washed out. (E) (F) Antagonism surmountable by 100-fold increase in dose of histamine and of the yeast extract. (Doses expressed as the final concentration per milliliter of the drug or extract in bath.)

aline released by amines such as tyramine. In pargyline-treated rats, L-α-methyldopa, an inhibitor of dopa decarboxylase, which prevents the formation of dopamine from dopa, completely blocked the pressor response of intravenously injected ethanol-soluble fractions of bean pods; the pressor effect of dopa was similarly blocked but that of dopamine was unaffected. This led Hodge *et al.* (1964) to conclude that hypertensive crises in patients who had eaten bean pods and who were being treated with pargyline, were due to the conversion of L-dopa to dopamine, a pressor amine normally inactivated by amine oxidase.

III. Metabolism of Amines and Related Substances in Foodstuffs

A. Aromatic Monoamines Such as Tyramine

An enzyme catalyzing the oxidative deaminations of tyramine was described by Hare (1928) and named "tyramine oxidase." The probability that only one oxidase, amine oxidase, dealt with a large number of aliphatic and aromatic amines, the aromatic amines including tyramine, ephedrine, and adrenaline was debated by Blaschko *et al.* (1937a). Excellent reviews on amine oxidase are provided by Blaschko (1952) and Davison (1958) from which much of the following is taken.

It is the ionized form of the amine, i.e., the form which is not readily absorbed from the gut, that reacts with the enzyme; amines which are not ionized to any extent are not oxidized. The overall reaction in the presence of catalase is

$$R—CH_2\overset{+}{N}R\,R'R'' + \tfrac{1}{2}O_2 \rightarrow R\cdot CHO + \overset{+}{N}H_2R'R''$$

The aldehyde formed may then be oxidized further to the corresponding carboxylic acid. Aromatic amines, like aniline, in which the amino group is directly attached to the ring, are not attacked by amine oxidase; benzylamine is oxidized by amine oxidase. With increasing length of side chain the rate of oxidation increases. β-Phenylethylamine is oxidized more rapidly than benzylamine and γ-phenylpropylamine more rapidly than β-phenylethylamine (Beyer and Morrison, 1945). Not only phenolic compounds with the hydroxyl group in the *para* position, as in tyramine, but also *meta*-phenolic amines like phenylephrine are oxidized; the *meta* and *ortho* analogs of tyramine are substrates of amine oxidase (Randall, 1946). Of the diphenolic derivatives, adrenaline, noradrenaline, and dopamine are oxidized by amine oxidase. Substitution of the terminal amino group in aromatic amines can also affect oxidation. However, unless the compound is rapidly *N*-methylated or *N*-acetylated after absorption from the bowel, this factor is unlikely to be important with respect to amines in foodstuffs. Any substrate of amine oxidase, because it has affinity for the enzyme, may interfere with the oxidation of another substrate. Such substrate competition could be relevant with a food such as cheese which contains a number of amines deaminated by amine oxidase.

Recently it has transpired that indirectly acting amines such as amphetamine or tyramine are metabolized by microsomal enzymes (Axelrod, 1954,

1955) as well as by monoamine oxidase in mitochondria. The microsomal enzyme inhibitor SKF-525A (Brodie, 1956, Kato *et al.*, 1964) does not inhibit monoamine oxidase (Dubnick *et al.*, 1963) and lacks the pharmacological effects of monoamine oxidase inhibitor (Axelrod *et al.*, 1954; Fouts and Brodie, 1955). The finding therefore that the pressor effects of intravenous tyramine or amphetamine were enhanced in cats pretreated with SKF-525A indicated that nonspecific microsomal enzymes also degraded these amines (Rand and Trinker, 1968).

B. Aliphatic Monoamines and Diamines

Many aliphatic amines of the series $CH_3 \cdot (CH_2)_n \cdot NH_2$ are substrates for the enzyme (Alles and Heegaard, 1943; Blaschko *et al.*, 1937a; Kohn, 1937). Rate of oxidation and affinity vary with the number of carbon atoms in the carbon chain, and with increasing length of chain the rate of oxidation increases, a maximum being reached with 5 or 6 carbon atoms.

Diamines $NH_2(CH_2)_nNH_2$ are not oxidized by amine oxidase; the presence of the second amino group interferes with substrate specificity by lowering the affinity. Diamines such as cadaverine and putrescine, both present in cheese, are not substrates, therefore, for amine oxidase but for another enzyme, diamine oxidase (Zeller, 1942).

C. Tryptamine and 5-Hydroxytryptamine

Deamination of tryptamine by monoamine oxidase was shown by Blaschko *et al.* (1937a). They also demonstrated that tryptamine competes with tyramine as a substrate for the enzyme; tyramine and tryptamine are present together in certain cheeses. 5-HT is also deaminated by amine oxidase (Blaschko, 1952).

D. Histamine

The following processes are believed to be involved in the inactivation of physiological quantities of histamine although the importance of some of the mechanisms has not been rigorously established (Schayer, 1959): (1) Oxidation by diamine oxidase to produce imidazoleacetaldehyde, (2) methylation on the ring nitrogen remote from the side chain to produce 1-methyl-4-(β-aminoethyl)imidazole, (3) oxidation by monoamine oxidase or monoamine oxidase-like enzymes to produce imidazoleacetaldehyde, (4) acetylation of the amino group to produce acetylhistamine, (5) methylation of the amino group of the side chain to produce *N*-methylhistamine and *N*,*N*-dimethylhistamine, and (6) catabolism by uncharacterized enzymes such as histaminase.

The stages in histamine metabolism are shown in Fig. 2. The two main routes are by oxidation to imidazoleacetaldehyde and by methylation to

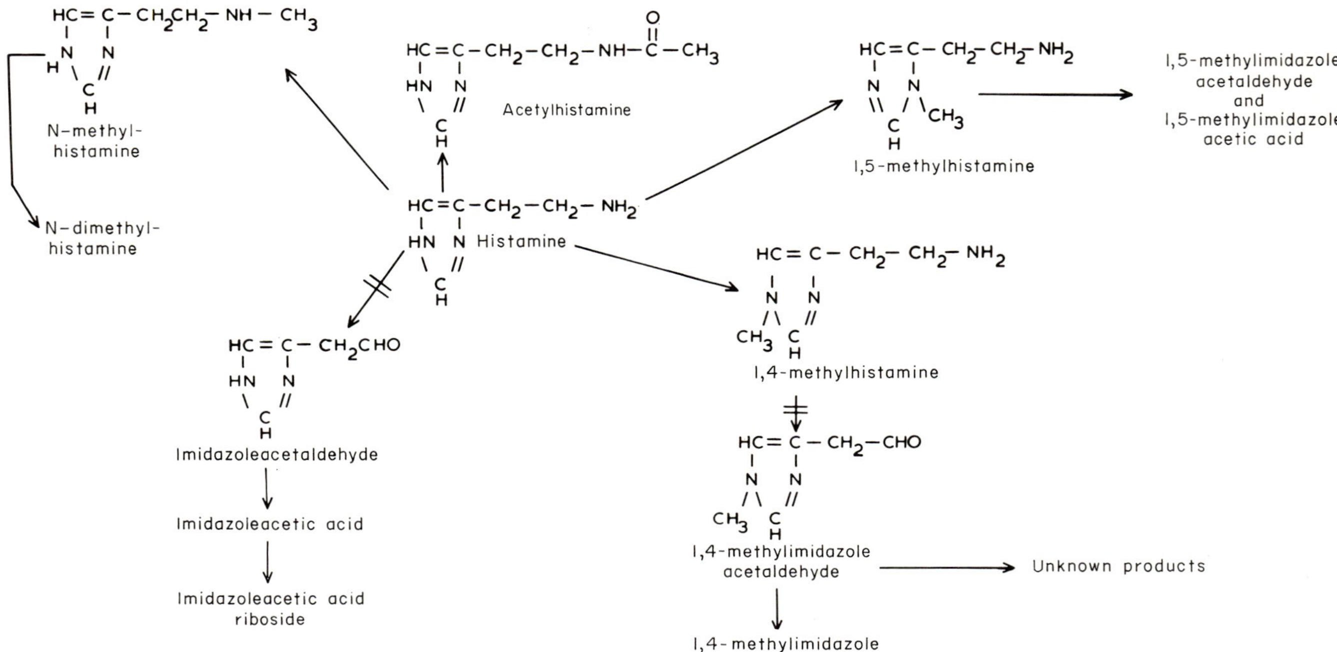

FIG. 2. Stages in histamine catabolism. The main routes are oxidation to imidazoleacetaldehyde and ring methylation to 1,4-methylhistamine. Arrows with double bars are the pathways thought to involve monoamine oxidase. (Adapted from Schayer, 1959.)

1,4-methylhistamine. Indeed, in mammals 60 to 80% of the metabolites of histamine are derived from oxidative deamination (Schayer, 1959). Other mechanisms such as acetylation or methylation of the terminal nitrogen are of subsidiary importance. Amine oxidase is involved in both the main routes. It converts 1,4-methylhistamine to the corresponding aldehyde and plays a minor role in the conversion of histamine to imidazoleacetaldehyde. Inhibitors of monoamine oxidase could therefore interfere with either of these stages, although the metabolism of 1,4-methylhistamine is the one most likely to be affected since diamine oxidase is primarily involved in the conversion of histamine to imidazoleacetaldehyde. There are species differences in the metabolism of histamine. In cats and dogs methylation of the ring nitrogen is the predominant mechanism, whereas in mice, oxidation is prepotent; in rats, both mechanisms are equally important (Schayer, 1959).

Monoamine oxidase inhibitors may interfere with histamine metabolism in yet another way. Thus inhibitors of the hydrazine and hydrazide type, but not those of the phenylcyclopropylamine variety, inhibit *in vitro* and *in vivo* not only monoamine oxidase but also diamine oxidase (Burkard *et al.*, 1962; Shore and Cohn, 1960). Their finding puts a different complexion on the problem, because yeast extracts such as Marmite contain large amounts of histamine (Blackwell and Marley, 1966a). In a species in which oxidation was the main mechanism for histamine metabolism, ingestion of a histamine-containing food could be disastrous. In cats, despite methylation of the ring nitrogen being the predominant means of histamine metabolism, absorption of histamine from the small bowel was facilitated by pretreatment with inhibitors of the hydrazine and hydrazide variety (Blackwell and Marley, 1966a); in addition, some systemic effects of histamine were potentiated in cats pretreated by these inhibitors (Blackwell and Marley, unpublished). The amine oxidases of cat liver act on histamine and methylhistamine (Kobayashi, 1958).

E. L-Dopa

The decarboxylation of L-dopa (L-3,4-dihydroxyphenylalanine) to dopamine is catalyzed by two enzymes: the mammalian L-dopa decarboxylase (Holtz *et al.*, 1938) and the bacterial L-tyrosine decarboxylase (Epps, 1944). The two enzymes differ in their affinity for L-tyrosine; this is probably the "natural substrate" of the bacterial enzyme but it is not attacked by the mammalian enzyme. Dopamine so formed is then converted to noradrenaline and adrenaline.

IV. Distribution of Monoamine Oxidase in the Body

Amine oxidase is widely distributed in the body of vertebrates and invertebrates being present in the mitochondria. Particularly high concentrations are present in the intestinal wall. In sheep, for example, the rumen, abomasum, duodenum, and ileum contain large amounts of amine oxidase; in the duodenum and ileum, the muscular coat is richer in enzyme than is the mucous membrane (Blaschko, 1952). There is species difference in distribution, and according to Davison (1958) enzyme activity is not detectable in the rat intestine. It is, however, present in large amounts in human small intestine (Mustala *et al.*, 1969). That intraduodenal doses of tyramine are without effect on blood pressure unless the rat has been pretreated with an amine oxidase inhibitor (Blackwell and Marley, 1964, 1966b) may indicate that in this species the enzyme is present in large amounts in the liver and/or lungs so that inactivation of tyramine occurs before it reaches the systemic circuit. Species difference in concentration of hepatic enzyme also applies, and the guinea pig liver has particularly high enzymatic activity.

The relative significance of intestinal and liver monoamine oxidase in cats was investigated by Natoff (1965a). Intravenous injection of tyramine (0.2 mg/kg) evoked a mean pressor response of 85 mm Hg, whereas intraportal injection produced only half this effect (44 mm Hg), a response unaffected by nialamide. Hence, although intraportal injections of tyramine were less effective on blood pressure than those given intravenously, they were not enhanced by inhibition of liver monoamine oxidase. The role of hepatic monoamine oxidase in this species would appear subsidiary to that of the intestinal enzyme in amine metabolism. To the extent either that histamine is inactivated by monoamine oxidase or that monoamine oxidase inhibitors interfere with diamine oxidase, the same conclusions apply. Thus in cats with an extracorporeal circulation which superfused an isolated guinea pig ileum (Vane, 1964), a tissue extremely sensitive to circulating histamine, histamine (55 μmole/kg) injected intraduodenally was without effect on the tone of the superfused ileum, whereas as little as 0.02 μmole/kg histamine injected into the splenic vein maximally contracted the superfused ileum (Blackwell and Marley, 1966a). The time course of recovery from amine oxidase inhibition also points to the greater importance of gut over liver enzyme in inactivating amines. Thus, amine oxidase inhibition following oral administration of tranylcypromine to mice was at its peak 1 to 2 hours later in the duodenum and liver, but, whereas inhibition of liver enzyme persisted for more than 4 hours, that in the intestine had 80% recovered in this time (Natoff, 1965b).

The serious systemic effects of amines in food develop once they have been absorbed from the gut and passed through the liver. The brunt of these effects are borne by the cardiovascular system. Thompson and Tickner (1951) studied the distribution of amine oxidase in blood vessels. Enzyme activity was found in blood vessels of guinea pigs, rabbits, rats, and of man. In rabbits, the species most extensively examined, monoamine oxidase activity was high in the aorta and renal arteries but lower in most peripheral arteries. Enzymatic activity was low in veins. The little enzymatic activity in skeletal muscle may be mostly accounted for by the enzyme present in the blood vessels of the tissue. The heart also contains amine oxidase. Bernheim and Bernheim (1945) studied the disappearance of tyramine in the presence of slices of heart tissue from different animals. In guinea pigs, rabbits, and rats, tyramine disappeared rapidly, whereas in cats and dogs the disappearance was slower. The human heart also contains amine oxidase (Langemann, 1944), but blood is without such activity.

In the suprarenal gland amine oxidase is present in the medulla as well as the cortex (Bhagvat *et al.*, 1939; Langemann, 1951). The enzyme occurs in other glands, e.g., in the thyroid (Bhagvat *et al.*, 1939) and Harderian glands of rabbits (A. Spinks, quoted in Blaschko, 1952). It has been found in lungs (Blaschko *et al.*, 1937b) including those of man (Langemann *et al.*, 1943) and in the spleen (Bhagvat *et al.*, 1939). Amine oxidase occurs in the testes (Bhagvat *et al.*, 1939), prostate gland, and seminal vesicles (Zeller and Joel, 1941). In the uterus, activity is high (Bhagvat *et al.*, 1939), but seems to be related to the functional state of the organ; enzymatic activity is often low in the uteri of virgin rabbits (B. M. Schofield, quoted in Blaschko, 1952). In a sheep which had been pregnant for 113 days, amine oxidase was present in the placenta and chorion but there was little activity in the amnion (Blaschko, 1952). The human placenta (Luschinsky and Singher, 1948) and that of other mammals (Thompson and Tickner, 1949) contain amine oxidase.

Pugh and Quastel (1937) were the first to study amine oxidase in nervous tissue, particularly the brain. The human brain also contains amine oxidase (Birkhäuser, 1940). The white matter does not contain much enzyme and the basal ganglia have greater activity than the cortex. Amine oxidase has also been found in ganglia (Blaschko, 1952).

A fact which may partly invalidate much of this earlier work on tissue concentration has been the more recent observation that monoamine oxidase is a binary complex of enzymes with different tissue distributions, substrate specificity and inhibitor sensitivity (Hall *et al.*, 1969; Hall and Logan, 1969; Huszti *et al.*, 1969).

V. Classification and Chemical Structure of Some Monoamine Oxidase Inhibitors

Amine oxidase inhibitors are conventionally divided into hydrazides (R·CO·NH·NH·R), hydrazines (R·NH·NH·R), and amines. Some inhibitors that are or have been in clinical use and have also been employed in studying the food interactions in animals are shown in Fig. 3. The list is not intended to be exhaustive but only to cover those inhibitors mentioned in the text. The resemblance of most of the compounds to β-phenethylamine is striking; indeed,

MONOAMINE OXIDASE INHIBITORS IN CLINICAL USE

APPROVED NAMES	PROPRIETARY NAMES	STRUCTURAL FORMULA
IPRONIAZID	MARSILID	(pyridyl)–$CONH{-}NH{-}CH(CH_3)_2$
ISOCARBOXAZID	MARPLAN	(phenyl)–$CH_2NHNH{-}C{=}O$ (isoxazole ring, N, O, CH_3)
NIALAMIDE	NIAMID	(phenyl)–$CH_2NH{-}C({=}O){-}CH_2CH_2NH{-}NH{-}C{=}O$–(pyridyl)
PIVHYDRAZINE	TERSAVID	$CH_3{-}C(CH_3)_2{-}CONH{\cdot}NH{-}CH_2$–(phenyl)
PHENIPRAZINE	CAVODIL CATRON	(phenyl)–$CH_2\,CH(CH_3){-}NH\,NH_2$
PHENOXYPROPAZINE	DRAZINE	(phenyl)–$OCH_2\,CH(CH_3){-}NH\,NH_2$
PHENELZINE	NARDIL	(phenyl)–$CH_2\,CH_2\,NH\,NH_2$
MEBANAZINE	ACTOMOL	(phenyl)–$CH(CH_3){-}NH\,NH_2$
PARGYLINE	EUTONYL	(phenyl)–$CH_2{-}N(CH_3){-}CH_2\,C{\equiv}CH$
TRANYLCYPROMINE	PARNATE	(phenyl)–$CH{-}CH{-}NH_2$ (ring closed by CH_2, printed CH_3)

FIG. 3. Names, synonyms, and chemical structure of some monoamine oxidase inhibitors.

in describing the high biological activity of certain aralkylhydrazines, reference is commonly made to their being *isosteres* of β-phenethylamine, the parent structure of the sympathomimetic amine family. However, the isosteric relation between amines and the "corresponding" hydrazines is more complex than first thought (Bloom, 1963). For example, benzylhydrazine is more active than β-phenethylhydrazine as an inhibitor of monoamine oxidase (Biel *et al.*,

1959; Chessin *et al.*, 1959; Zeller *et al.*, 1959) and especially of dopamine-β-oxidase (Creveling *et al.*, 1962), enzymes whose normal substrates possess two-carbon side chains. On the other hand, β-phenethylhydrazine and β-phenisopropylamine, *but not benzylhydrazine*, possess the pressor and excitant properties of β-phenethyl- and β-phenisopropylamine (Chessin *et al.*, 1959; Eltherington and Horita, 1960). Despite many similarities between the actions of sympathomimetic drugs and those of monoamine oxidase inhibitors, some of which will be subsequently considered, their properties might be more suitably considered analogous than homologous.

VI. Absorption of Amines and Amino Acids from the Intestine

Acidic but not basic drugs are rapidly absorbed from the stomach (Brodie and Hogben, 1957); this is because the gastric mucosa is selectively permeable to undissociated forms of drugs (Travel, 1940). Consequently, basic substances such as histamine, 5-HT, or tyramine present in the foodstuffs would be ionized at the acid pH of the stomach and therefore not absorbed whereas in the duodenum and distal gut the alkaline pH would convert them to the unionized form which is lipid soluble and more easily absorbed. The position with L-dopa differs in that it is a zwitterion and so partly ionized in the stomach and in the intestine. Absorption from the bowel may be due to a specific amino acid transport system for dopa or to those for closely allied amino acids since these transport systems are partly nonselective. To achieve maximal pharmacological effects with amine-containing foodstuffs it would obviously be more expedient to inject them intraduodenally than into the stomach. Once the amines have crossed the intestinal wall, they are carried in the portal blood to the liver and thence to the lungs before having access to the systemic circuit. Because monoamine oxidase occurs in high concentration in the gut wall, liver, and lungs, even the intraduodenal injection of amines in the absence of enzyme inhibition would be unlikely to lead to their absorption and appearance in systemic blood unless the amount was sufficiently large to swamp the deaminating mechanisms.

In man, for example, 20 to 80 mg tyramine taken by mouth was without effect (Sollman, 1957); similar doses given orally or rectally were asymptomatic, whereas given intravenously or subcutaneously to avoid the main sites of inactivation by monoamine oxidase they markedly raised systolic blood pressure and induced tachycardia with increased amplitude of the T wave in the electrocardiogram (Sollman, 1957). In contrast, perhaps because it was given on an empty stomach, Dale and Dixon (1909) found that 10 mg tyramine hydrochloride produced a rise in blood pressure with "fullness of the head, flushing of the face, and a powerful heart beat." In subjects liable to migraine, headache, nausea, and vomiting were precipitated by tyramine (100 mg) taken by mouth (Hanington, 1967). Because migraine is a hereditary disorder, it was suggested that migraine sufferers might have a genetic enzyme deficiency (probably of monoamine oxidase) leading occasionally to absorption of amines from the intestine. Certainly, absorption of tyramine from the intestine is enormously facilitated in patients receiving amine oxidase inhibitors. Thus hypertensive attacks followed ingestion of 4 gm of a yeast extract Marmite (containing tyramine 2.5 mg/gm extract) in patients taking an inhibitor but not following the same amount of the extract (and of tyramine) when the inhibitor was withdrawn (Blackwell *et al.*, 1967). The effects of tyramine given intravenously to man were also potentiated. In four patients given pargyline, tyramine 0.9 to 5.7 mg/hour infused intravenously raised blood pressure 25 to 65 mm Hg, whereas 55 to 86 mg/hour was needed for equivalent pressor effects in the same patients before pargyline (Horwitz *et al.*, 1964). An enhanced response to intravenous tyramine does not necessarily indicate that the amine would be absorbed in significant amounts from the intestine. For example, in rats given a single intraduodenal dose of tranylcypromine (500 μg), the pressor action of tyramine (10 μg) was greatly enhanced, but intraduodenal tyramine (2.5 mg) was without effect (Blackwell and Marley, 1964).

The amount of tyramine required to elevate blood pressure in rats, cats, guinea pigs, and fowls was substantially greater than for man. In rats, tyramine (25 mg/kg) given into the stomach was ineffective although arterial blood pressure rose 23 mm Hg following 50 mg/kg (Tedeschi and Fellows, 1964); 10 mg/kg tyramine injected intraduodenally in rats and cats did not alter blood pressure (Blackwell and Marley, 1964, 1966b). After treatment of rats, cats, or fowls with a monoamine oxidase inhibitor, tyramine 6 mg/kg given intraduodenally now produced rises in blood pressure of up to 100 mm Hg (Blackwell and Marley, 1964, 1966b; Tedeschi and Fellows, 1964) which were accompanied in cats by contraction of the nictitating membranes. The emergence of sympathomimetic effects soon after intraduodenal injection of tyramine or a tyramine-containing food suggests but does not prove absorption of tyramine from the intestine. However, in cats pretreated with an amine oxidase inhibitor, tyramine was not detected in the blood in the absence of food administration but at the zenith of sympathomimetic effects produced by 10 gm/kg of cheese or yeast extract given intraduodenally, plasma tyramine concentrations were 0.009 and 0.008 μmole/ml respectively—sufficient to account for the pharmacological effects (Blackwell and Marley, 1966a,b).

A crucial point with yeast extracts such as Marmite which contain tyramine was to establish whether histamine was also absorbed. In man, up to 225 mg histamine orally have been well tolerated, although 10 mg given intravenously had profound effects. Large quantities of histamine introduced into the stomach elicited mild symptoms of intoxication in guinea pigs but were without effect in dogs (Koessler and Hanke, 1924). The conclusions were that a small amount of histamine was absorbed from the gut, but most of the histamine was rendered inert while passing through the intestinal wall. Using an extremely sensitive method for detecting absorption of histamine-^{14}C from the dog gastrointestinal tract, Duncan and Waton (1968) found that, despite destruction in the lumen and gastrointestinal wall, histamine entered the portal blood from all parts of the digestive tract. The amount of histamine injected into the lumen was similar to that normally present 2 hours after a meat meal. Meakins and Harington (1923) suggested that histamine was absorbed from the small intestine of the cat because of a sharp fall in blood pressure within seconds of placing histamine in the gut. Contraction of the uterus *in situ* and respiratory disturbance also occurred, but the time of onset was not stipulated. There are objections to using a fall of blood pressure as an index of histamine absorption. For example, fluids such as saline introduced into the bowel can elicit dramatic falls in blood pressure. If arterial tone is low, then, as found by Dale and Laidlaw (1919), the immediate effect of injecting a large intravenous dose of histamine is to raise blood pressure. A rise in blood pressure following a large intraduodenal dose of histamine is shown in Fig. 5A.

A more satisfactory method for evaluating absorption of histamine from a yeast extract injected intraduodenally was a technique devised by Vane (1964), in which the pharmacological effects could be recorded simultaneously with the demonstration that histamine was being absorbed from the intestine. This precluded the need to measure by chemical methods the amount of histamine in the blood. In this technique, a strip of guinea pig ileum was superfused by carotid blood in an extracorporeal circulation of chloralosed cats. The guinea pig ileum was relaxed under these circumstances but contracted to circulating histamine and did so 10 to 20 minutes after placing yeast extract or histamine in the small intestine of some control cats (Figs. 4A and 5A) but *immediately* in cats pretreated with mebanazine (Figs. 4B and 5C). The technique had many advantages not least in that the superfused ileum was considerably more sensitive than the blood pressure to histamine injected intravenously. Contraction of the superfused ileum was abolished by the histamine antagonist mepyramine (Figs. 4B and 5C), an antagonism surmountable by larger doses of histamine. The effects were attributed to absorption of histamine from the yeast extract, which was apparently facilitated by amine oxidase inhibition. The results were unlikely to be due to histamine release caused by substances absorbed from the extract, inasmuch as they were still obtained by intraduodenal injection of the extract into cats similarly prepared but in addition pretreated for 1 month with increasing doses of the histamine liberator compound 48/80, by which time the compound no longer evoked signs of histamine release. In the untreated cats in which absorption of histamine from the intestine was deemed not to have occurred because of the

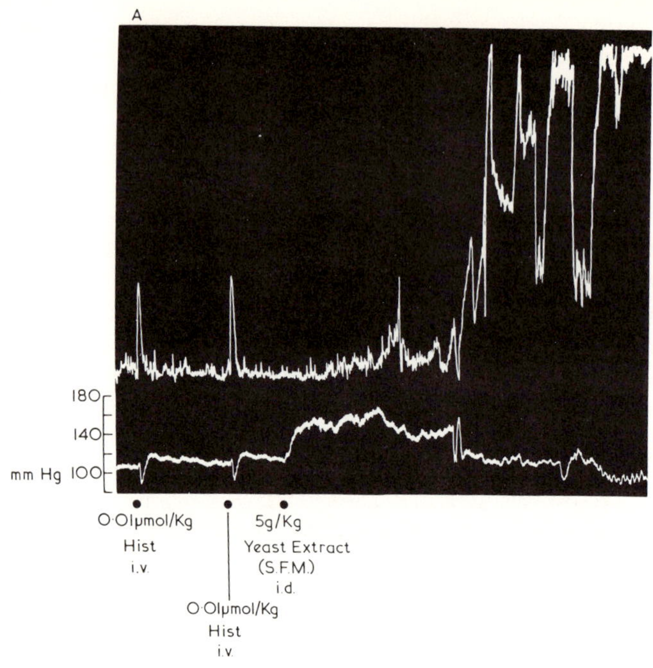
A
180
140
mm Hg 100
0·01µmol/Kg
Hist
i.v.
0·01µmol/Kg
Hist
i.v.
5g/Kg
Yeast Extract
(S.F.M.)
i.d.

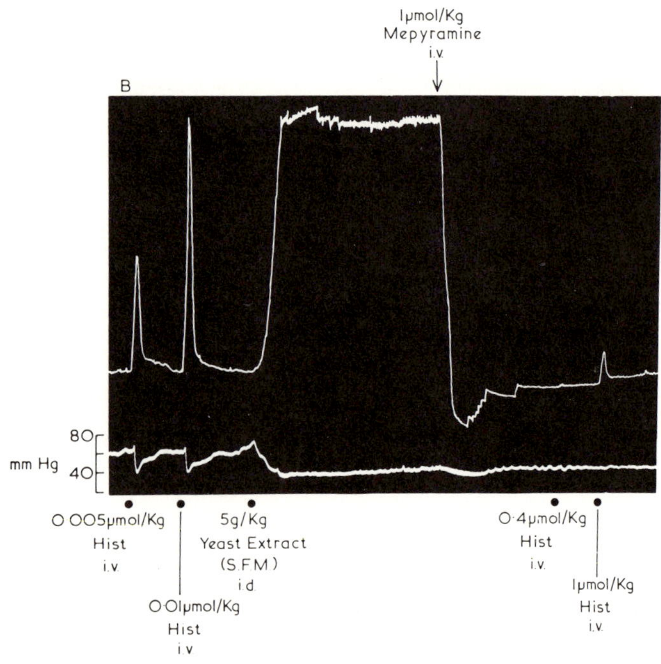
1µmol/Kg
Mepyramine
i.v.
B
80
mm Hg 40
0·005µmol/Kg
Hist
i.v.
0·01µmol/Kg
Hist
i.v.
5g/Kg
Yeast Extract
(S.F.M.)
i.d.
0·4µmol/Kg
Hist
i.v.
1µmol/Kg
Hist
i.v.
min

lack of effect on the superfused guinea pig ileum, injections of histamine into the splenic vein contracted the superfused ileum, pointing to the variability of histamine absorption from the gut in different cats, and to the intestinal wall rather than the liver as the site of histamine inactivation.

Hypertensive crises have also been provoked by broad beans. In a man treated with pargyline (Hodge *et al.*, 1964), the attack was reproduced by feeding the bean pods but not the seeds. Untreated subjects evinced no blood pressure changes after eating 375 gm of bean pods, but two others taking pargyline developed hypertensive attacks after 200 to 300 gm of pods. Although dopamine was not measured in the blood, the phenomena were attributed to conversion of dopa to dopamine, itself a substrate for monoamine oxidase. Certainly, the pressor effects of dopamine are potentiated in man by amine oxidase inhibition (Horwitz *et al.*, 1960).

Although there do not appear to have been untoward incidents in patients receiving amine oxidase inhibitors who have ingested 5-HT-containing foods, experiments in animals with radioactive 5-HT are relevant to the absorption from the intestine. Thus, 5-hydroxyindoleacetic acid-^{14}C appears in the intestinal mucosa and in the portal venous blood following injection of 5-hydroxytryptamine-^{14}C into the intestinal lumen of cats (Lembeck *et al.*, 1964). Pretreatment of cats with nialamide resulted in the appearance of unchanged 5-hydroxytryptamine-^{14}C in the portal blood—additional evidence for the importance of intestinal monoamine oxidase as a detoxication mechanism.

VII. Effects of Amines Absorbed from Foodstuffs in the Intestine and Reaching the Systemic Circulation

In this section it is assumed, for animals and man, that the active substance in the food had been absorbed from the intestinal lumen and reached the systemic circulation. There, it would have access to tissues in which enzymes affected by the monoamine oxidase inhibitors had been partially or entirely inactivated.

FIG. 4. Responses of a guinea pig ileum (upper trace in each panel) to superfused blood from the carotid artery and of the blood pressure (lower trace) in anesthetized (chloralose) cats A of 3.4 kg and B of 3.0 kg. Adrenal glands were excluded from the circulation by ligatures in both cats. (A) Contraction of the blood superfused guinea pig ileum beginning 12 minutes after the intraduodenal injection of the yeast extract salt-free Marmite (SFM in gm/kg) with initial rise and then fall in blood pressure. (B) *Immediate* contraction of the superfused ileum and fall of blood pressure produced by the yeast extract salt-free Marmite injected intraduodenally 90 minutes after the intraduodenal injection of mebanazine (120 μmole/kg). Contraction of the superfused ileum was abolished by mepyramine (1μmole/kg i.v.). Histamine (Hist, in μmole/kg) injected intravenously to ascertain sensitivity of ileum; i.v., intravenous; i.d., intraduodenal. (Reproduced from Blackwell and Marley, 1966a.)

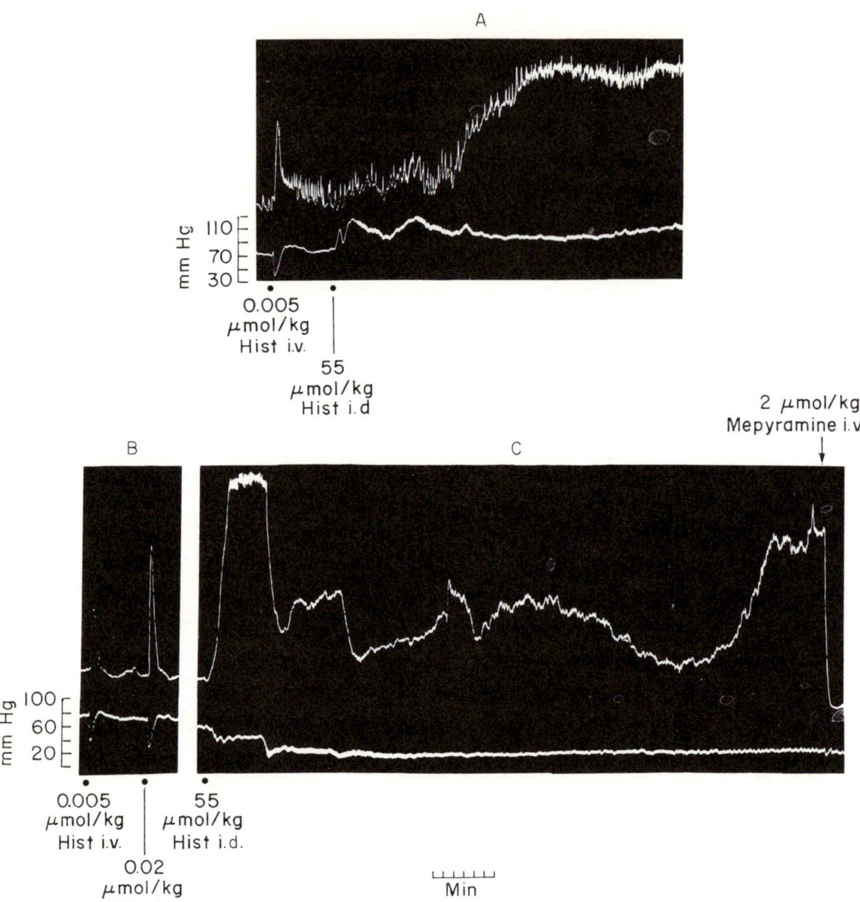

FIG. 5. Responses of a guinea pig ileum (upper trace in panels) to superfused blood from the carotid artery and of the blood pressure (lower trace in panels) in anesthetized (chloralose) cats, A of 3.0 kg and B, C of 3.2 kg. Adrenal glands were removed in both cats. (A) Contraction of the superfused guinea pig ileum beginning 12 minutes after the intraduodenal injection of histamine (Hist.) (B) Control responses of the superfused ileum and of the blood pressure to histamine injected intravenously. (C) *Immediate* contraction of the superfused ileum and fall of blood pressure produced by histamine injected intraduodenally 60 minutes after the intraduodenal injection of mebanazine (120 μmole/kg). Contraction of the superfused ileum was abolished by mepyramine.

A. Animals

Unless otherwise stated the following results have been taken from experiments by Blackwell and Marley (1964, 1966a,b, and unpublished) and Blackwell *et al.* (1965). In most instances, the foodstuff injected into the intestine (usually duodenum) had been tested and found to contain significant amounts of tyramine and/or histamine. The animals had been adequately pretreated with a monoamine oxidase inhibitor unless indicated to the contrary. For intravenous injection of cheese or yeast extract, the food was homogenized with saline. The homogenate was centrifuged at 0°C and the supernatant used for injection—these are termed cheese or yeast supernatants. For intraduodenal injections, the foodstuff was homogenized with saline or water and given intraduodenally through an indwelling cannula, the pylorus having been ligated. The numerous yeast products on the market, some of which were tested, are collectively termed yeast extracts.

1. *Cardiovascular System*

Intravenous injection of cheese supernatant into pithed rats and anesthetized or spinal cats produced a rise in blood pressure much prolonged by pretreatment with a monoamine oxidase inhibitor (compare Fig. 6A,B). Intraduodenal injection of cheese (5 or 10 gm/kg) in cats, rats, and fowls was followed within a few minutes by increase in carotid arterial pressure, reaching a maximum within the ensuing 10 to 20 minutes. The usual rise was 30 to 60 mm Hg; the maximum rise in eight cats tested was 90 mm Hg, although pressor responses in excess of this were obtained in pithed rats. An illustration of a blood pressure rise of 160 mm Hg in a cat pretreated with nialamide and injected with 5 gm/kg Emmenthal cheese is given by Natoff (1965b).

The blood pressure effects lasted at least 20 minutes and persisted as long as 120 minutes before they were abolished by a chemical antagonist such as phenoxybenzamine (Fig. 6B), Hydergine, or chlorpromazine. In Fig. 6C,D, the pressor effects of intraduodenal cheese and tyramine, respectively, in rats pretreated with mebanazine were unaffected by cocaine, methysergide, and hyoscine but abolished by chlorpromazine. Phenethylamine and tryptamine, substrates of monoamine oxidase, are also present in certain cheeses (Asatoor *et al.*, 1963). Their absorption from the intestine would contribute to a rise in blood pressure, although their pressor potency is less than that of tyramine. Cheese also contains the diamines cadaverine and putrescine which are not metabolized by amine oxidase (Blaschko, 1952). Cadaverine, in a dose exceeding that in cheese, did not alter blood pressure when injected intraduodenally in cats pretreated with a monoamine oxidase inhibitor. In our experiments, Camembert or Cheddar cheese were used; in those of Natoff (1964), Camembert or Emmenthal were used.

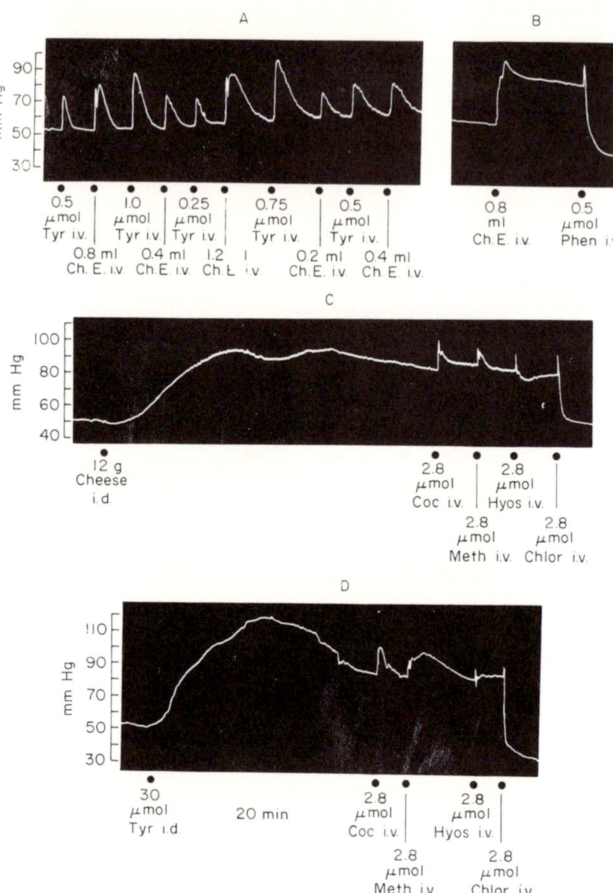

FIG. 6. Responses of the blood pressure in pithed rats to show the pressor activity of cheese or tyramine injected intravenously or intraduodenally. (A) Pithed rat, pressor activity of various intravenous doses of cheese supernatant (Ch.E. in ml) compared with those of intravenous tyramine (Tyr, in μmole). (B) Pithed rat given mebanazine (30 μmole/kg i.v.) 90 minutes previously. Cheese supernatant injected intravenously produced rise of blood pressure lasting 22 minutes until antagonized by intravenous phenoxybenzamine (Phen in μmoles). (C) Pithed rat given mebanazine (120 μmole/kg i.p. 5 hours previously and 60 μmole/kg i.v. 20 minutes beforehand). Cheese (12 gm) injected into the duodenum produced a rise in blood pressure completely antagonized by intravenous chlorpromazine (Chlor in μmole). Cocaine (Coc), methysergide (Meth), and hyoscine (Hyos) were ineffective (all doses in μmole, i.v.). (D) Pithed rat given mebanazine (30 μmoles/kg i.p. 90 minutes previously. Tyramine injected into the duodenum produced a rise in blood pressure completely antagonized by intravenous chlorpromazine; intravenous cocaine, methysergide, and hyoscine were ineffective. (Reproduced from Blackwell and Marley, 1966b.)

The effects of yeast supernatant injected intravenously differed from those of cheese. For example, in untreated cats a fall in carotid arterial pressure simultaneous with an increase in jugular venous pressure followed intravenous injections of histamine or of yeast supernatant (compare Fig. 7 with Fig. 6A). Substantial quantities of tyramine were in the extract, but injection of tyramine was without effect on jugular venous pressure and raised arterial pressure; presumably the histamine-like effects preponderated over the sympathomimetic. It has recently been shown (Allen and Rand, 1969) that pretreatment

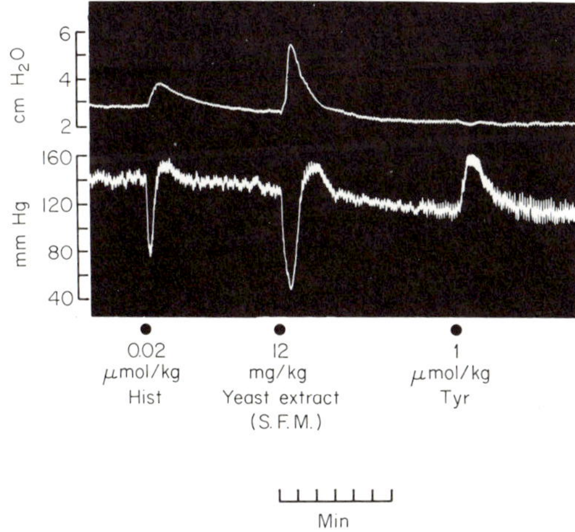

Fig. 7. Effect of intravenous injections of histamine, yeast extract, and tyramine on jugular venous pressure (upper trace) and arterial blood pressure (lower trace). Cat 4.2 kg; chloralose anesthesia. Both adrenal glands were excluded from the circulation by ligatures. Histamine (Hist, in μmole/kg) and yeast extract (SFM, salt-free Marmite, in mg/kg) produced an immediate fall of arterial blood pressure accompanied by an increase in jugular venous pressure. Tyramine (Tyr, in μmole/kg) raised the arterial pressure but was without effect on jugular venous pressure. (Reproduced from Blackwell and Marley, 1966a.)

with three different monoamine oxidase inhibitors potentiated the action of histamine injected intravenously on cat blood pressure. In our experiments, seven of 14 cats pretreated with mebanazine, nialamide, or tranylcypromine injection intraduodenally of the extract Marmite evoked an average fall in blood pressure of 35 mm Hg lasting over 60 minutes, again presumably because histamine-like effects preponderated. Absorption of histamine from the intestine and the influence of amine oxidase inhibition on this is discussed elsewhere. In three of the 14 pretreated cats, there was a decline in blood pressure lasting 3 to 10 minutes, followed by a rise in pressure lasting over

60 minutes. In the other four cats, sympathomimetic effects were paramount, blood pressure increasing 30 to 70 mm Hg. The usual electrocardiographic change elicited by intraduodenal injection of cheese or Marmite in cats pretreated with a monoamine oxidase inhibitor was a moderate bradycardia accompanying the rise in blood pressure. In two cats, dissociation between the auricular (P wave) and ventricular (Q R S) complexes developed with frequent ventricular extrasystoles.

2. *Nictitating Membrane and Iris*

Contraction of the nictitating membrane occurred in cats pretreated with a monoamine oxidase inhibitor and given intraduodenal cheese or yeast extract; the contraction after yeast extract is shown in Fig. 8. This contraction was elicited after acute, but not chronic, removal of the corresponding superior cervical and vagal nodose ganglia; under similar conditions mydriasis occurred after acute, but not chronic, removal of the ganglia. These findings, together with previous evidence suggested an indirect action on these tissues mediated via noradrenaline release from the postganglionic sympathetic trunk, compatible with absorption and circulation of tyramine or allied amine from the foodstuff. Following bretylium given to an untreated cat and in sufficient dose to abolish contractions of the nictitating membrane on tetanizing the superior cervical trunk, responses to cheese supernatant or to tyramine injected intravenously were enhanced, suggesting that the noradrenaline released was from a store in the nerve, different from that liberated by nerve impulses.

Particularly strong contractions of the nictitating membrane were observed after introduodenal injection of yeast extracts. This was ascribed to the summation of histamine and tyramine activities,. because histamine contracts the nictitating membrane both by ganglionic action and by evoking adrenal medullary secretion. The evidence for this was derived from two types of experiment. In the first, the effects of intravenous tyramine, yeast supernatant, histamine, and adrenaline were tested in cats with the superior cervical and vagal nodose ganglia extirpated on one side, but intact on the other; the adrenal medullae had also been removed. The membrane with the ganglia intact contracted to the four substances but the acutely denervated membrane only to tyramine and adrenaline (Fig. 8A). The second type of experiment differed in that the cat was pretreated with an amine oxidase inhibitor and the adrenal medullae were present. Yeast extract injected intraduodenally contracted both membranes, the acutely denervated more than the innervated (Fig. 8B). Because a ganglionic action of histamine was precluded, the denervated membrane presumably responded to both circulating tyramine and the adrenal medullary catecholamines.

A feature with both the cheese and yeast extract experiments was that, although the pressor response was readily abolished by selective antagonists at

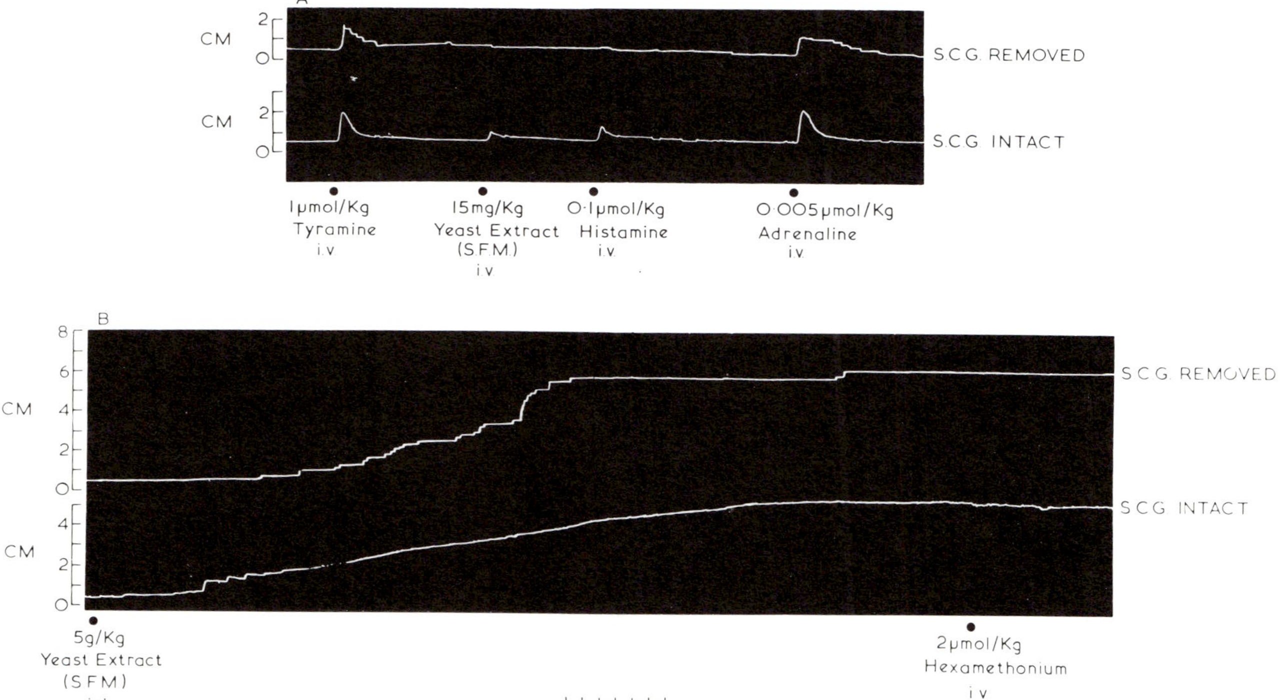

FIG. 8. Responses of the nictitating membranes with the superior cervical and nodose ganglia removed (upper trace in each panel) and with the ganglia intact. (A) Contractions of the membrane with the ganglia intact to intravenous injections of tyramine, histamine, and adrenaline (all in μmole/kg) and to the yeast extract salt-free Marmite (SFM in mg/kg) but contraction of the membrane with the ganglia removed only to tyramine and to adrenaline. (B) Contraction of both membranes to salt-free Marmite (5 gm/kg) injected intraduodenally 120 minutes after mebanazine (120 μmole/kg, i.d.). No effect of hexamethonium injected intravenously. (Reproduced from Blackwell and Marley, 1966a.)

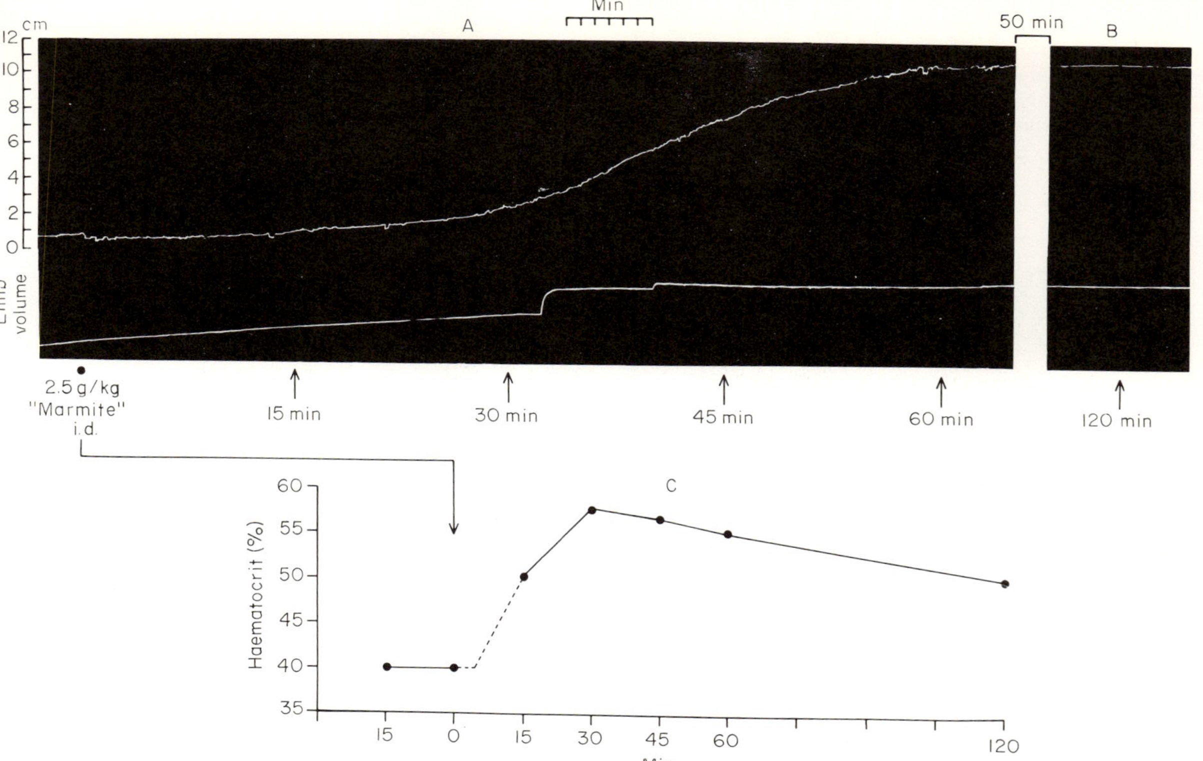

Fig. 9. Responses of the nictitating membrane and limb volume (A, B) and hematocrit (C) to the yeast extract Marmite injected intraduodenally into a 2.0 kg anesthetized (chloralose) cat given mebanazine (120 μmole/kg i.d.) 120 minutes previously. Upstroke on limb volume record indicates increase in volume. There was a 50-minute interval between A and B. (Reproduced from Blackwell and Marley, 1966a.)

α-receptors for catecholamines such as phenoxybenzamine or ergotamine, contraction of the nictitating membrane was only partly reduced.

3. *Limb Volume and Hematocrit*

After intraduodenal injection of the yeast extract Marmite in a cat pretreated with mebanazine, an increase in limb volume and a rise in hematocrit ensued, accompanied by contraction of the nictitating membranes. These effects are shown in Fig. 9, from which it can be seen that the hematocrit rose from a control value of 40% to 50% by 15 minutes and to 57% by 30 minutes; the rise in hematocrit preceded any marked change in limb volume and tone of the nictitating membrane. The effects on the nictitating membrane and limb volume were still as marked at 120 minutes (Fig. 9B), but the hematocrit had fallen to 50%. Histamine given intravenously raises the hematocrit (Dale and Laidlaw, 1919) and the rise in hematocrit of Fig. 9 was attributed to the effects of histamine absorbed from the intestine. From subsequent experiments (Blackwell and Marley, unpublished) it became clear that tyramine absorbed into the circulation from the intestine could also elevate the hematocrit, although to a lesser extent than histamine. Unless the cat had been pretreated with an amine oxidase inhibitor, intraduodenal injection of the yeast extract was without effect on the hematocrit.

4. *Respiration*

Insignificant changes in respiration were recorded with foodstuffs other than yeast extracts. Bronchoconstriction in guinea pigs was readily obtained with the yeast extract Marmite. Bronchoconstriction elicited by intravenous injections of this yeast extract (SFM) or histamine (Fig. 10A) was antagonized by mepyramine (Fig. 10B) an antagonism surmounted by increased doses of these substances (Fig. 10C). Bronchoconstriction was also elicited by intraduodenal injections of the yeast extract (Fig. 10D) or histamine (Fig. 10E) and was abolished or substantially reduced by mepyramine.

5. *Gastric Secretion*

Gastric secretion was unaffected by cheese but increased by yeast extracts. These experiments were made in cats and the extract was injected intraduodenally distal to the ligated pyloroduodenal junction, which prevented reflux of injectate into the stomach. The esophagus was tied at its junction with the stomach, the vagi divided in the neck, and gastric juice collected from a wide cannula tied into the most dependent part of the gastric greater curvature. As shown in Fig. 11B,C,D, within 10 to 25 minutes of giving the yeast extract Marmite (2 to 10 gm/kg) intraduodenally to cats treated with an amine oxidase inhibitor, the volume of gastric secretion increased two- to tenfold, with an

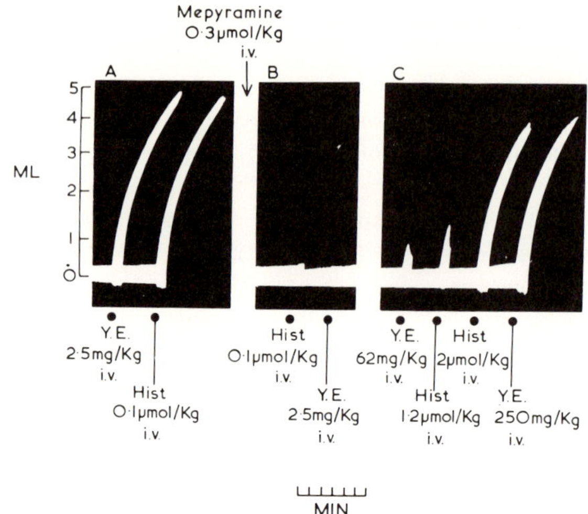
Mepyramine
0·3μmol/Kg
i.v.
A
B
C
ML
5
4
3
2
1
0
Y.E.
2·5mg/Kg
i.v.
Hist
0·1μmol/Kg
i.v.
Hist
0·1μmol/Kg
i.v.
Y.E.
2·5mg/Kg
i.v.
Y.E.
62mg/Kg
i.v.
Hist
1·2μmol/Kg
i.v.
Hist
2μmol/Kg
i.v.
Y.E.
250mg/Kg
i.v.
MIN

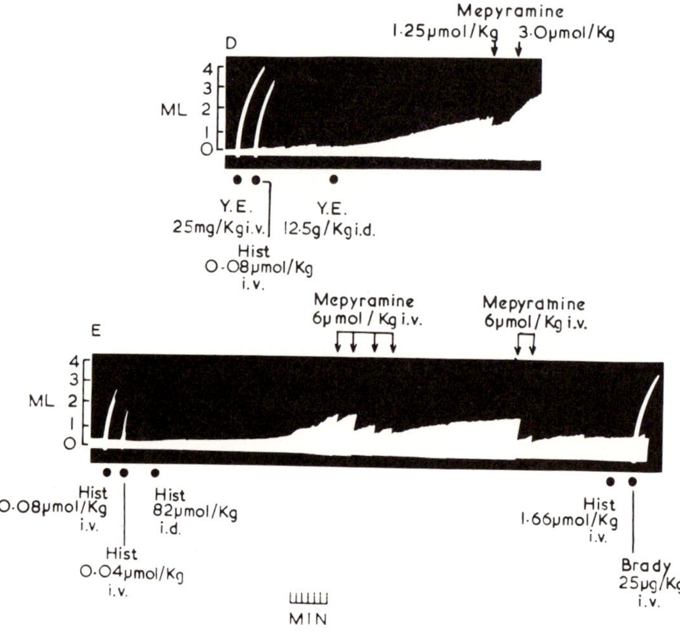
Mepyramine
1·25μmol/Kg
3·0μmol/Kg
D
ML
4
3
2
1
0
Y.E.
25mg/Kg i.v.
Hist
0·08μmol/Kg
i.v.
Y.E.
12·5g/Kg i.d.
Mepyramine
6μ mol / Kg i.v.
Mepyramine
6μmol / Kg i.v.
E
ML
4
3
2
1
0
Hist
0·08μmol/Kg
i.v.
Hist
0·04μmol/Kg
i.v.
Hist
82μmol/Kg
i.d.
Hist
1·66μmol/Kg
i.v.
Brady
25μg/Kg
i.v.
MIN

increase in total acid and the appearance of and subsequent increase in free acid. For example, in the experiment Fig. 11B, the free acid which had been undetectable in the control secretion rose to between 0.4 and 0.5 gm, of hydrochloric acid per 100 ml, 100 minutes after giving the extract. The secretion, which was initially mucous and sticky, became a pale amber watery fluid. These histamine-like effects were observed in cats anesthetized with chloralose (Fig. 11B and D) and in a spinal cat (Fig. 11C). In a control cat given only the yeast extract, the secretion was unaffected until mebanazine was injected into the duodenum when, as illustrated in Fig. 11A, the volume of juice secreted increased and free acid appeared. The volume of gastric juice secreted and the content of free acid usually remained high until the end of the experiment 110 to 140 minutes after giving the yeast extract, indicating that a histamine-like substance was being continuously absorbed from the duodenum into the circulation or that its effect was prolonged, or both. The amine oxidase inhibitor itself did not cause secretion, since in experiments Fig. 11B,C and D (in which the inhibitor had been injected 40 to 75 minutes) secretion was minimal for the following 45 to 80 minutes and did not contain free acid until the yeast extract was given. The increased secretion produced by the yeast extract was obtained after treating cats with the hydrazide nialamide (Fig. 11D), the hydrazine mebanazine (Fig. 11B and C), and the amine tranylcypromine (not shown in Fig. 11).

Drugs which interfere with histamine catabolism modify its effects on gastric secretion (Ghosh and Schild, 1958; Amure and Ginsburg, 1964); indeed gastric secretion in rats, measured in terms of pH of gastric perfusate, and provoked by histamine was enhanced by iproniazid (Amure and Ginsburg, 1964). Presumably the effects of histamine absorbed from the extract in the above

---

FIG. 10. Three guinea pigs; resistance of lungs to inflation (*in vivo*). Guinea pig 1: (A) Maximal resistance to inflation produced by intravenous injection of the yeast extract salt-free Marmite (SFM, in mg/kg) and of histamine (Hist, in μmole/kg.) Between A and B, mepyramine (0.3 μmole/kg) was injected intravenously. (B) Antagonism of the effects of histamine and of yeast extract, progressively surmounted (C) by increasing doses of the substances. Guinea pigs 2 and 3: Comparison of the effects of yeast extract (D) and of histamine (E) given intraduodenally. (D) Resistance to inflation produced initially by intravenous injections of the yeast extract salt-free Marmite (Y.E. in mg/kg) and by histamine (Hist, in μmole/kg) and then by the yeast extract injected intraduodenally which produced progressive increase in resistance to inflation unaffected by intravenous mepyramine (1.25 and 3.0 μmole/kg) and with fatal termination. (E) Increase in resistance to inflation produced initially by intravenous injection of histamine. Progressive increase in resistance to inflation elicited by the intraduodenal injection of histamine antagonized by intravenous mepyramine (six doses of 6 μmole/kg). An intravenous dose of histamine was now ineffective although bradykinin (Brady, in μg/kg) still elicited maximal resistance to inflation. (Reproduced from Blackwell and Marley, 1966a.)

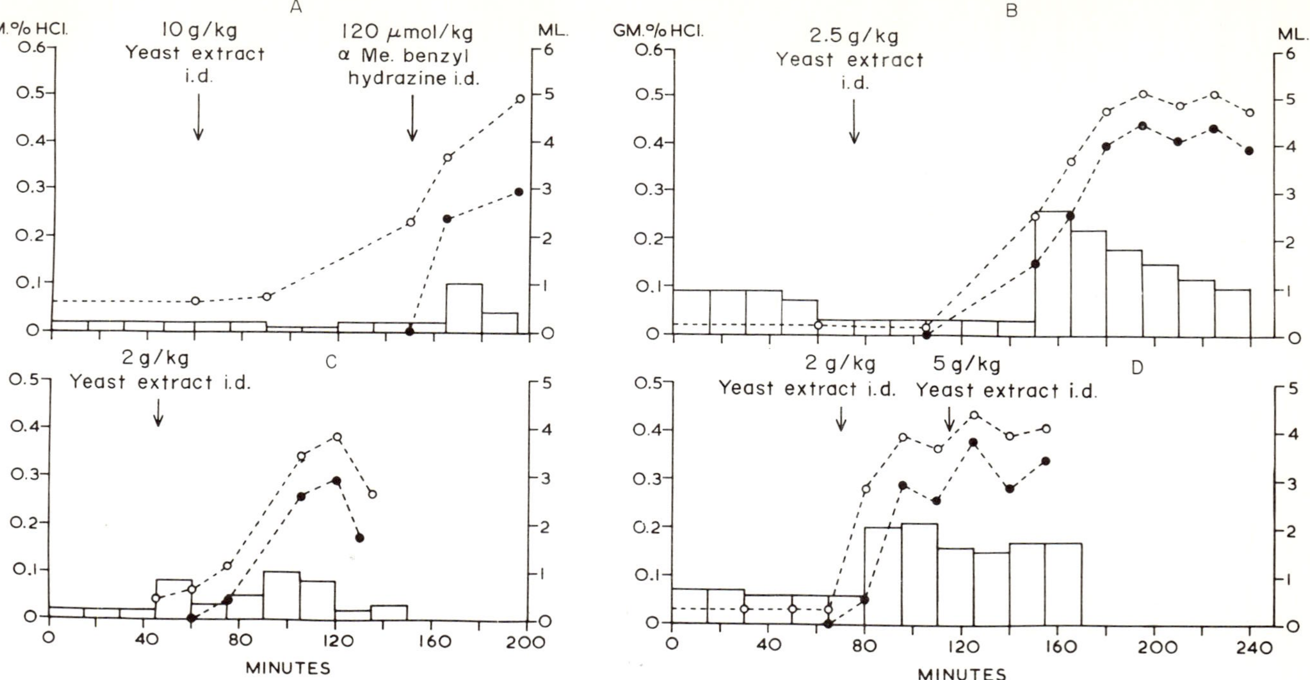

FIG. 11. Histograms of gastric secretion and graphs of free and total acidity produced by the yeast extract Marmite in a spinal cat of 2.2 kg (C) and in anesthetized (chloralose) cats of 2.0 kg (A), 2.5 kg (B), and 2.1 kg (D), respectively. Gastric secretion is expressed as milliliters on the right of each graph; free acidity (filled circles) and total acidity (empty circles) are expressed as grams of hydrochloric acid per 100 ml on the left of each graph. In (A) the yeast extract Marmite 10 gm/kg was given intraduodenally 90 minutes before mebanazine (α-methylbenzylhydrazine 120 μmole/kg i.d.); in (B) and (C) the yeast extract was given 120 minutes after mebanazine (120 μmole/kg i.d.); and in (D) 120 minutes after nialamide (76 μmole/kg i.d.).

experiments on cats were modified by amine oxidase inhibitors. That this could be the case was demonstrated in two ways.

In the first (Fig. 12A), the effects of single intravenous doses of histamine (0.75 μmole/kg) on volume and acidity of gastric secretion were shown to be augmented and prolonged 30 minutes after injecting mebanazine (α-Me·B·H). The increased effects of histamine could not be attributed to enhanced sensitivity produced by repeated doses of histamine, for the volume of and duration of secretion was smaller with the second than with the first control histamine injection. That gastric secretion was unaffected by larger doses (2 μmole/kg i.v.) of *N*-acetylhistamine or 1.4 methylhistamine suggested that the phenomena were not due to interference in metabolic pathways inactivating histamine by ring methylation or *N*-acetylation.

In other cats, the effects of histamine absorbed from the bowel was simulated by infusing histamine intravenously at 0.05 μmole/min/kg for 30 minutes (Fig. 12B). As shown in the figure, once the effects of the control infusion had waned, a second infusion of histamine 60 minutes after mebanazine had a substantially greater effect on volume of secretion and a much prolonged action on its acidity. Similar results were obtained after a diamine oxidase inhibitor, aminoguanidine (Fig. 12C).

6. *Lower Limb Flexor Reflex*

In cats pretreated with nialamide and given the yeast extract Marmite intraduodenally, changes in spinal reflex activity were observed. Thus a single shock to the central end of a divided posterior tibial nerve, instead of eliciting a brief twitch of the ipsilateral anterior tibialis, produced a twitch with rhythmic oscillations as the twitch decayed. Next, extensor-flexor movements of the limbs developed, superimposed on the reflex twitch. These limb movements were not evoked by the stimulus to the posterior tibial nerve, as they also occurred when the nerve was not stimulated. Spinal cord excitability was increased, because with each shock to the posterior tibial nerve there was a marked extensor thrust not previously present, indicating stimulus irradiation.

These effects appeared to be due to a combination of absorption of histamine from the yeast extract and pretreatment with a monoamine oxidase inhibitor, because without the inhibitor histamine depressed peak twitch tension (Fig. 13A). The same dose of histamine 90 minutes after mebanazine increased peak tension from 0.2 to 0.5 kg lasting 1 minute (Fig. 13C); there was no subsequent diminution of peak tension. As shown in Fig. 13D, in which the recording drum was speeded up at the onset of the increase in peak tension, twitch duration was prolonged (compare Fig. 13D with B) and small oscillations appeared on the decaying slope of the twitch. What is not clear from Fig. 13D, is that there was a delay of 30 seconds between injecting histamine and increased peak

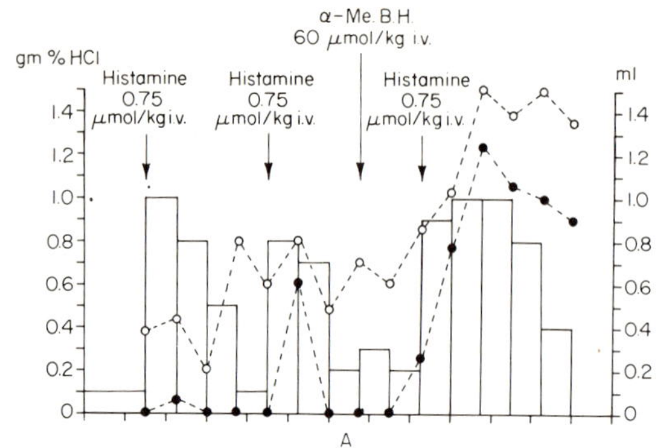
α-Me. B.H.
60 μmol/kg i.v.
gm % HCl
Histamine
0.75
μmol/kg i.v.
Histamine
0.75
μmol/kg i.v.
Histamine
0.75
μmol/kg i.v.
ml
0
0.2
0.4
0.6
0.8
1.0
1.2
1.4
A

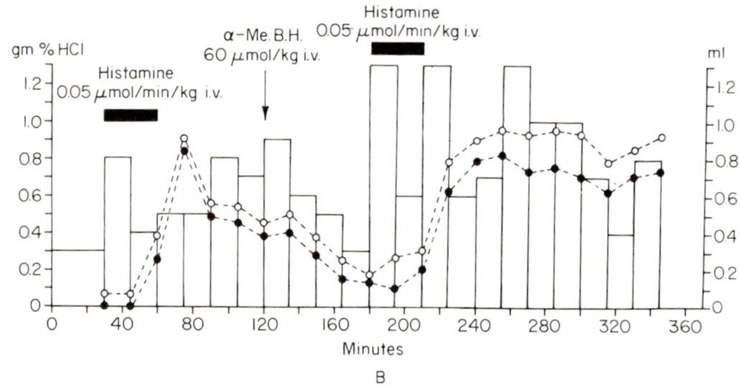
Histamine
0.05 μmol/min/kg i.v.
α-Me. B.H.
60 μmol/kg i.v.
gm % HCl
Histamine
0.05 μmol/min/kg i.v.
ml
0
0.2
0.4
0.6
0.8
1.0
1.2
0
40
80
120
160
200
240
280
320
360
Minutes
B

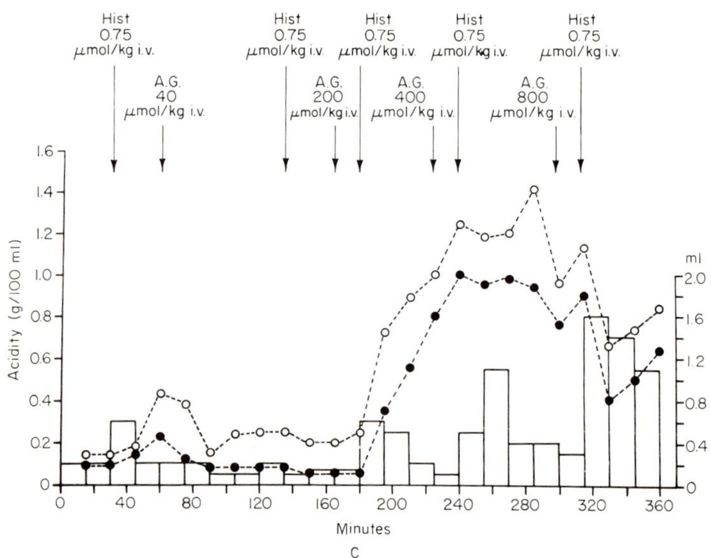
Hist
0.75
μmol/kg i.v.
A.G.
40
μmol/kg i.v.
Hist
0.75
μmol/kg i.v.
A.G.
200
μmol/kg i.v.
Hist
0.75
μmol/kg i.v.
A.G.
400
μmol/kg i.v.
Hist
0.75
μmol/kg i.v.
A.G.
800
μmol/kg i.v.
Hist
0.75
μmol/kg i.v.
Acidity (g/100 ml)
0
0.2
0.4
0.6
0.8
1.0
1.2
1.4
1.6
ml
0
0.4
0.8
1.2
1.6
2.0
0
40
80
120
160
200
240
280
320
360
Minutes
C

tension. This is shown in Fig. 13E, in which limb movements elicited by histamine are superimposed on changes in twitch tension. The delayed effect of histamine on the spinal cord reflex contrasts with its immediate effect of blood pressure and was found in all tests. The effect was obtained both with the dihydrochloride and the acid phosphate histamine salts, but not with the metabolites (1,4-methylhistamine or *N*-acetylhistamine (up to 1.5 μmole/kg i.v.). Similar effects were also obtained with histamine after treating cats with aminoguanidine, a diamine oxidase inhibitor. This finding and the potentiation of histamine effects on gastric secretion by aminoguanidine might suggest, as aminoguanidine is an inhibitor of diamine oxidase, that the enhanced effects of histamine following monoamine oxidase inhibitors were due to inhibition of diamine oxidase. Tyramine is also present in yeast extracts, but in doses up to 5.0 μmole/kg i.v. either before or after monoamine oxidase inhibition it was either ineffective or it depressed the flexor reflex.

7. *Electromyogram*

An unexpected finding was that electromyographic potentials were enhanced in cats pretreated with an amine oxidase inhibitor and given yeast extract. The effects on the electromyogram, blood pressure, and nictitating membrane are illustrated in Fig. 14. The electromyograms were taken from the thigh adductor muscles of a spinal cat given nialamide (76 μmole/kg intraduodenally) 150 minutes previously. The control record (at A) shows minimal electromyographic activity. After administration of the yeast extract Marmite (5 gm/kg i.d.), a small blood pressure rise and large contraction of the nictitating membrane ensued; 24 minutes later (at C) the electromyographic potentials were more marked and continuous although limb movements had not yet appeared. Subsequently, limb movements developed accompanied by huge electromyographic potentials (at D and E). The periods between limb move-

---

FIG. 12. Histograms of gastric secretion and graphs of free and total acidity provoked by histamine in two cats (A, B) before and after a monoamine oxidase inhibitor mebanazine (α-MeB,H) and one cat (C) given a diamine oxidase inhibitor aminoguanidine (AG). Gastric secretion expressed as milliliters on right of each graph; free acidity (black circles) and total acidity (open circles) expressed as gram % HCl on left of each graph. (A) Cat 4.2 kg; chloralose. Increase in volume of gastric secretion with first intravenous injection of histamine; second intravenous injection of histamine produced increase of free acid as well as of gastric secretion. Histamine injected intravenously 30 minutes after mebanazine (60 μmole/kg i.v.) produced much longer increase in gastric secretion and increase in free acid. (B) Cat 2.5 kg; chloralose. More sustained increase in free acid and volume of gastric secretion produced by intravenous infusion of histamine for 30 minutes after injecting the cat with mebanazine (60 μmole/kg i.v.) 90 minutes previously. (C) Cat 1.5 kg; chloralose. Volume of gastric secretion and total and free acidity provoked by histamine were enhanced by aminoguanidine.

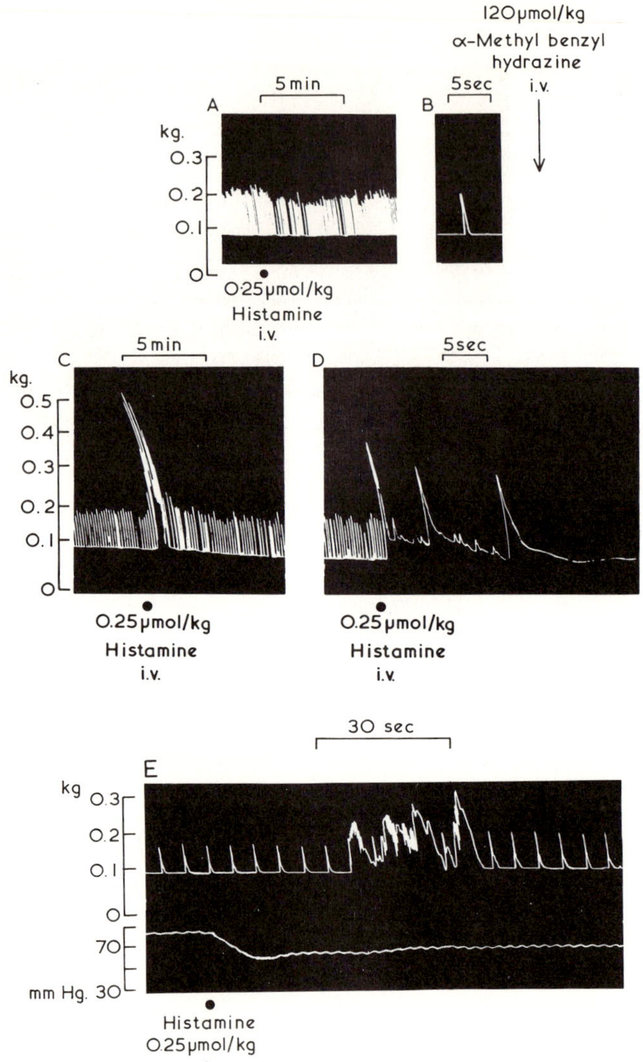

Fig. 13. Record of reflex tibialis twitch in a 3.0-kg spinal cat (A to D) and a 2.8-kg spinal cat (E), each with additional cord transection at the thoracico-lumbar junction and the adrenal glands removed. Blood pressure also recorded in E. (A) Control injection of histamine showing slight depression of peak tension. (B) Single twitch on fast moving drum. Between B and C, injection of mebanazine (α-methylbenzylhydrazine, 120 μmole/kg i.v.). (C) Increase in peak and basal tensions produced by histamine 90 minutes after mebanazine. (D) Prolonged duration of twitch evoked by histamine and shown on fast moving drum (compare with B). (E) Immediate lowering of arterial blood pressure and delayed effect on reflex tibialis twitch due to histamine given 90 minutes after mebanazine (60 μmole/kg i.v.).

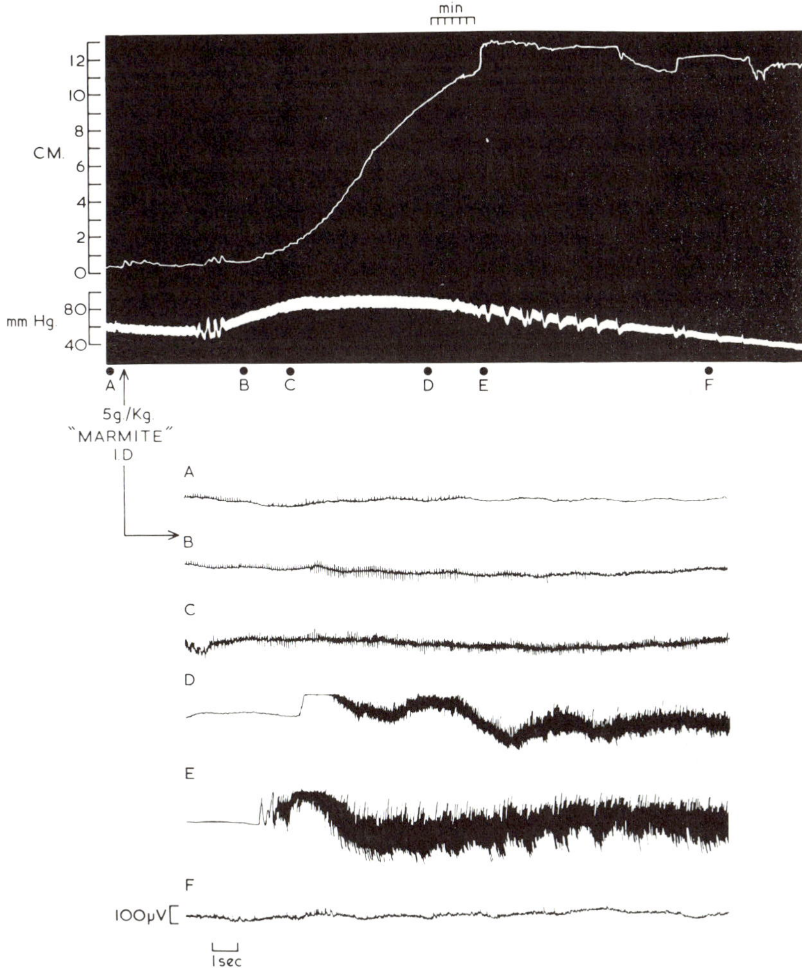

FIG. 14. Responses of the acutely denervated nictitating membrane, the blood pressure, and electromyogram in a spinal cat 3.5 kg, to the yeast extract Marmite (5 gm/kg) given intraduodenally 150 minutes after the intraduodenal injection of nialamide (76 μmole/kg). Contraction of the nictitating membrane (upper trace) develops 18 minutes after injecting the yeast extract, and is sustained. Blood pressure (middle trace) rises 30 mm Hg. Electromyographic records (lower traces). (A) Control: alternating phases of minimal electromyographic activity and quiescence. (B) (C) Progressive increase in amplitude and quantity of muscle potentials 17 and 24 minutes after Marmite. (D) (E) Large electromyographic potentials accompanying limb movements at 43 and 51 minutes (F) Electromyographic activity abating at 82 minutes. (Reproduced from Blackwell and Marley, 1966a.)

ments were accompanied by electromyographic silence. The limb movements and electromyographic potentials ultimately waned (at F).

The electromyographic changes appeared attributable to a combination of histamine absorbed from the yeast extract and to monoamine oxidase inhibition. In three spinal cats, histamine (0.25 μmole/kg i.v.) had little or no effect on the electromyogram. After mebanazine (120 μmole/kg i.v. given 30 minutes previously), which did not affect the electromyogram, histamine evoked electromyographic potentials lasting 1 minute. There was a delay in onset of just over 2 minutes. The electromyographic effects were not apparently due to the formation of histamine metabolites 1,4-methylhistamine or *N*-acetylhistamine because a sixfold increase in dose (1.5 μmole/kg i.v.) of these substances did not affect the electromyogram; nor were the effects due to a direct action of histamine on muscle because they could not be obtained from a chronically denervated limb. Tyramine (up to 5 μnole/kg i.v.), the other major amine in yeast extracts, was without effect on the electromyogram.

B. Man

The syndrome provoked by cheese or other foodstuffs in subjects taking amine oxidase inhibitors has been described by a number of investigators (Bethune *et al.*, 1964; Blackwell, 1963; Blackwell *et al.*, 1967; Cooper *et al.*, 1964; Davies, 1963; Foster, 1963; Glazener *et al.*, 1964; Hedberg *et al.*, 1966; Hodge *et al.*, 1964; Nuessle *et al.*, 1965). Headache and hypertension in patients taking amine oxidase inhibitors had been previously observed without there being suspicion that food might be partly responsible (Brown and Waldron, 1962; Clark, 1961; Davies, 1959; Ogilvie, 1955). Indeed, there are likely to be other foodstuffs so far unrecognized that could provoke hypertensive crises, and a feature in our series (Blackwell *et al.*, 1967) was that almost half the patients had dietary fads, i.e., were vegetarians or were on weight-reducing or high-protein diets.

Three modes of presentation were described by de Villiers (1966): (1) headache of great severity which may merge into the second mode, (2) in which the cardivascular manifestations predominate simulating the crises seen in phaechromocytoma, and (3) occurrence of intracranial hemorrhage. The headache develops suddenly, most often in the evening when the subject is at rest. Prior to the headache, or accompanying it, the patient experienced a forceful increase in heart beat ("palpitations") accompanied by throbbing of the blood vessels in the neck. The headache, invariably distinguished from those due to migraine or to tension, was first confined to the occiput or temporal regions, but later became generalized. Blood pressure was raised in those patients in whom it was measured during the early part of the attack. The threshold at which severe throbbing headache commenced varied, but the systolic pressure was usually in the region of 200 mm Hg or more, the headache remitting as the blood pressure fell and recurring if pressure rose again. The attacks lasted from 10 minutes to 6 hours, during which the hypertension and headache fluctuated. Change in pulse rate and rhythm included bradycardia with the rise in blood pressure, tachycardia, pulsus bigeminus, and fibrillation. Exercise aggravated the reaction and conversely "Patients who were in bed during an attack suffered less than those who were up and about" (Davies, 1963). The patient sometimes felt flushed or perspired profusely; nausea and vomiting were frequent. Neck stiffness and photophobia also occurred. Chest pain simulating angina pectoria and even acute heart failure have been described with pulmonary oedema (Songco, 1961; Womack, 1963). An intensely itchy skin eruption occurred in one patient less than an hour after eating a sandwich containing slightly seasoned cheese (Bichel, 1968).

Recovery was complete unless cardiac failure, subarachnoid, or cerebral haemorrhage supervened, complications which have proved fatal. In some patients the hypertensive attack was followed by hypotension (systolic pressure below 90 mm Hg) for 1 or 2 days. In others, the headache persisted although greatly diminished being ascribed to impaction of one or more "apophyseal" joints, following intense cervical spasm associated with the headache (Bethune *et al.*, 1964).

There are certain puzzling features about the reactions. For example, a particular foodstuff can precipitate an attack in a subject who had previously eaten or subsequently eats large amounts of the food with impunity. Leaving aside the variation in amine content of foods, this could be attributed to partial recovery of intestinal amine oxidase and should therefore be a function of the interval since the previous dose of inhibitor. Measurement of monoamine oxidase activity in biopsy specimens from the intestinal mucosa in man showed that the enzyme is 85% inhibited after 2 weeks' treatment with nialamide, pargyline, or isocarboxazid (Mustala *et al.*, 1969), but Levine and Sjoerdsma (1963) found a high rate of recovery of the intestinal enzyme within 18 hours of the last dose of inhibitor. The influence of duration of treatment with the monoamine oxidase inhibitor (MAOI) and also the importance of the size and proximity of the antecedant dose of inhibitor before food ingestion were carefully studied in a volunteer (Blackwell *et al.*, 1967).

Tests were made on a subject treated with phenelzine 15 mg t.d.s. for several weeks. During this time she had eaten large quantities of a yeast extract on frequent occasions with no ill effects. First, phenelzine was discontinued for 5 days and then the dose doubled to 30 mg t.d.s. After the first dose of phenelzine, the extract (10 gm dissolved in 250 ml water) was taken by mouth 90 minutes later. (The yeast extract came from the same sample in all tests, and assay on the blood pressure of a pithed rat showed it to contain a pressor substance equivalent in activity to 2.3 mg tyramine per gram of extract.)

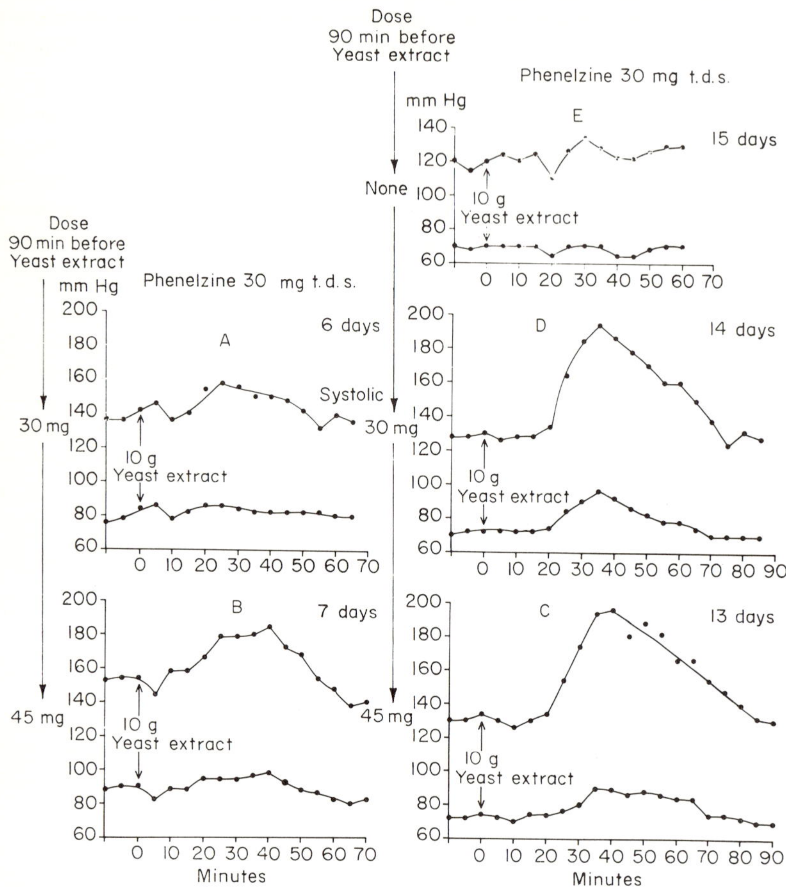

FIG. 15. Effects on blood pressure of a yeast extract (10 gm orally) in a patient treated with phenelzine (30 mg t.d.s.). Magnitude of response dependent on duration of treatment and size of antecedant dose of phenelzine. (A) six days treatment and phenelzine 30 mg 90 minutes before test—small pressor effect. (B) (C) Seven and 13 days treatment, respectively, and phenelzine 45 mg 90 minutes before test—blood pressure response larger in C than B. (E) Fifteen days treatment, but phenelzine omitted before test. No effect of yeast extract, although after 14 days treatment (D) with phenelzine 30 mg before test, a good pressor effect had been elicited with yeast extract. (Reproduced from Blackwell *et al.*, 1967.)

This first dose of yeast extract was ineffective on the subject's blood pressure. After 6 days of phenelzine the same amount of extract given under identical conditions produced a small rise in blood pressure (test A, Fig. 15). On the following day (test B) the morning dose of phenelzine was raised to 45 mg and the blood pressure response was doubled in amplitude and prolonged (compare A with D, preceding dose of phenelzine 30 mg; and B with C, preceding dose of phenelzine 45 mg). On day 15 when the morning dose of phenelzine was omitted (Fig. 15E), hardly any change in blood pressure occurred. Because the extract contained tyramine and a constant amount was given throughout, the lack of effect when the dose of phenelzine was omitted could be attributed to some recovery of intestinal amine oxidase activity. In these tests the extract was always taken after a fast of one night so that dilution of the amine by stomach contents would not be a complication. Another source of variability might be the specificity of a particular inhibitor to selectively affect the enzyme at one site. It has recently been shown that a developmental drug appears to affect the brain monoamine oxidase more than other tissues (Huszti *et al.*, 1969) and such a drug might prove less likely to permit access of amines through the intestinal wall.

Assuming that the dose of inhibitor is kept constant, duration of treatment is not apparently crucial for the reactions since they have occurred for the first time in patients taking inhibitors for only a few days or after many months. It was at first assumed that attacks would be more likely in those subjects who had received lengthy treatment because of greater accumulation of catecholamines in the sympathetic nerves. The evidence was against this as a major factor because the excretion of vanillylmandelic acid was normal in the urine collected from three patients in the 24 hours following a hypertensive attack (Blackwell *et al.*, 1967). Moreover, in cats, a species in which noradrenaline stores are not increased by amine oxidase inhibitors (von Euler and Hellner-Bjorkman, 1955), cheese or yeast extracts given intraduodenally had sympathomimetic effects including raised blood pressure.

Bram (1963) suggested that patients taking monoamine oxidase inhibitors and who experienced headaches following ingestion of food precipitants were those with "a predisposition to cerebrovascular insufficiency" and a previous history of headaches. This has not been substantiated, and indeed severe headache was as prevalent in a group of psychiatric patients taking amine oxidase inhibitors and who ate foods containing amines as it was in those who abstained from them. The headache was unlike anything the individual had experienced previously and in most instances was typical of that associated with a sudden major elevation in blood pressure (Wolff, 1963). The rise in blood pressure required to evoke headache varies among patients, and this too could account for some of the inconsistencies. In the series of Blackwell *et al.* (1967), a rise of 60 mm Hg systolic pressure produced severe head pain in some subjects, whereas a 70 mm Hg rise in others caused no concern. Even a rise of 120 mm Hg systolic pressure can be asymptomatic (Hodge *et al.*, 1964).

VIII. Failure to Obtain Sympathomimetic Effects with Foods Containing Significant Amounts of Tyramine

This aspect has been to a certain extent anticipated in other sections of the review. It applies to circumstances under which pretreatment with a monoamine oxidase inhibitor had been adequate and the foodstuff contained ample tyramine. The investigations were made in cats, although the findings are relevant to unexplained aspects of food reactions in man. Because the blood pressure effects of histamine and tyramine in yeast extracts may cancel each other when other sympathomimetic phenomena prevail, failure to obtain sympathomimetic effects was preferred as a criterion to failure to elicit a rise in blood pressure.

In our earlier experiments, failure to obtain sympathomimetic effects with foods was observed after a single large dose of an inhibitor with sympathomimetic properties, e.g., tranylcypromine. Subsequently, a similar lack of effect was encountered after repeated doses of hydrazine inhibitors when food was administered soon after the previous dose of inhibitor. The lack of reaction was attributed to tachyphylaxis to indirectly acting sympathomimetic amines engendered by the inhibitor as a consequence of its similar chemical structure. This is easy to comprehend in the case of tranylcypromine but less so for the hydrazines. Because of the tachyphylaxis, not only was tyramine absorbed from the intestine ineffective but normally pressor intravenous doses of β-phenethylamine, phenylethanolamine, or tyramine were without effect or lowered blood pressure and did not contract the nictitating membrane: directly acting amines such as noradrenaline retained their pressor action (Blackwell and Marley, 1966b).

Conversely, when tachyphylaxis to tyramine had been induced then cheese or yeast extracts failed to provoke sympathomimetic effects. Because amine oxidase inhibition is long-lasting but tachyphylaxis wanes more rapidly, the sympathomimetic effects of cheese or yeast extracts could be obtained after tachyphylaxis had developed if sufficient time was allowed before re-administering the foods.

IX. Interaction between and Autopotentiation of Monoamine Oxidase Inhibitors

About 30% of hypertensive crises in patients taking monoamine oxidase inhibitors cannot be attributed to interactions with foodstuffs (Cooper *et al.*,

1964); the majority of such unexplained incidents occur with tranylcypromine (Marks, 1965) but phenelzine has also been incriminated (Sjöqvist, 1965). A number of monoamine oxidase inhibitors have sympathomimetic properties and resemble β-phenethylamine in chemical structure (Fig. 3). Presumably in addition to the similarity in structure, their mode of action is similar. Indeed, pressor effects in dogs of pheniprazine or tranylcypromine have been attributed to release of noradrenaline from sympathetic postganglionic nerves because the effects were abolished by phentolamine (Gillespie, 1960; Spencer *et al.*, 1960). Conceivably then, these inhibitors serve as substrates for the very enzyme they inhibit and once monoamine oxidase was inhibited, their sympathomimetic effects would be much prolonged. Autopotentiation of this kind could account for some of the unexplained hypertensive crises in patients taking tranylcypromine, a compound with marked sympathomimetic properties. That this is feasible is shown in Fig. 16A, demonstrating a marked pressor reaction to intraduodenal tranylcypromine in a rat pretreated for 10 days with tranylcypromine, the same dose being ineffective in a control untreated rat. A tranylcypromine tablet of 10 mg contains 56 μmole of drug—that is, slightly less than 1 μmole/kg by mouth for an average-sized man. The recommended daily dose is 10 to 60 mg, that is, about 1 to 6 μmole/kg, so this dose in the rat does not greatly exceed that in man. Potentiation and autopotentiation of the pressor effects of mebanazine in cats and rats have also been noted (Blackwell and Marley, 1966b; Fig. 16B). Phenelzine and pheniprazine likewise potentiate their own sympathomimetic action on the nictitating membranes in cats because of their ability to inhibit monoamine oxidase (Clineschmidt and Horita, 1967).

Some facets of these interactions between monoamine oxidase inhibitors were studied further using pithed rats. Nialamide was the amine oxidase inhibitor preferred for pretreatment because it does not have sympathomimetic effects, nor do such effects emerge after pretreatment with a monoamine oxidase inhibitor. Unless stated, pretreatment consisted of nialamide (76 μmole/kg intraperitoneally) daily for 8 days prior to the experiment. The pressor effects of intravenous doses of phenelzine and of tyramine in an untreated rat are shown in Fig. 17A,B, and they should be compared with those after pretreatment with nialamide in which enhanced pressor responses to intravenous phenelzine were obtained (Fig. 18A,B). Intraduodenal doses of phenelzine (4 and 16 μmole/kg), which did not affect blood pressure in an untreated rat, now had substantial pressor actions (Fig. 17C,D). The total daily dose of phenelzine in man is about 2.5 μmole/kg. The pressor reactions appeared to be mediated by noradrenaline release, because they were abolished by phenoxybenzamine (Fig. 17D; Fig. 18C,D,E), and by pretreatment with guanethidine (Fig. 18H,I). Pretreatment with guanethidine was 50 μmole/kg i.p. daily for 3 days followed by a single dose of nialamide (76 μmole/kg i.p.)

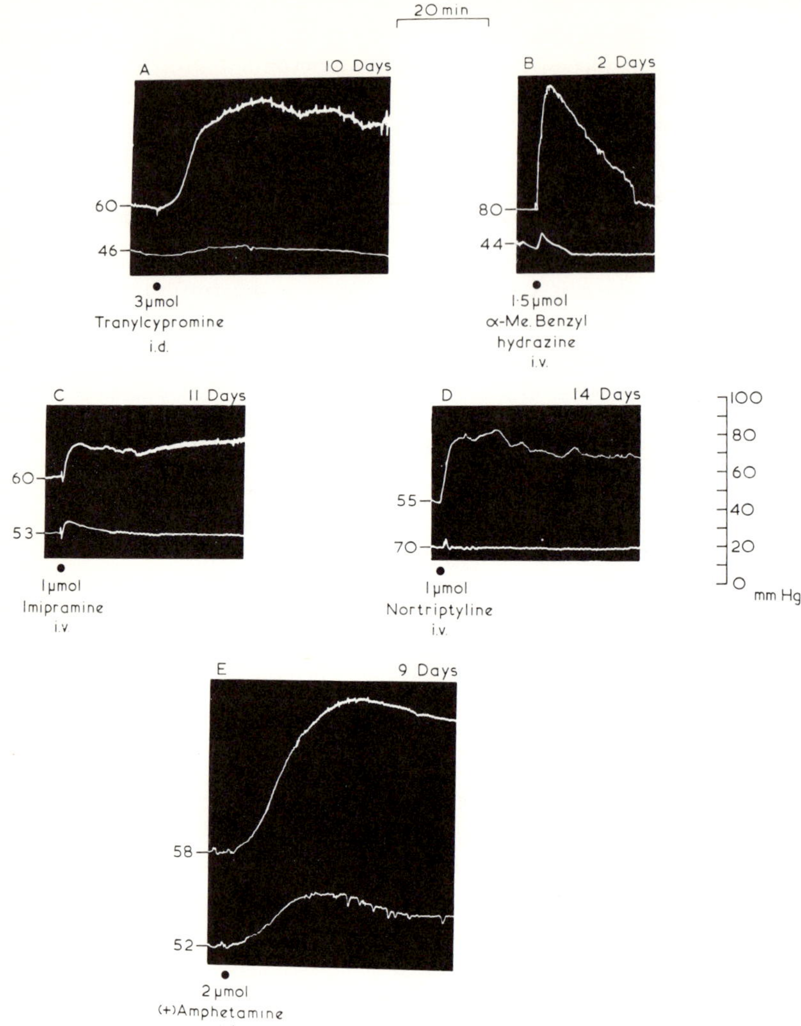

FIG. 16. Interaction between monoamine oxidase inhibitors and various amines measured by blood pressure responses in pithed rats. In each panel, upper trace is response after pretreatment with a monoamine oxidase inhibitor and lower trace is the response in a control rat. (A) Reponse to control dose of tranylcypromine (3 μmole/kg i.d.) (lower trace) and same dose after 10 days pretreatment with tranylcypromine (10 μmole/kg i.p. daily). (B) Response to control dose (lower trace) of mebanazine (α-methylbenzylhydrazine) (1.5 μmole/kg i.v.) and same dose after 2 days pretreatment with mebanazine (120 μmole/kg i.p. daily). (C) Response to control dose (lower trace) of imipramine (1 μmole/kg i.v.) and same dose after 11 days pretreatment with mebanazine (120 μmole/kg i.p. daily). (D) Response to control dose (lower trace) of nortryptyline (1 μmole/kg i.v.) and same dose after 14 days pretreatment with mebanazine (120 μmole/kg i.p. daily). (E) Response to control dose (lower trace) of dexamphetamine (2 μmole/kg i.d.) and same dose after 9 days pretreatment with mebanazine (120 μmole/kg i.p. daily).

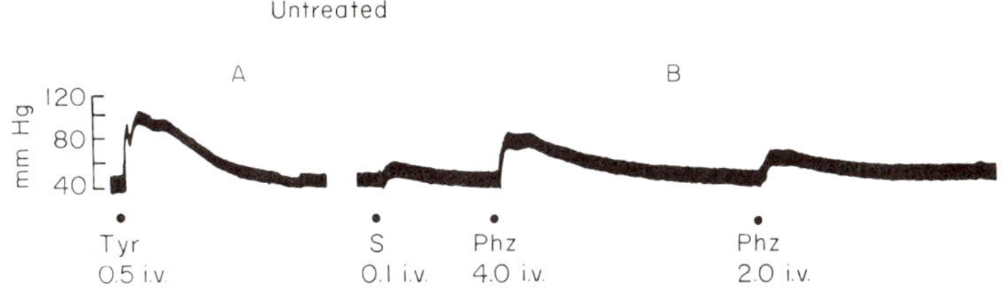

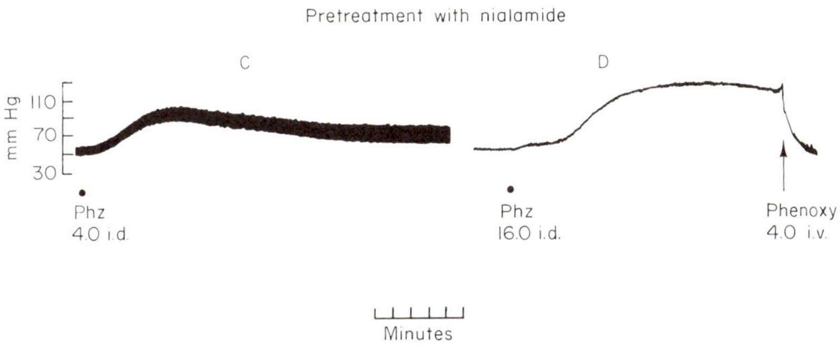

FIG. 17. Blood pressure of three pithed rats. In the first (A, B), a control untreated rat, blood pressure effects of tyramine (Tyr) and phenelzine (Phz) are compared. These doses of tyramine and phenelzine were ineffective when injected into the duodenum (not shown). In the second (C) and third (D) rats pretreated with nialamide (76 μmole/kg given daily for 8 days) intraduodenal doses of phenelzine now have prolonged pressor effects abolished by phenoxybenzamine (Phenoxy) given intravenously. Doses in μmole/kg.

2 hours before the experiment. The pressor effects of phenelzine were more difficult to abolish by guanethidine than were those due to tyramine (Fig. 18F,G).

The effect of another inhibitor, pheniprazine, with marked sympathomimetic properties is shown in Fig. 19. Pheniprazine had pressor effects when given intravenously (Fig. 19A) but not when given intraduodenally (Fig. 19C,D). After pretreatment with nialamide, a smaller intravenous dose produced a much larger rise in blood pressure (Fig. 19B) and an intraduodenal dose significantly elevated blood pressure, an effect abolished by phenoxybenzamine (Fig. 19E). These doses are substantially higher than the daily oral

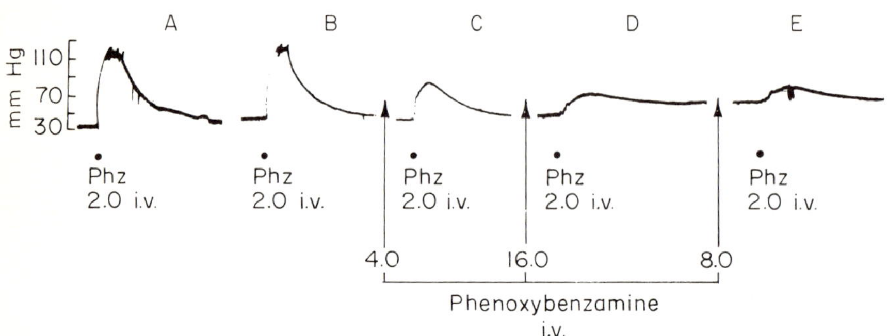

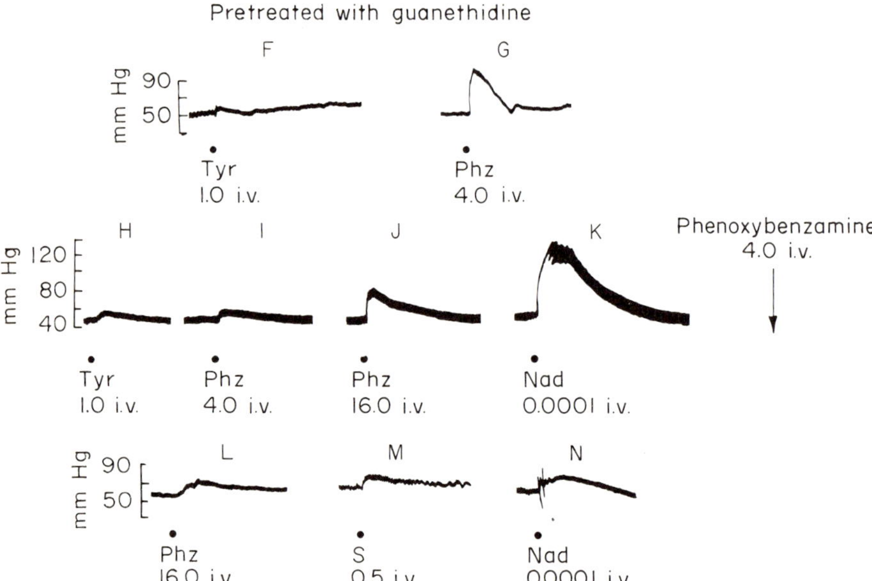

FIG. 18. Blood pressure responses of three pithed rats. In the first (A to E) pretreated with nialamide (76 μmole/kg i.p. daily for 8 days) large pressor effects were obtained with phenelzine (Phz) given intravenously (compare with those in an untreated rat Fig. 17B). These effects were progressively reduced (C, D, E) by successive doses of phenoxybenzamine. The second (F, G) and third (H to N) rats were pretreated with guanethidine (50 μmole/kg i.p. daily for 3 days) followed by a single dose of nialamide (76 μmole/kg i.p.) 2 hours before the experiment. (F) (G) Effects of tyramine (Tyr) more reduced than that of phenelzine. (H) (I) (J) Effects of tyramine abolished and those of phenelzine reduced although that of noradrenaline (Nad) was present (K). (L) (N) Effects of phenelzine and noradrenaline abolished by phenoxybenzamine. All doses in μmole/kg and given intravenously.

dose in man of about 1.0 μmole/kg. Phenoxypropazine had pressor activity in untreated pithed rats (Fig. 20A) which was markedly enhanced by pretreatment with nialamide (Fig. 20C). In support of the pressor effects of phenoxypropazine being due to its ability to release noradrenaline, the blood pressure responses were reduced by phenoxybenzamine (Fig. 20B,D) and tachyphylaxis

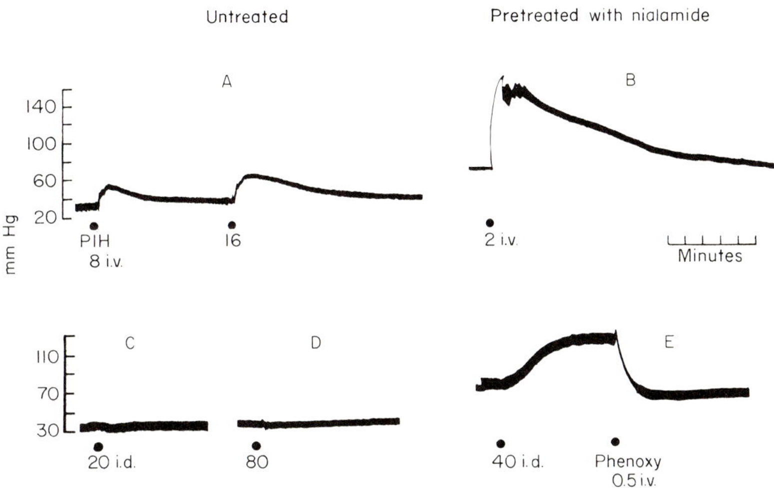

FIG. 19. Blood pressure responses in three rats, two (A, C, D) not pretreated, and two (B, E) pretreated with nialamide (76 μmole/kg i.p. daily for 8 days). (A) Small pressor effects to pheniprazine (P.I.H.) given intravenously, and (C, D) no effect of larger doses given intraduodenally. After pretreatment with nialamide the effect of intravenous pheniprazine (B) was greatly enhanced and intraduodenal pheniprazine (E) now raised blood pressure, an effect abolished by phenoxybenzamine (Phenoxy). All doses in μmole/kg.

developed with repeated doses (Fig. 20E,F,G). Again, these doses are substantially higher than the total daily recommended dose in man of about 1.5 μmole/kg. Hydrazides did not affect blood pressure after pretreatment with nialamide. Hence Pivazide in intravenous doses up to 120 μmole/kg, many times the therapeutic dose in man, was without effect, as was nialamide 76 μmole/kg i.v.

Of the compounds tested, only tranylcypromine and phenelzine showed significant autopotentiation of their pressor activity in doses comparable to those used in man. It may be significant that these are the two drugs which have been incriminated in the majority of hypertensive crises.

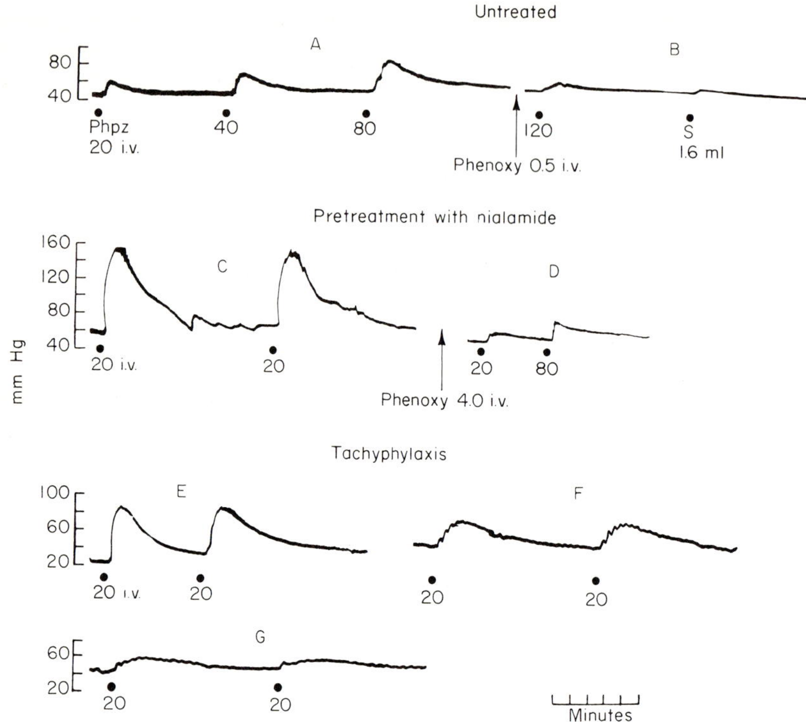

FIG. 20. Blood pressure responses of three pithed rats, one (A, B) not pretreated and two (C to D and E to G) pretreated with nialamide (76 μmole/kg i.p. daily for 8 days). (A) Pressor effects of phenoxypropazine (Phpz) abolished (B) by phenoxybenzamine (Phenoxy). (C) Enhanced pressor effects of phenoxypropazine after pretreatment with nialamide again abolished (D) by phenoxybenzamine. (E–G) Tachyphylaxis to repeated doses of phenoxypropazine. E: First and second doses; F: seventh and eighth doses; G: twelfth and thirteenth doses. All doses in μmole/kg and given intravenously.

X. Other Interactions with Monoamine Oxidase Inhibitors

The effects produced by interactions of monoamine oxidase inhibitors with sympathomimetic amines resemble those due to excessive dosage with these amines; a less marked similarity occurs in interactions with some iminodibenzyl drugs.

A. Interactions between Sympathomimetic Drugs and Monoamine Oxidase Inhibitors

In these interactions and despite their dramatic character both the amine oxidase inhibitor and sympathomimetic drug were given in a *therapeutic dose*. The sympathomimetic drugs incriminated were amphetamine (optical activity not always specified), dexamphetamine, *N*-methylamphetamine, *m*-hydroxynorephedrine, methylphenidate, phenylpropanolamine; the monoamine oxidase inhibitors involved included those with intrinsic sympathomimetic activity, e.g., tranylcypromine and phenelzine, and those lacking such properties, e.g., iproniazid and isocarboxazid (Bethune *et al.*, 1964; Boudin *et al.*, 1966; Cuthbert *et al.*, 1969; Dally, 1962; Horler and Wynne, 1965; Humberstone, 1969; Levy and Michel-Ber, 1968; Lewis, 1965; Lloyd and Walker, 1965; Low-Beer and Tidmarsh, 1963; Mason, 1962; Nymark and Nielson, 1963; Mason and Bueckle, 1969; Sherman *et al.*, 1964; Stark, 1962; Tonks and Livingston, 1963; Tonks and Lloyd, 1965; Zeck, 1961).

The interactions resemble those with cheese. There was a similar sudden onset of occipital headache ranging from severe to "devastating," often but not invariably associated with raised blood pressure; palpitations (slow or rapid pulse), profuse sweating, sometimes chest pain, and even acute pulmonary edema ensued. The extent to which the blood pressure was elevated can be gauged from Dally (1962), who noted that after intravenous injection of *N*-methylamphetamine (dose not given) to a subject treated until 8 days previously with phenelzine, arterial pressure rose immediately from 120/80 mm Hg to 280/150 mm Hg and had not returned to normal 24 hours later. Photophobia, nausea, and vomiting often presaged intracranial hemorrhage. Physical signs included mydriasis, extrasystoles, pulsus bigeminus, hyperreflexia, extensor plantar responses, and even opisthotonus and hemiplegia. Hyperpyrexia (up to 109.4°F or 43°C) has also been recorded (Lewis, 1965). The mental state may show minimal impairment, such as nominal dysphasia or temporal disorientation with subsequent amnesia for the episode. Other patients became comatose and died. Postmortem findings included cerebral edema and subarachnoid or cerebral hemorrhage (Dorrell, 1963; de Villiers, 1966). The importance of hypertensive crises as a cause of subarachnoid hemorrhage in patients taking amine oxidase inhibitors was indicated by this association in 13 patients (3.9%) of a series of 883 subjects with subarachnoid hemorrhage admitted to a neurosurgical unit between 1962 and 1964 (de Villiers, 1966). The danger of these combinations of drugs are underlined by tests in animals. In grouped mice pretreatment when phenelzine potentiated fivefold the lethal effect of amphetamine or *N*-methylamphetamine (Brownlee and Williams, 1963), while pretreatment with pargyline increased toxicity two- to threefold (Everett *et al.*, 1963). A study on the LD_{50} of amphetamine in mice before and after six different monoamine oxidase inhibitors (O'Dea and Rand, 1969) showed that they all increased the toxicity of amphetamine independent of chemical type and intrinsic toxicity. Tranylcypromine was more potent, possibly due to an impairment of liver microsomal enzymes. Another possibility would be augmentation of pressor activity. The marked potentiation of the pressor effect of dexamphetamine (2 μmole/kg intraduodenally and equivalent to about 20 mg in a 60-kg man) given to a pithed rat pretreated with tranylcypromine (2 μmole/kg i.p. for 9 days) is shown in Fig. 16E.

The signs and symptoms of the drug combinations are also reminiscent of those in addicts following ingestion of *large* doses of amphetamine—usually 60 mg (1 mg/kg) or more (Connell, 1958; Herman and Nagler, 1954; Kalant, 1966; Marley, 1960)—or phenmetrazine (Abély *et al.*, 1963; Bartholomew and Marley, 1959; Evans, 1959), except that headache was a less conspicuous complaint. In non-addicted subjects who took a large dose of amphetamine (100 to 325 mg amphetamine sulfate), headache was an early and intense feature (Gericke, 1945; Poteliakhoff and Roughton, 1956); hyperpyrexia (109°F or 42.75°C) has also been reported (Jordan and Hampson, 1960). Such doses have elicited cerebral edema, subdural and subarachnoid hemorrhage, or cerebral hemorrhage (Gericke, 1945; Jordan and Hampson, 1960; Pontrelli, 1942; Poteliakhoff and Roughton, 1956). Rather similar symptoms of both central excitation and peripheral cardiovascular effects can occur after overdose of the inhibitors alone which most resemble amphetamine (Davies, 1970; Reid and Kerr, 1969).

B. Interactions between Iminodibenzyl Compounds and Monoamine Oxidase Inhibitors

Although their pharmacological properties differ considerably, the iminodibenzyl compounds bear a superficial structural resemblance to the sympathomimetic amines insofar as they possess a ring structure attached to a short aliphatic chain terminating in an amino group. After amine oxidase inhibition a syndrome has been elicited by some of the iminodibenzyl compounds which partly resembles the interactions with sympathomimetic drugs. Hyperpyrexia is marked; other features include agitation, delirium, coma, extreme generalized muscular rigidity, and convulsions. These have been evoked in patients on maintenance therapy with amine oxidase inhibitors (nialamide, pargyline, phenelzine, tranylcypromine) and in those who in most cases had received three or less doses of imipramine (Brachfield *et al.*, 1963; Hills, 1965; Lockett and Milner, 1965; Luby and Domino, 1961; McCurdy and Kane, 1964; Singh, 1960; Stanley and Pal, 1964); a similar interaction has been described between monoamine oxidase inhibitors and amitriptyline (Jarecki, 1963). Fatal hyperthermia ensued on infusing imipramine or amitriptyline intravenously in rabbits pretreated with a monoamine oxidase inhibitor (Loveless and Maxwell, 1965; Nymark and Nielson, 1963); trimipramine failed to provoke hyperpyrexia so this response is not characteristic of all iminodibenzyl drugs (Loveless and Maxwell, 1965). A pressor reaction to these compounds has not been noted, but that this might occur is indicated in Fig. 16C,D, which shows a rise in blood pressure to imipramine and nortriptyline respectively in rats pretreated with tranylcypromine.

XI. Conclusion

"An important and interesting pharmacological advance has been made by those who have investigated the profound effects of many amine-containing foodstuffs when eaten by patients taking monoamine oxidase inhibiting drugs" (Editorial, 1965). The advance was perhaps more apparent than real, since Bhagvat *et al.* had suggested in 1939 that the high concentration of amine oxidase in the gut and liver was to prevent amines taken up from the alimentary canal from reaching the general circulation. The consequence of inhibiting monoamine oxidase could therefore have been predicted and indeed Blaschko (1952) had speculated whether "uptake of amines, such as tyramine, from the intestine is an event that is likely to occur on a large scale." Had one these words in mind when amine oxidase inhibitors were subsequently introduced into therapeutics then the interactions with foods could perhaps have been avoided. Here, pre-eminently then, is one of those curious and all-too-frequent situations in which foreknowledge becomes inexplicably dissociated from forewarning.

References

Abély, P., Rondepiere, N., and Gellman, C. (1963). *Ann. Med. Psychol.* **121**, 593.

Allen, G. S., and Rand, M. J. (1969). *J. Pharm. Pharmacol.* **21**, 317.

Alles, G. A., and Heegaard, E. V. (1943). *J. Biol. Chem.* **147**, 487.

Amure, B. O., and Ginsburg, M. (1964). *Brit. J. Pharmacol. Chemother.* **22**, 520.

Asatoor, A. M., Levi, A. J., and Milne, M. D. (1963). *Lancet* **ii**, 733.

Axelrod, J. (1954). *J. Pharmacol. Exp. Ther.* **110**, 315

Axelrod, J. (1955). *J. Biol. Chem.* **214**, 753.

Axelrod, J., Reichenthal, J., and Brodie, B. B. (1954). *J. Pharmacol. Exp. Therap.* **112**, 49.

Bartholomew, A. A., and Marley, E. (1959). *Psychopharmacologia* **1**, 124.

Bernheim, F., and Bernheim, M. L. C. (1945). *J. Biol. Chem.* **136**, 425.

Bethune, H. C., Culpan, R. H., and Ogg, G. J. (1964). *Amer. J. Psychiat.* **121**, 245.

Beyer, K. H., and Morrison, H. S. (1945). *Ind. Eng. Chem.* **37**, 143

Bhagvat, K., Blaschko, H., and Richter, D. (1939). *Biochem. J.* **33**, 1338.

Bichel, J. (1968). *Lancet* **ii**, 877.

Biel, J. H., Nuhfer, P. A., and Conway, A. C. (1959). *Ann. N.Y. Acad. Sci.* **80**, 568.

Birkhäuser, H. (1940). *Helv. Chim. Acta* **23**, 1071.

Blackwell, B. (1963). *Lancet* **i**, 849.

Blackwell, B., and Mabbitt, L. A. (1965). *Lancet* **1**. 938.

Blackwell, B., and Marley, E. (1964). *Lancet* **i**, 530.

Blackwell, B., and Marley, E. (1966a). *Brit. J. Pharmacol. Chemother.* **26**, 142.

Blackwell, B., and Marley, E. (1966b). *Brit. J. Pharmacol. Chemother.* **26**, 120.

Blackwell, B., Marley, E., and Mabbitt, L. A. (1965). *Lancet* **1**, 940.

Blackwell, B., Marley, E., Price, J., and Taylor, O. (1967). *Brit. J. Psychiat.* **113**, 349.

Blackwell, B., Mabbitt, L. A., and Marley, E. (1969). *J. Food Sci.* **34**, 47.

Blaschko, H. (1945). *Advan. Enzymol.* **5**, 67

Blaschko, H. (1952). *Pharmacol. Rev.* **4**, 415.

Blaschko, H., Richter, D., and Schlossman, H. (1937a). *Biochem. J.* **31**, 2187.
Blaschko, H., Richter, D., and Schlossman, H. (1937b). *J. Physiol.* (*London*) **91**, 13P.
Bloom, B. M. (1963). *Ann. N.Y. Acad. Sci.* **107**, 878.
Boudin, G., Lauras, A., and Poirier, J. (1966). *Presse Med.* **74**, 43.
Brachfield, J., Wirtschafter, A., and Wolfe, S. (1963). *J. Amer. Med. Assoc.* **186**, 1172.
Bram, G. (1963). *Brit. Med. J.* **ii**, 1407.
Brock, A. J. (1929). "Greek Medicine," p. 49. Dent, London.
Brodie, B. B., and Hogben, C. A. M. (1957). *J. Pharm. Pharmacol.* **9**, 345.
Brodie, B. B. (1956). *J. Pharm. Pharmacol.* **8**, 1.
Brown, D. D., and Waldron, D. H. (1962). *Practitioner* **189**, 83.
Brownlee, G., and Williams, G. W. (1963). *Lancet* **i**, 669.
Bruce, D. W. (1960). *Nature* (*London*) **188**, 147.
Burkard, W. P., Gey, K. F., and Pletscher, A. (1962). *Biochem. Pharmacol.* **11**, 177.
Chessin, M., Dubnick, B., Leeson, G. K., and Scott, C. C. (1959). *Ann. N.Y. Acad. Sci.* **80**, 597.
Clark, J. A. (1961). *Lancet* **i**, 618.
Clineschmidt, V., and Horita, A. (1967). *Brit. J. Pharmacol. Chemother.* **30**, 67
Connell, P. (1958). "Amphetamine Psychosis," Maudsley Monograph No. 5. Chapman & Hall, London.
Cooper, A. J., Magnus, R. V., and Rose, M. J. (1964). *Lancet* **i**, 527.
Creveling C. R., van der Schoot, J. B., and Udenfriend, S. (1962). *Biochem. Biophys. Res. Commun.* **8**, 215.
Cuthbert, M. F., Greenberg, M. P., and Morley, S. W. (1969) *Brit. Med. J.* **i**, 393.
Dale, H. H., and Dixon, W. E. (1909). *J. Physiol.* (*London*) **39**, 25.
Dale, H. H., and Laidlaw, P. P. (1919). *J. Physiol.* (*London*) **52**, 355.
Dally, P. J. (1962). *Lancet* **i**, 1235.
Davies, B. E. (1959). *J. Soc. Gen. Med. Lisbon* **123**, 163.
Davies, B. E. (1963). *Lancet* **ii**, 691.
Davies, G. (1970). *Med. J. Aust.* **1**, 85.
Davison, A. N. (1958). *Physiol. Rev.* **38**, 729.
Dawson, R., and Porter, J. W. G. (1962). *Brit. J. Nutr.* **16**, 27.
de Villiers, J. C. (1966). *Brit. J. Psychiat.* **112**, 109.
Dixon, W. E. (1913). *Proc. Roy. Soc. Med.* **6**, 1.
Dorrell, W. (1963). *Lancet* **i**, 388.
Dubnick, B., Morgan, F. D., and Phillips, G. E. (1963). *Ann. N.Y. Acad. Sci.* **107**, 914.
Duncan, J. G. C., and Watson, N. G. (1968). *J. Physiol.* (*London*) **198**, 505.
Editorial (1965). *Lancet* **i**, 945.
Eltherington, L. G., and Horita, A. (1960). *J. Pharmacol. Exp. Ther.* **128**, 7.
Epps, H. M. R. (1944). *Biochem. J.* **38**, 242.
Evans, J. (1959). *Lancet* **ii**, 152.
Everett, G. M., Wiegane, R. C., and Rinaldi, F. U. (1963). *Ann. N.Y. Acad. Sci.* **107**, 1069.
Findlay, L. (1911). *Quart. J. Med.* **4**, 489.
Foster, A. R. (1963). *Lancet* **ii**, 587.
Fouts, J. R., and Brodie, B. B. (1955). *J. Pharmacol. Exp. Ther.* **115**, 68.
Foy, J. M., and Parratt, J. R. (1960). *J. Pharm. Pharmacol.* **12**, 360.
Foy, J. M., and Parratt, J. R. (1961). *J. Pharm. Pharmacol* **13**, 382.
Gale, F. E. (1940). *Biochem. J.* **34**, 392.
Gericke, O. L. (1945). *J. Amer. Med. Ass.* **128**, 1098.
Gerold, M. (1968). *Arzneim.-Forsch.* **18**, 1198.
Ghosh, M. N., and Schild, H. O. (1958). *Brit. J. Pharmacol. Chemother.* **13**, 54.

Gillespie, L. (1960). *Ann. N.Y. Acad. Sci.* **88**, 1011.

Glazener, F. S., Morgan, A., Simpson, J. M., and Johnson, P. K. (1964). *J. Amer. Med. Ass.*, **188**, 754.

Hall, D. W. R., and Logan, B. W. (1969). *Biochem. Pharmacol.* **18**, 1955.

Hall, D. W. R., Logan, B. W., and Parsons, G. H. (1969). *Biochem. Pharmacol.* **18**, 1447.

Hanington, E. (1967). *Brit. Med. J.* **ii**, 550.

Hare, M. L. C. (1928). *Biochem. J.* **22**, 968.

Harley, V. (1913). *Proc. Roy. Soc. Med.* **6**, 1.

Hedberg, D. L., Gordon, M. W., and Glueck, B. C. (1966). *Amer. J. Psychiat.* **122**, 933.

Herman, M., and Nagler, S. H. (1954). *J. Nerv. Ment. Dis.* **120**, 268.

Hills, N. F. (1965). *Brit. Med. J.* **i**, 859

Hodge, J. V., Nye, E. R., and Emerson, G. W. (1964). *Lancet* **i**, 1108.

Holtz, P., Heise, R., and Ludtke, K. (1938). *Naunyn-Schmiedebergs Arch. Exp. Pathol. Pharmakol.* **191**, 87.

Horler, A. E., and Wynne, N. A. (1965). *Brit. Med. J.* **ii**, 460.

Horwitz, D., Goldberg, L. I., and Sjoerdsma, A. (1960). *J. Lab. Clin. Med.* **56**, 747.

Horwitz, D., Lovenberg, W., Engelman, K., and Sjoerdsma, A. (1964). *J. Amer. Med. Ass.* **188**, 1108.

Humberstone, P. M. (1969). *Brit. Med. J.* **i**, 846.

Huszti, A., Fekete, M., and Hajos, A. (1969). *Biochem. Pharmacol.* **18**, 2293.

Jarecki, H. G. (1963). *Amer. J. Psychiat.* **120**, 189.

Jordan, S. C., and Hampson, F. (1960). *Brit. Med. J.* **ii**, 844.

Kalant, O. J. (1966). "Alcoholism and Drug Addiction Research Foundation." Univ. of Toronto Press, Toronto.

Kato, R., Chiesara, E., and Vassanelli, P. (1964). *Biochem. Pharmacol.* **13**, 179.

Kayaalp, S. O., Kaymakcalan, S., and Oezer, A. (1968). *Arzneim.-Forsch.* **18**, 1195.

Keil, W., and Kritter, H. (1934). *Naunyn-Schmiedebergs Arch. Exp. Pathol. Pharmakol.* **175**, 736.

Kimata, M. (1961). *In* "Fish as Food" (G. Borgstrom, ed.), Vol. 1, p. 329. Academic Press, New York.

Kobayashi, Y. (1958). *Arch. Biochem. Biophys.* **77**, 275.

Koessler, K. K., and Hanke, M. T. (1924). *J. Biol. Chem.* **59**, 889.

Kohn, H. I. (1937). *Biochem. J.* **31**, 1693.

Langemann, H. (1944). *Helv. Physiol. Acta* **2**, 367.

Langemann, H. (1951). *Brit. J. Pharmacol. Chemother.* **6**, 318.

Langemann, H., Roulet, F., and Zeller, E. A. (1943). *Klin. Wochenschr.* **22**, 42.

Lembeck, F., Winne, D., and Sewing, K.-F. (1964). *Lancet* **i**, 933.

Levine, R. J., and Sjoerdsma, A. (1963). *Ann. N.Y. Acad. Sci.* **107**, 966.

Levy, J., and Michel-Ber, E. (1968). *In* "Toxicity and Side Effects of Psychotropic Drugs" (S. B. de C. Baker, J. R. Boissier, and W. Koll, eds.), Vol. 9, p. 212. Excerpta Med. Found. Amsterdam.

Lewis, E. (1965). *Brit. Med. J.* **i**, 1671.

Liebig, J. (1846). *Ann. Chem. Pharm.* **57**, 127.

Lloyd, J. T. A., and Walker, D. R. H. (1965). *Brit. Med. J.* **ii**, 168.

Lockett, M. F., and Milner, G. (1965). *Brit. Med. J.* **i**, 921.

Loveless, A. H., and Maxwell, D. R. (1965). *Brit. J. Pharmacol. Chemother.* **25**, 158.

Low-Beer, G. A., and Tidmarsh, D. (1963). *Brit. Med. J.* **ii**, 683.

Luby, E. D., and Domino, E. F. (1961). *J. Amer. Med. Ass.* **177**, 68.

Luschinsky, H. L., and Singher, H. O. (1948). *Arch. Biochem.* **19**, 95.

Lyall, N. (1963). *Food Trade Rev.* **33**, 57.

McCurdy, R. L., and Kane, F. J. (1964). *Amer. J. Psychiat.* **121**, 397.
Marks, J. (1965). *In* "The Scientific Basis of Drug Therapy in Psychiatry" (J. Marks and C. M. B. Pare, eds.), p. 191. Macmillan (Pergamon), New York.
Marley, E. (1960). *J. Ment. Sci.* **106**, 76.
Mason, A. (1962). *Lancet*, **1**, 1073.
Mason, A. M. S., and Buekle, R. M. (1969). *Brit. Med. J.* **i**, 845.
Meakins, J., and Harington, C. R. (1923). *J. Pharmacol. Exp. Ther.* **20**, 45.
Melnykowycz, J., and Johannson, K. R. (1955). *J. Exp. Med.* **101**, 507.
Metchnikoff, E. (1903). "The Nature of Man" (P. G. Mitchell, ed. and transl.), pp. 72, 253. Heinemann, London.
Mustala, O., Solantunturi, E., and Tarpila, S. (1969). *Acta Med. Scand.* **185**, 145.
Natoff, I. L. (1964). *Lancet* **i**, 532.
Natoff, I. L. (1965a). *Excerpta Med. Int. Congr. Ser.* **81**, 158.
Natoff, I. L. (1965b). *Med. Proc.* **11**, 101.
Nuessle, W. F., Norman, C., and Miller, H. E. (1965). *J. Amer. Med. Ass.* **192**, 726.
Nymark, M., and Nielson, I. M. (1963). *Brit. Med. J.* **ii**, 524.
O'Dea, K., and Rand, M. J. (1969). *Eur. Pharm. J.* **6**, 115
Ogilvie, C. (1955). *Quart. J. Med.* **24**, 175.
Pettinger, W. A., Soyangco, F. G., and Oaks, I. A. (1968). *Clin. Pharmacol. Ther.* **9**, 442.
Pontrelli, E. (1942). *G. Clin. Med.* **23**, 591.
Poteliakhoff, A., and Roughton, B. C. (1956). *Brit. Med. J.* **i**, 26.
Proc. Roy. Soc. Med. (1913). **6**, 11.
Pugh, C. E. M., and Quastel, J. H. (1937). *Biochem J.* **31**, 286.
Rand, M. J., and Trinker, F. R. (1968). *Brit. J. Pharmacol. Chemother.* **33**, 287.
Randall, L. O. (1946). *J. Pharmacol. Exp. Ther.* **83**, 216.
Reid, D. D., and Kerr, W. C. (1969). *Med. J. Aust.* **2**, 1214.
Schayer, R. W. (1959). *Physiol. Rev.* **39**, 116.
Sealock, R. R. (1949). *Biochem. Prep.* **1**, 25.
Sherman, M., Hauser, G. C., and Glover, B. J. (1964). *Amer. J. Psychiat.* **120**, 1019.
Shore, P. A., and Cohn, V. (1960). *Biochem. Pharmacol.* **5**, 91.
Singh, H. (1960). *Amer. J. Psychiat.* **117**, 360.
Sjöqvist, F. (1965). *Proc. Roy. Soc. Med.* **58**, 967.
Sollman, T. (1957). "A Manual of Pharmacology," 11th Ed., p. 513. Saunders, Philadelphia, Pennsylvania.
Somerville, D. (1913). *Proc. Roy. Soc. Med.* **6**, 1.
Songco, M. F. (1961). *Amer. J. Psychiat.* **118**, 360
Spencer, J. N., Porter, M., Froehlich, H. L., and Wendel, H. (1960). *Fed. Proc. Fed. Amer. Soc. Exp. Biol.* **19**, 277.
Stanley, B., and Pal, N. R. (1964). *Brit. Med. J.* **ii**, 1011.
Stark, D. C. C. (1962). *Lancet*, **i**, 1405.
Stern, I. J., Hollifield, R. D., Wilk, S., and Buzard, J. A. (1967). *J. Pharmacol. Exp. Ther.* **156**, 492.
Tabor, H. (1954). *Pharmacol Rev.* **6**, 299.
Tanner, W. E. (1946). "Arbuthnot Lane, His Life and Work. Baillière, London.
Tedeschi, D. H., and Fellows, E. J. (1964). *Science* **144**, 1225.
Thompson, R. H. S., and Tickner, A. (1949). *Biochem. J.* **45**, 125.
Thompson, R. H. S., and Tickner, A. (1951). *J. Physiol. (London)* **115**, 34.
Tonks, C. M., and Livingston, D. (1963). *Lancet* **i**, 1323.
Tonks, C. M., and Lloyd, A. T. (1965). *Brit. Med. J.* **i**, 589.
Travel, J. (1940). *J. Pharmacol. Exp. Ther.* **69**, 21.

Udenfriend, S., Lovenberg, W., and Sjoerdsma, A. (1959). *Arch. Biochem. Biophys.* **85**, 48.

Van Slyke, L., and Hart, B. (1903). *Amer. Chem. J.* **30**, 8.

Vane, J. R. (1964). *Brit. J. Pharmacol. Chemother.* **23**, 360.

von Euler, U. S., and Hellner-Bjorkman, S. (1955). *Acta Physiol. Scand.* **33**, Suppl. 118, 21.

Wilson, G. S., and Miles, A. A. (1955). *In* "Topley and Wilson's Principles of Bacteriology and Immunity" (G. S. Wilson and A. A. Miles, eds.), p. 2251. Arnold, London.

Wolff, G. H. (1963). "Headache and Head Pain," p. 746. Oxford Univ. Press, London and New York.

Womack, A. M. (1963). *Brit. Med. J.* **ii**, 366.

Zeck, P. (1961). *Med. J. Aust.* **2**, 607.

Zeller, E. A. (1942). *Advan. Enzymol. Relat. Subj. Biochem.* **2**, 93.

Zeller, E. A., and Joel, C. A. (1941). *Helv. Chim. Acta* **24**, 968.

Zeller, E. A., Blanskma, L. A., Burkard, W. P., Pacha, W. L., and Lazanas, J. C. (1959). *Ann. N.Y. Acad. Sci.* **80**, 583.

AUTHOR INDEX

Numbers in italics show the page on which the complete reference is listed.

C

D

E

F

H

M

N

O

P

Q

R

T

SUBJECT INDEX

E

F

G

H

I

J

L

Q

R

S

T

V

X

Y